CRASH COURSE
Renal System

Renal System

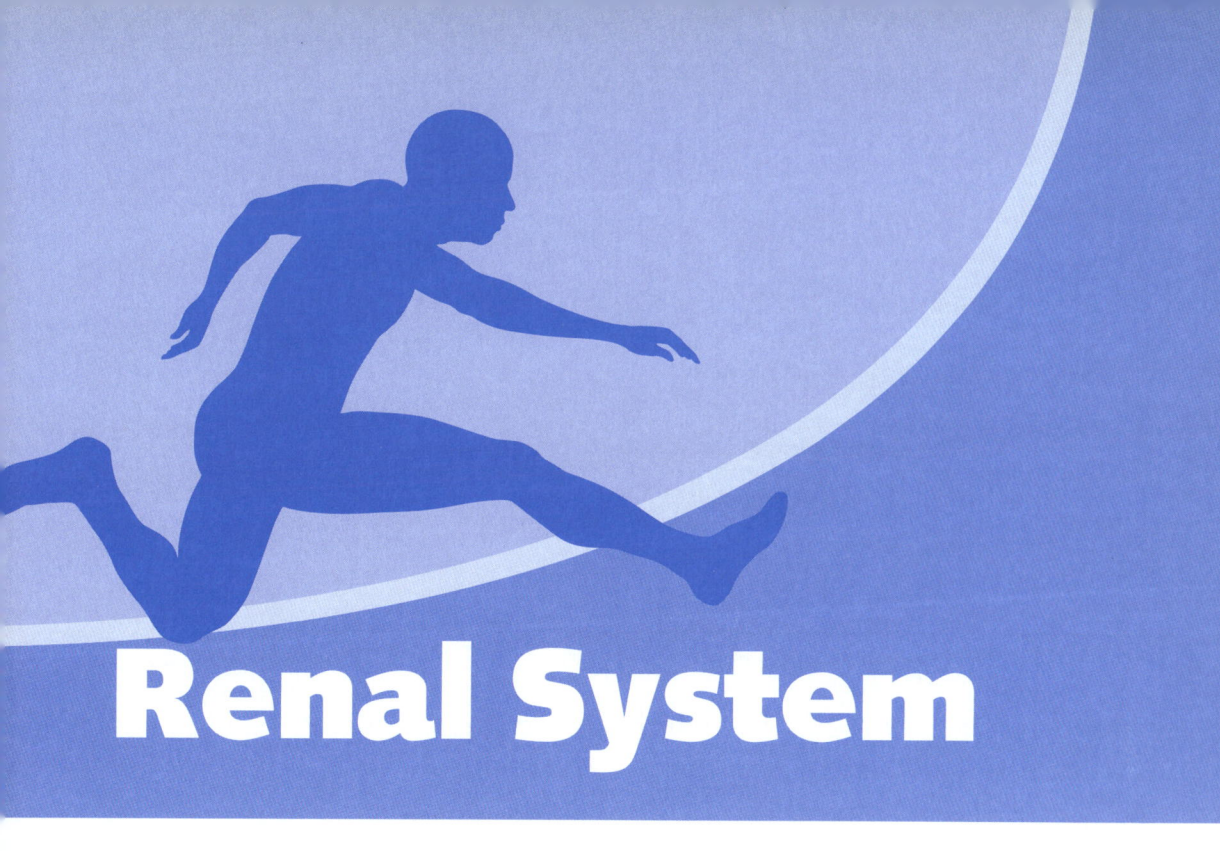

Frazier Stevenson, MD
Associate Professor, Department of Internal Medicine
University of California at Davis
Davis, California

UK edition authors
Shreelatta Datta, Nisha Mirpuri, and Pratiksha Patel

UK series editor
Dan Horton-Szar

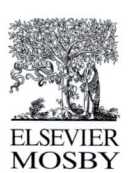

ELSEVIER
MOSBY

ELSEVIER
MOSBY

1600 John F. Kennedy Blvd.
Ste 1800
Philadelphia, PA 19103-2899

CRASH COURSE: RENAL SYSTEM   ISBN 0-323-03560-4
Copyright 2005, Elsevier, Inc. All right reserved.

All rights reserved. No part of this publication may be reproduced or transmitted in any form or by any means, electronic or mechanical, including photocopying, recording, or any information storage and retrieval system, without permission in writing from the publisher. Pemissions may be sought directly from Elsevier's Health Sciences Rights Department in Philadelphia, PA, USA: phone: (+1) 215 239 3804, fax: (+1) 215 239 3805, e-mail: healthpermissions@elsevier.com. You may also complete your request on-line via the Elsevier homepage (http://www.elsevier.com), by selecting "Customer Support" and then "Obtaining Permission."

Notice

Knowledge and best practice in this field are constantly changing. As new research and experience broaden our knowledge, changes in practice, treatment and drug therapy may become necessary or appropriate. Readers are advised to check the most current information provided (i) on procedures featured or (ii) by the manufacturer of each product to be administered, to verify the recommended dose or dormula, the method and duration of administration, and contraindications. It is the responsibility of the practitioner, relying on their own experience and knowledge of the patient, to make diagnoses, to determine dosages and the best treatment for each individual patient, and to take all appropriate safety precautions. To the fullest extent of the law, neither the Publisher nor the Author assumes any liability for any injury and/or damage to persons or property arising out of or related to any use of the material contained in this book.

The Publisher

First Edition 1998. Second Edition 2003.

Library of Congress Cataloging-in-Publication Data

Stevenson, Frazier.
  Renal sysem/Frazier Stevenson.—1st ed.
    p. ; cm.—(Crash course)
  ISBN 0-323-03560-4
  1. Kidneys—Diseases. I. Title. II. Series.
  [DNLM: 1. Kidney Diseases. WJ 300 S847r 2005]
  RC902.S73 2005
  16.6'1—dc26   2004063174

Acquisitions Editor: Alex Stibbe
Project Development Manager: Stan Ward
Publishing Services Manager: David Saltzberg
Designer: Andy Chapman
Cover Design: Richard Tibbets
Illustration Manager: Mick Ruddy

Printed in China

Last digit is the print number: 9 8 7 6 5 4 3 2 1

**Working together to grow
libraries in developing countries**

www.elsevier.com | www.bookaid.org | www.sabre.org

ELSEVIER   BOOK AID International   Sabre Foundation

Preface

This book intends to provide a focused review of renal and genitourinary anatomy, physiology, and pathophysiology suitable for students reviewing for board exams. Renal physiology and pathophysiology are traditionally subjects that strike fear into the hearts of the most intrepid medical students (and experienced physicians). In these fields it is particularly difficult for learners to separate forest from trees: overconcentration on detail frequently obscures global understanding of volume regulation, acid-base homeostasis, and other critical renal functions. Since this book is intended as a review for NBME boards, I have attempted to walk the fine line between oversimplification (which falsely clarifies) and obfuscation by encyclopedic detail (which satisfies completists but confuses the rest of us). Cutting-edge research and detailed explanations have been de-emphasized for the sake of brevity and clarity.

All experienced teachers turn to student-generated explanations for the best insight into what really needs to be taught—the students of UC Davis have provided me with such teaching insights through the years.

The book retains the traditional *Crash Course* chapter divisions in the interest of series uniformity, although these divisions did create some difficulties. It is not easy to discuss the structure of the nephron segments without segueing into function; thus, there is some preliminary discussion of renal function in Chapter 2. Rather than discussing the electrolyte disorders in "The Kidneys in Disease," I chose to incorporate them into the discussions of normal renal physiology in Chapter 3, since I believe that the two must be discussed and understood together. This organization allows the book to divide nicely into the following chapter divisions: 1, basics; 2, anatomy; 3, physiology and electrolyte disorders; 4, renal pathology; 5, lower genitourinary pathophysiology; 6, renal signs and symptoms that overlap the above groupings; and lastly, 7 and 8, diagnostic principles. I hope that the structure and content help students to master this challenging material for both their board examinations and their subsequent medical practice.

Frazier Stevenson, M.D.

Acknowledgments

I would like to thank these people for their inspiration and contribution to this text:

The British authors of the earlier edition of this text, who wrote an outstanding review of the field and made my job easy.

Dr. Jane Yeun, whose description and clarification of renal disease for our students has been a model for teaching this subject, and for many of the descriptions in this text.

The medical students of UC Davis, whose questions teach me how to teach nephrology.

Dr. Marty Cogan, along with the past and present nephrology faculty at UCSF and UC Davis, for their ideas and insights into teaching nephrology.

The faculty of Pomona College, who taught me the art, science, and value of teaching.

My parents, two of the world's best teachers, who serve as role models for all that I do.

Contents

Preface v
Acknowledgments vii

Part I: Basic Medical Science of the Renal and Urinary Systems 1

1. **Basic Principles** 3
   Overview of the kidney and urinary tract 3
   Fluid compartments of the body 3

2. **Organization of the Kidneys** 13
   Development of the kidneys 13
   General organization of the kidneys 13
   Glomerular structure and function 20
   Transport processes in the renal tubule 22
   The proximal tubule 24
   The loop of Henle 29
   The distal nephron 29

3. **Renal Function** 33
   The glomerular filtration rate (GFR): regulation and disorders 33
   Reduced GFR: renal failure 38
   Body fluids: regulation and clinical disorders 43
   Regulation and clinical disorders of serum osmolality 51
   Regulation and clinical disorders of body fluid pH 60
   Potassium: regulation and clinical disorders 68
   Calcium, phosphate, and magnesium: regulation and clinical disorders 70
   Uric acid: regulation and clinical disorders 76
   Renal regulation of erythropoiesis 76

4. **The Kidneys in Disease** 79
   Congenital abnormalities of the kidney 79
   Cystic diseases of the kidney 79
   Diseases of the glomerulus 82
   Diseases of the tubules and interstitium 90
   Diseases of the renal blood vessels 93
   Neoplastic disease of the kidney 95
   Renal responses to systemic disorders 97

5. **The Lower Urinary Tract** 103
   Organization of the lower urinary tract 103
   Micturition 108
   Congenital abnormalities of the urinary tract 111
   Urinary tract obstruction 114
   Renal calculi 116
   Inflammation and infection of the urinary tract 117
   Neoplastic disease of the ureters and bladder 121
   Disorders of the prostate 124

Part II. Clinical Assessment 129

6. **Common Presentations of Renal Disease** . . . 131
   Introduction 131
   Hematuria 131
   Proteinuria 131
   Pyuria 134
   Hypertension 135
   Dysuria 137
   Dyfunctional voiding 137

7. **History and Examination** 143
   Key historical points in renal disease 143
   Key physical exam points in renal disease 143

8. **Lab Investigation and Imaging** 147
   Testing the blood and urine 147
   Imaging and other investigations 147

Index 159

BASIC MEDICAL SCIENCE OF THE RENAL AND URINARY SYSTEMS

1. Basic Principles — 3
2. Organization of the Kidneys — 13
3. Renal Function — 33
4. The Kidneys in Disease — 79
5. The Lower Urinary Tract — 103

1. Basic Principles

Overview of the kidney and urinary tract

Structural organization of the kidney and urinary tract

The kidneys lie in the retroperitoneum on the posterior abdominal wall on either side of the vertebral column (T11–L3). The right kidney is displaced by the liver, so it is 12 mm lower than the left kidney. The adult kidney is approximately 11 cm long and 6 cm wide, with a mass of 140 g. Each kidney is composed of two main regions:
- An outer dark brown cortex.
- An inner pale medulla and renal pelvis.

The renal pelvis contains the major renal blood vessels and the origins of the ureter. Each kidney consists of 1 million nephrons, which span the cortex and medulla and are bound together by connective tissue containing blood vessels, nerves, and lymphatics.

The kidneys form the upper part of the urinary tract. The urine produced by the kidneys is transported to the bladder by two ureters. The lower urinary tract consists of the bladder and the urethra.

Approximately 1–1.5 liters of urine are produced by the kidneys each day. The volume and osmolality vary according to fluid intake and fluid loss.

The urinary tract epithelium is impermeable to water and solutes, unlike the nephrons in the kidney, so the composition of the urine is not altered as it is transported to the bladder. The bladder contents are emptied via the urethra, expulsion from the body being controlled by an external sphincter. Both the upper and lower urinary tract are innervated by the autonomic nervous system.

Figure 1.1 shows the anatomy of the kidneys and urinary tract.

Functions of the kidney and the urinary tract

1. **Excretion:** of waste products and drugs—this involves selective reabsorption and excretion of substances as they pass through the nephron.
2. **Regulation:** of body fluid volume and ionic composition. The kidneys have a major role in homeostasis (the maintenance of a constant internal environment) and are also involved in maintaining the acid–base balance.
3. **Endocrine:** the kidneys are involved in the synthesis of renin (which generates angiotensin I from angiotensinogen, and thus has a role in blood pressure and sodium balance), erythropoietin (which controls erythrocyte production) and prostaglandins (involved in vasodilation).
4. **Metabolism:** of vitamin D (converting 25-OH vitamin D into the metabolically active 1,25 form) and of low-molecular-weight proteins. The kidney is a major site for the catabolism of several hormones, such as insulin, parathyroid hormone, and calcitonin.

Fluid compartments of the body

Body fluids

Water is a major component of the human body. Approximately 60–65% of an adult male and 50–55% of an adult female is water (i.e., 45 L in a 70-kg male, 36 L in a 70-kg female). This difference is due to the fact that females have a higher proportion of body fat, which has a low water content.

The total body water (TBW) is divided into:
- Intracellular fluid (ICF), two-thirds of TBW (about 30 L in a 70-kg male).

Basic Principles

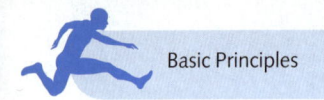

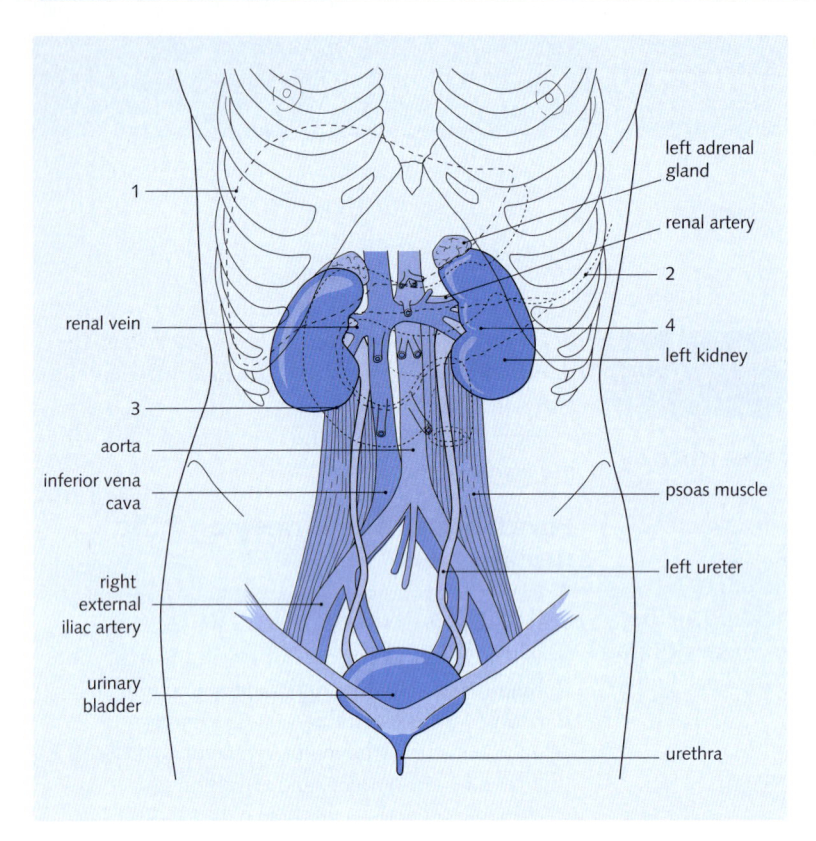

Fig. 1.1 Anatomy of the posterior abdominal wall showing the renal and urinary system. 1, Liver; 2, stomach; 3, second part of the duodenum; 4, pancreas.

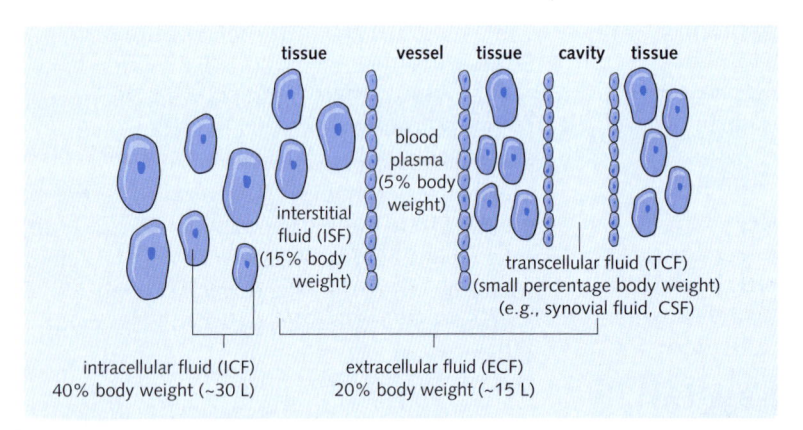

Fig. 1.2 Fluid compartments of the body.

- Extracellular fluid (ECF), one-third of TBW (about 15 L in a 70-kg male).

ECF is divided into:
- Plasma: ECF within the vascular system (i.e., the noncellular component of blood).
- Interstitial fluid: ECF outside the vascular system (and separated from plasma by the capillary endothelium).
- Transcellular fluid (TCF): ECF separated from plasma by the capillary endothelium and an additional epithelial layer that has specialized functions (e.g., synovial fluid, aqueous and vitreous humor, cerebrospinal fluid; Fig. 1.2).

Osmolarity and osmolality
Basic concepts
Osmosis is the net passage of a solvent through a semipermeable membrane from a less concentrated solution to a more concentrated solution. This occurs until both solutions reach the same concentration

Fig. 1.3 Osmolarity can be described as 1 mole of glucose added to water, dissolved to make up to 1 liter. Osmolality is the addition of 1 liter of water to one mole of glucose (adapted from Lote CJ: *Principles of renal physiology*, 4th ed. Kluwer Academic Publishers, 2000, pp. 4–5).

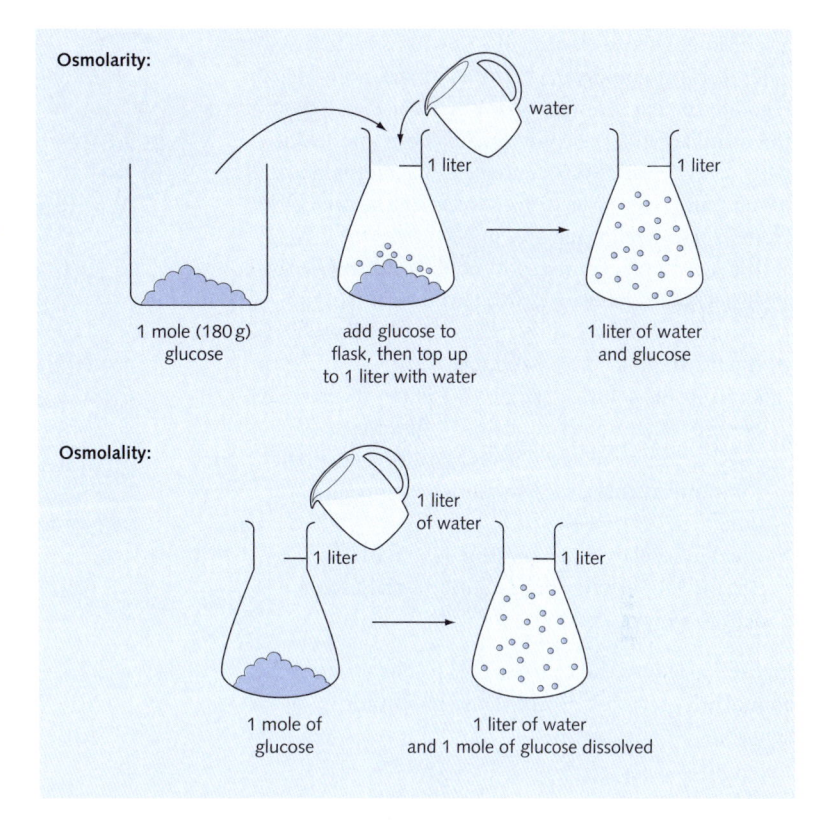

(equilibrium). The osmotic effect can be measured as an osmotic pressure.

Osmotic pressure is the pressure at which water is drawn into a solution across a semipermeable membrane. Thus, the more concentrated the solution (i.e., the higher the solute content), the greater the osmotic pressure. Hydrostatic pressure is the pressure that needs to be applied to the region containing the solute to prevent the net entry of water.

Osmolarity is the total solute concentration of a solution—the number of osmotically active particles in solution. The higher the osmolarity, the lower the water concentration. 1 osmole (Osmol) = 1 mole of solute particles.

Osmolarity vs. osmolality

Osmolarity measures the molar concentration of solute particles per liter of solution (mOsmol/L). *Osmolality* is the molar concentration of solute particles per kilogram of solvent (water) (mOsmol/kg H_2O). For the purposes of most human physiology, the two can be used interchangeably.

Figure 1.3 illustrates the differences between osmolality and osmolarity.

- Normal body fluid osmolality is between 285 and 295 mOsmol/kg H_2O (mosm/kg). Its main constituents are sodium and chloride.
- Urine osmolality may vary between 60 and 1400 mosm/kg. Its main constituents are urea, sodium, chloride, and potassium.

Plasma osmolality can be estimated from sodium ion (Na^+), urea (blood urea nitrogen [BUN]), and glucose concentrations using the formula:

Plasma osmolality = $2(Na^+) + BUN/2.8 + glucose/18$

where serum [Na] is in mEq/L, whereas BUN and glucose are in mg/dl.

Tonicity: movement of water across membranes

Changes in the extracellular osmolarity can cause cells to shrink or swell because water will move across the plasma membrane by osmosis into or out of the cells to maintain equilibrium. The tendency of

Basic Principles

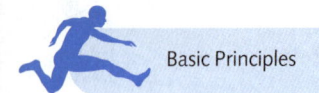

a solution to cause water shifts in cells is its *tonicity*. Therefore, an important function of the kidneys is to regulate the excretion of water in the urine so that the osmolarity of the ECF remains nearly constant despite wide variations in intake or extrarenal losses of salt and water. This prevents damage to the cells from excess swelling and shrinkage:

- If cells are placed in a solution over 295 mOsmol (hypertonic solution), they shrink as water moves out into the solution.
- If cells are placed in a solution of 285–295 mOsm/kg (isotonic solution, i.e., 0.9% saline), there is no net movement of water by osmosis and no swelling or shrinkage. This is because an isotonic solution has the same osmolarity as normal body fluid.
- If cells are placed in a solution less than 285 mOsmol (hypotonic solution), they swell as water enters from the solution.

Figure 1.4 shows the changes in the cells brought about by hypertonic, isotonic and hypotonic solutions.

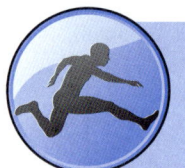

- Isoosmotic solutions have the same solution concentration per kilogram water.
- Isotonic solutions do not cause any change in cell volume (e.g., 285–295 mOsmol/L of nonpermeable solute).

Thus, some solutions that have osmolality different from plasma will be isotonic, since not all solutes cause water to shift across the cell membrane.

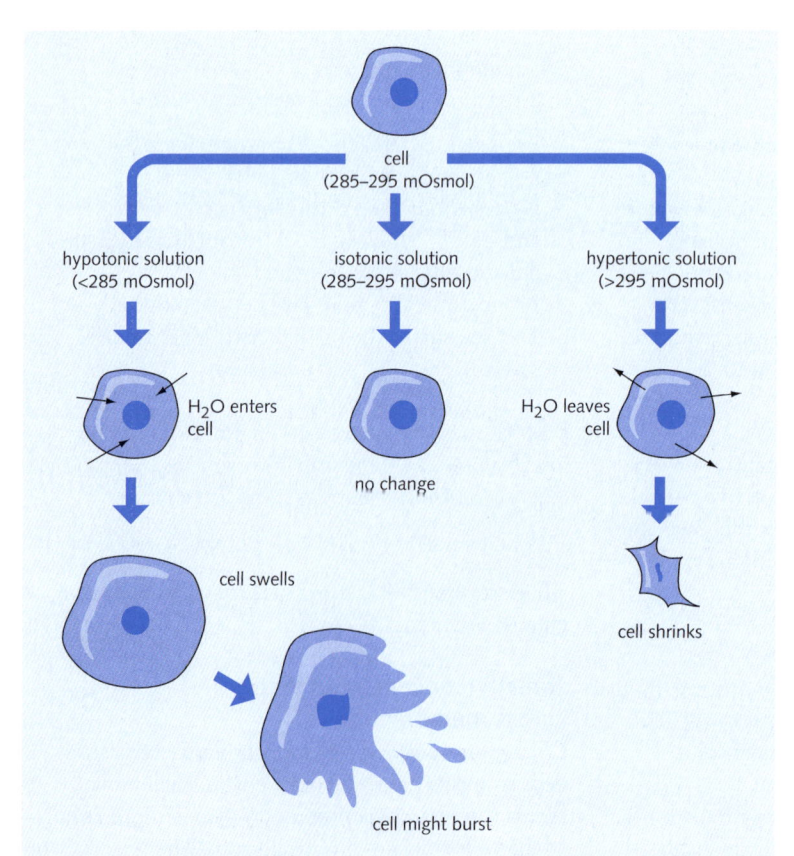

Fig. 1.4 Cell changes induced by hypotonic, isotonic, and hypertonic solutions.

Diffusion of ions across biological membranes
Passive transport
Biological membranes (e.g., cell membranes) are selectively permeable, allowing only small molecules and ions to diffuse through them. The concentration gradient and electrical gradient influence the movement of these molecules into or out of cells.

The rate of diffusion of different molecules depends upon their shape, size, weight and electrical charge. When solutions either side of a membrane contain diffusible ions only, ions move passively from an area of high ionic concentration down the electrical gradient to an area of lower ionic concentration. This occurs until equilibrium is reached, when the ion distribution on either side of the membrane will be as follows:

Side A (diffusible cations × diffusible anions)
= Side B (diffusible cations × diffusible anions)

The Gibbs–Donnan effect
Proteins are negatively charged molecules that are so large that they cannot diffuse across membranes. Thus, if proteins are present on one side of the membrane (side A), they act as anions and attract positive ions (cations) from side B. Cations diffuse across the membrane to the more negative side A, and thus maintain electrical neutrality. As a result, side A will not only contain non-diffusible proteins, but also the cations from side B—and therefore will have a greater number of total ions. Consequently, the osmotic pressure on side A will be greater. This encourages the entry of water, unless the osmotic pressure difference is counterbalanced by hydrostatic pressure on side B (Fig. 1.5).

Cell membranes are permeable to:
- Potassium ions (K^+).
- Chloride ions (Cl^-).
- Sodium ions (Na^+).

Active transport
Na^+ permeability across cell membranes is only 1/50th that of K^+ permeability. The primary active transport mechanism uses energy in the form of adenosine triphosphate (ATP) to actively pump Na^+ out of and K^+ into the cells against a concentration gradient. This sodium pump is composed of several proteins and lies within the cell membrane of all cells. Cl^- ions diffuse passively out of the cell across the cell membrane because there is an overall negative charge within the cell. This leads to a higher concentration of Cl^- ions outside the cells. At equilibrium, the cell has a net negative charge (−70mV).

According to the Gibbs–Donnan effect, there should be more ions inside the cell than outside because of the effects of anionic proteins. This is balanced in biological systems by the sodium pump as Na^+ is effectively nondiffusible.

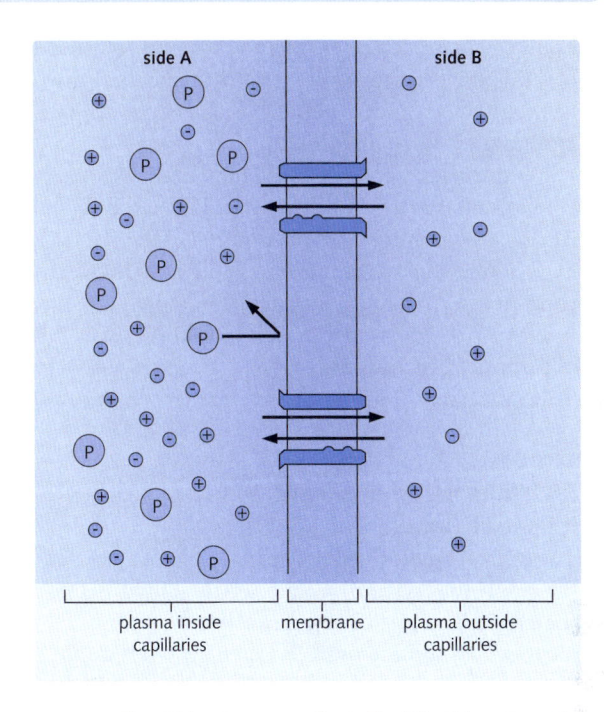

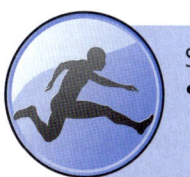

Fig. 1.5 The Gibbs–Donnan effect. ⊕, diffusible cation; ⊖, diffusible anion; P, impermeable molecule (e.g., protein).

Solute transport can be
- Passive—i.e., spontaneous, down an electrochemical gradient. This requires no energy.
- Active—i.e., against an electrochemical gradient. This is energy-dependent.

Fluid movement between body compartments
At any one moment, body fluid compartments have a relatively constant yet dynamic composition.

Basic Principles

Equilibrium is maintained by the continual transfer of fluid between the different compartments.

Exchange between ECF and ICF
Water diffuses freely across cell membranes so that equilibrium is reached between the ICF and ECF. Any change in the ionic concentration of the ICF or ECF is followed by the movement of water between these compartments.
- Na^+ is the most important extracellular osmotically active ion.
- K^+ is the most important intracellular osmotically active ion.

Exchange between plasma and interstitial fluid
The capillary endothelium separates plasma (within the circulatory system) from interstitial fluid (outside the circulatory system). Water and ions move between these two compartments—90% of ions by simple diffusion and 10% by filtration. Water and ion filtration between plasma and interstitial fluid relies on Starling forces, the balance between:
- Intracapillary hydrostatic pressure (which forces fluid out of the capillary) and
- Oncotic (or colloid osmotic) pressure, formed by proteins that are too large to cross the capillary endothelial cells, and therefore remain in the plasma (25 mmHg).

Hydrostatic pressure depends upon:
- Systemic blood pressure.
- Arteriolar resistance (which determines the extent to which blood pressure is transferred to the capillary).
- Venous blood pressure.

Oncotic pressure is produced by plasma proteins and the imbalance of ions—there are more ions (e.g., Na^+) within the capillary than outside. This is due to the presence of negatively charged proteins and the Gibbs–Donnan effect.

In the arterial end of the capillary the hydrostatic pressure of 32 mmHg exceeds the oncotic pressure of 25 mmHg, forcing fluid out of the capillary plasma into the interstitium. In the venous end of the capillary the hydrostatic pressure of 12 mmHg is less than the oncotic pressure, causing fluid to move out of the interstitium and re-enter the capillary plasma.

The movement of fluid across a capillary wall between the plasma and ISF is illustrated in Fig. 1.6.

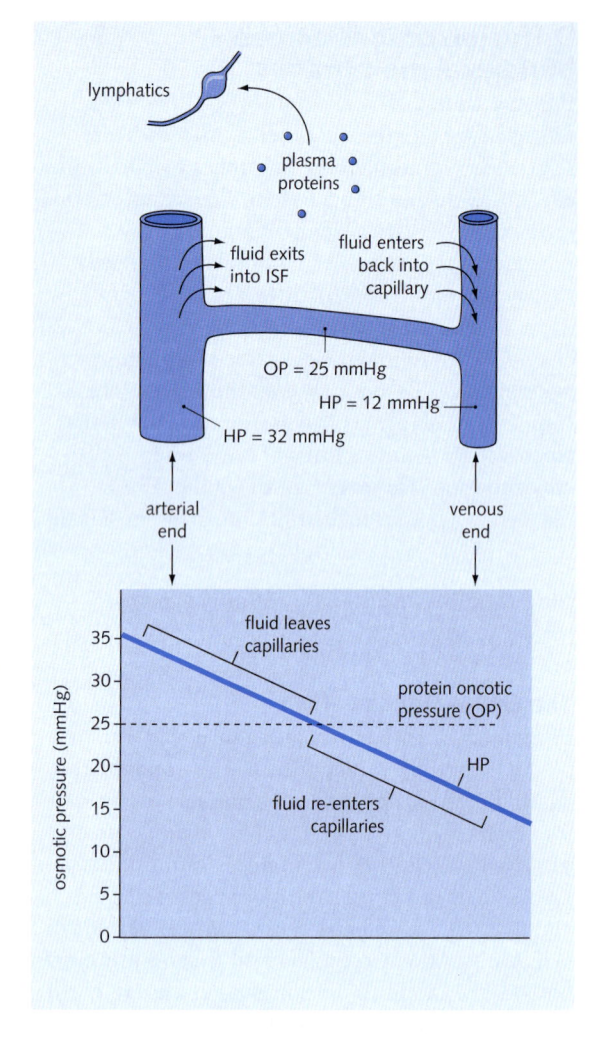

Fig. 1.6 Starling forces—factors involved in fluid exchange between the plasma and ISF across a capillary wall. HP, hydrostatic pressure; OP, oncotic pressure. *Note*: HP decreases from the arterial to the venous end of the capillary; OP is constant throughout.

Exchange between interstitial fluid and lymphatic vessels
Plasma proteins and fluid lost from the vascular system are filtered into the ISF, and taken up by the lymphatic system. This is composed of a network of lymphatic capillaries in all organs and tissues, which eventually drain into the venous system via the thoracic duct in the neck. These lymphatic capillaries are very permeable to protein and thus return both the fluid and plasma proteins to the circulatory system.

The ionic composition of the fluid compartments is shown in Fig. 1.7.

8

Fig. 1.7 Composition of the body fluid compartments.

Composition of fluid compartments

Component	Plasma	ECF	ICF*
Na^+ (mmol/L)	142	145	12
K^+ (mmol/L)	4	4.1	150
Cl^- (mmol/L)	103	113	4
HCO_3^- (mmol/L)	25	27	12
proteins (g/L)	60	0	25
osmolality (mOsm/kg H_2O)	280	280	280
compartment volume (L)	3.0	12.0	30

*ICF compartment is not the same throughout the body; it varies with different types of cells.

Water intake and output

Water intake (mL)		Water output (mL)	
drink	1500	lungs	400
food	500	skin	400
metabolism	400	feces	100
		urine	1500
total	2400	total	2400

Fig. 1.8 Distribution of daily water ingestion and losses.

Fluid and ion movement between the body and the external environment

There is a continuous exchange of body fluids with the external environment, but there must be a balance between intake and output, as body weight is consistent from day to day.

Daily water intake and output are shown in Fig. 1.8. Water lost from the lungs varies with the climate (e.g., in very dry climates over 400ml per day is lost). Insensible losses are those due to evaporation of water from the skin (i.e., not sweat). Sweating ("sensible perspiration") is an additional loss, which acts as a homeostatic mechanism to maintain constant body temperature. Urinary loss can be adjusted according to the needs of the body, and water intake. The amount of water lost in defecation can also vary, and is increased greatly in diarrhea. Daily water intake can fluctuate considerably and can be altered according to need (i.e. thirst mechanism). Water derived from metabolism is the result of oxidation of food. Despite these variations, the body's ionic concentration is maintained within the normal range by the kidney's homeostatic mechanisms, which include control of tubular reabsorption of filtered Na^+—and to a lesser extent K^+—as well as regulating water reabsorption.

Whereas water intake can be controlled, the minimum water loss from urine, lungs, skin and feces normally cannot fall below 1200mL/day. Thus, if there is no water intake, dehydration occurs, eventually resulting in death within a few days.

Measuring body fluid compartments
Dilution principle

The dilution principle is used to measure fluid volume if fluids cannot be directly measured or extracted from the container or compartment holding them. This allows measuring in situ. A substance that will mix completely and uniformly

Basic Principles

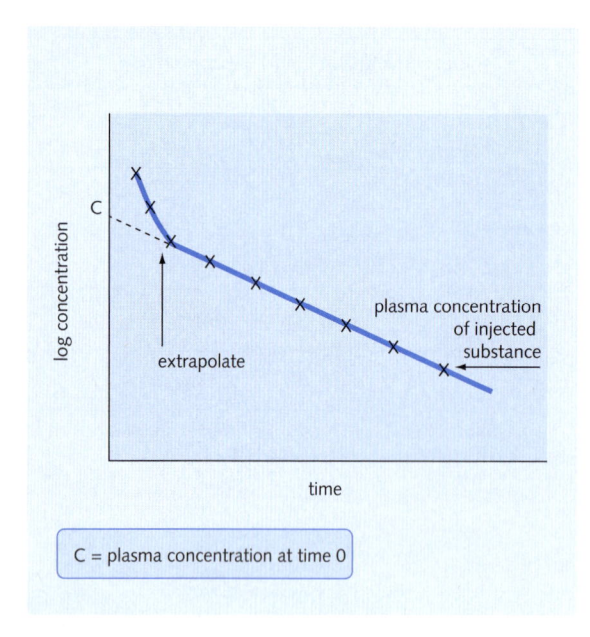

Fig. 1.9 The dilution principle: single injection method, showing the plasma concentration of an injected substance.

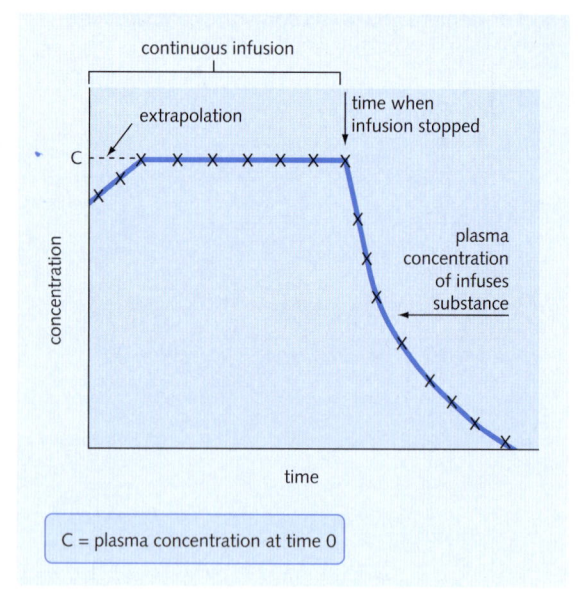

Fig. 1.10 The dilution principle: constant infusion method, showing the plasma concentration of an infused substance.

in the fluid compartment is used to allow all of the volume present to be measured (e.g., a dye). Allowances must be made for the excretion and metabolism of the selected indicator by the body.

$$V_D = \frac{Q_A - Q_H}{C}$$

Where V_D = volume of distribution; Q_A = quantity administered; Q_H = quantity metabolized; and C = concentration.

Two methods are used:
- Single injection method.
- Constant infusion method.

Single injection method
This is used for test substances with a slow rate of excretion from the compartment being measured, and is carried out as follows:
1. A known amount of test substance is injected intravenously.
2. Plasma concentration is determined at intervals.
3. A graph (log concentration against time scale) is plotted (Fig. 1.9).
4. The straight portion back to the start (i.e., time 0) is extrapolated—this gives the concentration of substance assuming it had distributed evenly and instantly.

Using this method:

Compartment volume =
   Amount injected/Concentration at zero time

Constant infusion method
This is used for test substances that are excreted rapidly and is carried out as follows:
1. A loading dose of the test substance is injected intravenously.
2. The test substance is infused at a rate to match the excretion rate.
3. Plasma concentration is measured at intervals.
4. When the substance comes to equilibrium, the plasma concentration is constant (Fig. 1.10).
5. The infusion is stopped and urine collected until all the test substance has been excreted.

Using this method:

Amount excreted = Amount present in the body at the time the infusion was stopped and:

Compartment volume (L) =
   $$\frac{\text{Amount excreted (mg)}}{\text{Plasma concentration (mg/L)}}$$

Figure 1.11 summarizes the methods used to measure the different fluid volumes.

Fig. 1.11 Summary of fluid compartments and their measurement in a person weighing 70kg.

Summary of fluid volume measurements in a 70kg individual		
Fluid volume	**Normal volume**	**Method of measurement**
plasma volume	3 L	radio-iodinated human serum albumin or Evans blue dye
blood volume	5 L	determined from the hematocrit
red cell volume	2 L	• measured from plasma volume and hematocrit • direct dilution
extracellular fluid (ECF)	15 L	indirect measurement using an injected substance (e.g., inulin)
intracellular fluid (ICF)	28 L	ICF = TBW − ECF − TCF
interstitial fluid (ISF)	12 L	calculated from ECF and plasma volume
total body water (TBW)	63% of total mass (men) 53% of total mass (women)	isotopes of water are used as markers
transcellular fluid (TCF)	20 L/day turnover in the gut	TCF = TBW − ECF − ICF

- Describe the location and composition of the kidneys.
- Summarize the main functions of the kidney.
- Name the different fluid compartments within the body, stating their relative proportions and values.
- Distinguish between osmolarity, osmolality, and tonicity.
- Explain how the following influence the distribution of ions across a semi-permeable membrane:
  (a) Concentration gradient.
  (b) Electrical gradient.
  (c) Proteins.
- What is the role of the lymphatic system in fluid movement?
- Describe the routes by which water and ions enter and leave the body, giving the relevant values.
- Outline the difference between the two methods used in the dilution principle.
- Discuss why it is important to use high-molecular-weight plasma proteins when measuring plasma volume.

2. Organization of the Kidneys

Development of the kidneys

The kidneys pass through three developmental stages (Fig. 2.1):
- **Pronephros:** the most primitive system, developing in the cervical region of the embryo during the fourth week of gestation. It is non-functional and regresses soon after its formation, leaving behind a nephritic duct.
- **Mesonephros:** develops in the lumbar region and functions for a short period. It consists of excretory tubules with their own collecting ducts known as mesonephric ducts. These drain into the nephritic ducts.
- **Metanephros:** develops in the sacral region at approximately 5 weeks of gestation and eventually forms the final adult kidneys. It becomes functional in the latter half of the pregnancy.

The functional unit of the kidney—the nephron—develops from the fusion of the:
- **Metanephric blastema**, which is derived from the nephrogenic cord (part of the intermediate mesoderm). This forms the nephron tubular system from the glomerulus to the distal tubule.
- **Ureteric bud**, which is an outgrowth of the mesonephric duct (this eventually dilates and splits to form the renal pelvis, calyces and collecting ducts).

The mesonephric tissue forms a cap over the ureteric bud (ampulla), which grows toward the metanephric blastema, dilates, and divides repeatedly. This eventually forms the pelvis, the major and minor calyces, and the collecting ducts of the kidneys. The ampulla differentiates into the nephron once fusion with the metanephric blastema is complete. A solid clump of cells near the differentiating ampulla is converted into a vesicle and fuses with the ampulla, eventually becoming a web of capillaries known as the glomerulus.

The metanephros initially relies on the pelvic branches of the aorta for its blood supply. Later, when the kidney ascends to the lumbar region, its primary blood supply is from the renal arteries, which branch from the aorta. Finally, the hilum of the kidney rotates from its anterior position to rest medially.

The ureters develop from the part of the ureteric bud between the pelvis and the vesicourethral canal (this develops from part of the hindgut known as the cloaca). They drain into the mesonephric ducts and the urogenital sinus. The urinary bladder develops from the mesoderm, and its epithelium is derived from both the mesoderm (the mesonephric ducts) and the endoderm (vesicourethral canal). This process is summarized in Fig. 2.2.

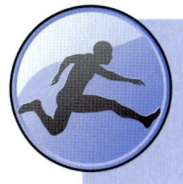

> Both the kidneys and the urinary system develop from the intermediate mesoderm (at the back of the fetal abdominal cavity).

General organization of the kidneys

Macroscopic organization
The anatomy of the kidneys is shown in Fig. 2.3. The relationships of the kidneys are as follows:
- **Anterior** (Fig. 2.4): to the right kidney: liver, 2nd part of the duodenum and the colon; to the left kidney: stomach, pancreas, spleen, jejunum, and descending colon.
- **Posterior:** diaphragm, quadratus lumborum, psoas, 12th rib, and three nerves (subcostal, iliohypogastric and ilioinguinal).
- **Medial:** hilum (a deep fissure containing the renal vessels, nerves, lymphatics and the renal pelvis);

Organization of the Kidneys

Fig. 2.1 The three embryological renal systems: pronephros, mesonephros, and metanephros.

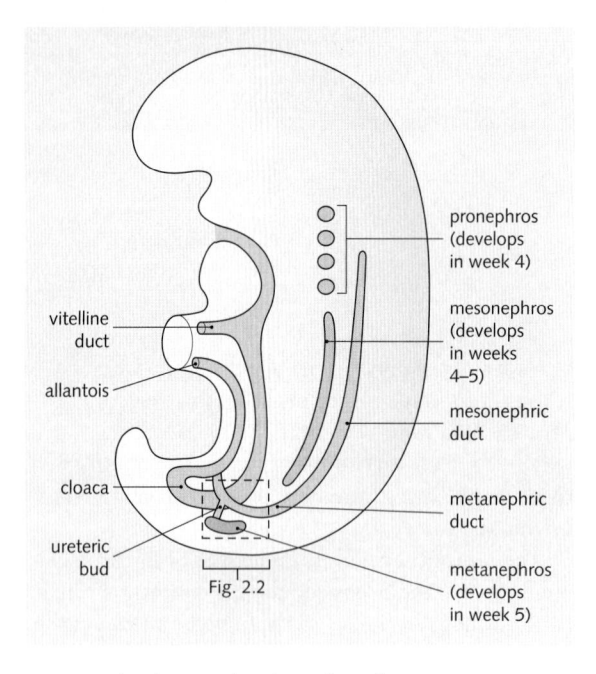

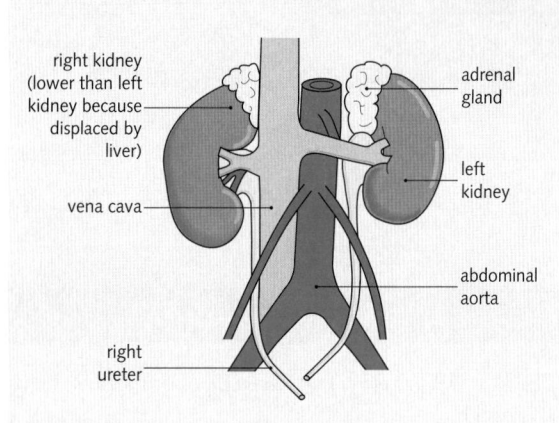

Fig. 2.3 Anatomy of the kidneys.

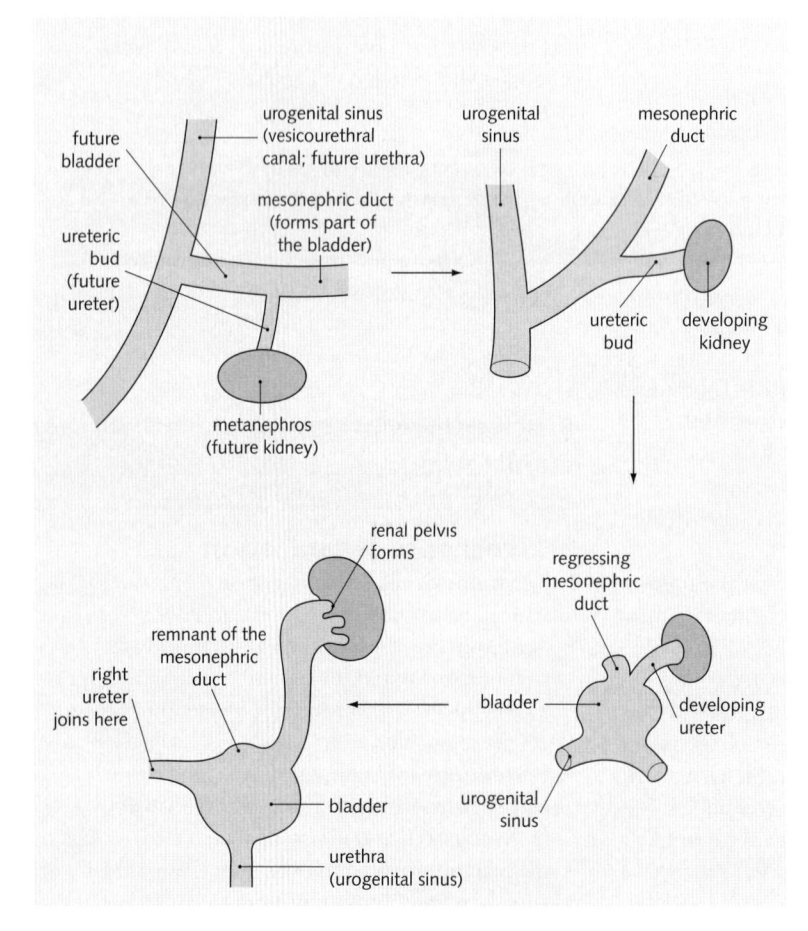

Fig. 2.2 Development of the kidneys, ureters, and bladder.

14

General organization of the kidneys

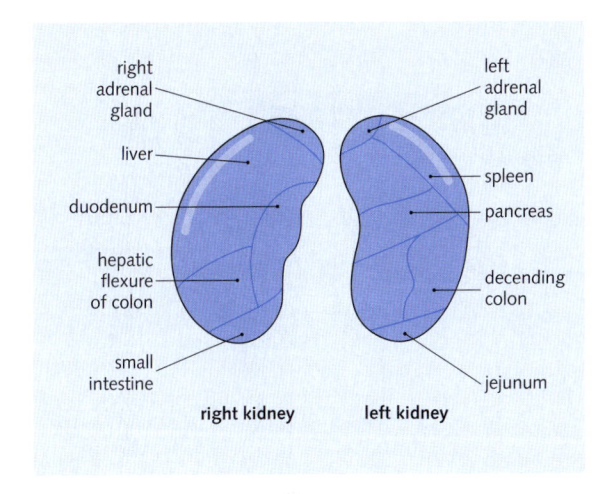

Fig. 2.4 Anterior relations of the kidney.

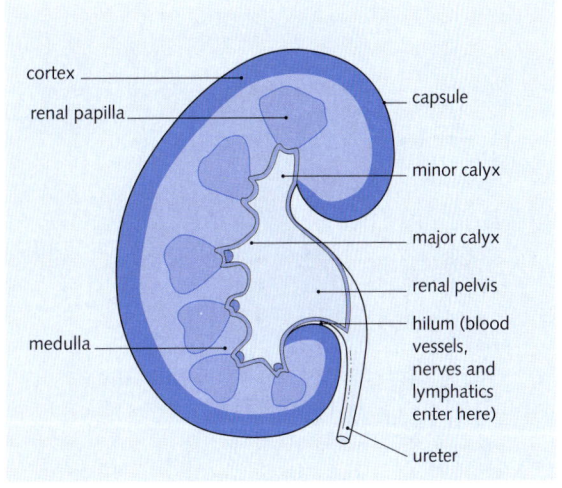

Fig. 2.5 Longitudinal section showing the macroscopic organization of the kidney.

to the left kidney: aorta; to the right kidney: inferior vena cava.
- **Superior:** adrenal gland.

The kidneys lie in a fatty cushion (perinephric fat) contained within the renal fascia. They have three capsular layers:
1. Fascial (renal fascia).
2. Fatty (perinephric fascia).
3. True (fibrous capsule).

Morphology and internal structure

Within the kidney, the ureter continues as the renal pelvis, which lies in a deep fissure called the hilum. The outer border of the renal pelvis divides into two or three major divisions (calyces). These subdivide into a number of minor calyces and are each indented by a papilla of renal tissue called the renal pyramid. It is here that the collecting tubules empty the urine. Along with the renal pelvis, the renal artery, vein, nerve and lymphatics all enter the medial border of the kidney at the hilum (Fig. 2.5).

The kidney is divided into two main layers:
1. Outer renal cortex (dark).
2. Inner renal medulla (paler).

The glomeruli in the cortex give it a granular appearance on histology.

The blood supply to the kidneys is from the right and left renal arteries, which branch directly off the abdominal aorta at the level of L1–2. The renal veins drain from the kidneys directly into the vena cava. Lymphatics drain to the para-aortic lymph nodes.

The kidney is innervated by sympathetic fibers mainly from the celiac plexus.

Nephrons

Each kidney has approximately one million nephrons. The nephron (Fig. 2.6) is the functional unit of the kidney and consists of:
1. A renal corpuscle: the glomerulus and its surrounding Bowman's capsule, emptying directly into the
2. Tubule (proximal tubule, loop of Henle, distal convoluted tubule and collecting duct).

There are two types of nephron, depending on the length of the loop of Henle:
1. **Cortical nephrons:** these have renal corpuscles in the outer part of the cortex, with a short loop of Henle.
2. **Juxtamedullary nephrons:** these have larger renal corpuscles in the inner third of the cortex, with long loops of Henle extending into the medulla.

In the human kidney, 85% of the nephrons are cortical nephrons and the remaining 15% are juxtamedullary nephrons.

Glomerulus

The glomerulus is formed by the invagination of a ball of capillaries into the Bowman's capsule, which is the blind end of a nephron. It has a diameter of approximately 200μm.

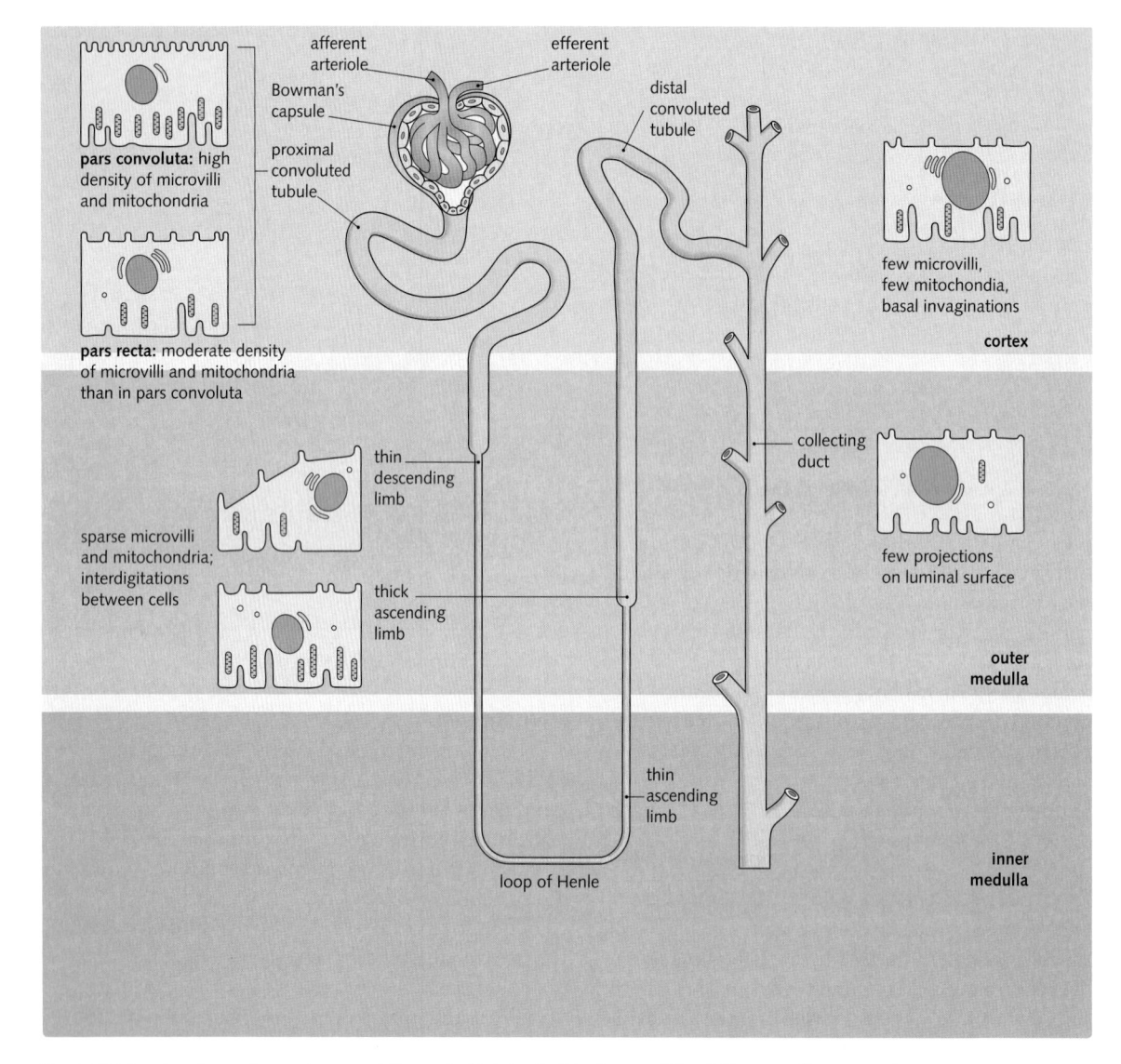

Fig. 2.6 The structure of a nephron and the main histological features of the different cell types within it.

The function of the glomerulus is to produce a protein-free filtrate from the blood in the glomerular capillaries. The capillaries are supplied by the afferent arterioles and drained by the efferent arterioles. The filtration membrane of the glomerulus is made up of three layers and is fundamental to kidney function.

Proximal tubule

The proximal tubule continues from the renal corpuscle. It is 15 mm long and 55 μm in diameter. Its wall is composed of a single layer of cuboidal cells, which interdigitate extensively and are connected by tight junctions at their luminal surfaces. The luminal edge of each cell is made up of millions of microvilli, forming a dense brush border that increases the surface area available for absorption of tubular filtrate. At the base of each cell there are infoldings of the cell membrane (see Fig. 2.6). The extracellular space between the cells is known as the lateral intercellular space.

The structure of the proximal tubule varies along its length:

- The first part is convoluted (pars convoluta), and cells have an increased density of microvilli and a greater number of mitochondria than cells in the

second straight part. This suggests a role in transport of substances across the lumen and the filtrate.
- The second straight part (pars recta) leads on to the first part of the loop of Henle (the thin descending limb).

Loop of Henle

The loop of Henle consists of a single layer of flattened squamous cells, which form a thin-walled, hairpin-shaped tube. The cells of the thin descending segment interdigitate sparingly and have few mitochondria and microvilli on the luminal surface (see Fig. 2.6). This segment ends at the tip of the hairpin loop.

The thin ascending segment is 2 mm long and 20 μm in diameter. Its structure is similar to the preceding part of the tubule (the pars recta), except that the cells have extensive interdigitations. This might have a role in the active transport and permeability properties of the cells. There is an abrupt transition between the thin and thick ascending segments, and the level of this transition depends upon the length of the loop.

The thick ascending segment is 12 mm in length and consists of a single layer of columnar cells. The luminal membrane is invaginated to form many projections, although there is no brush border and there are few infoldings of the basal membrane.

Distal convoluted tubule

The distal convoluted tubule is the continuation of the loop of Henle into the cortex, ending in the collecting ducts. The cells have very few microvilli, no brush border, and basal infoldings surrounding mitochondria that gradually decrease towards the collecting ducts (see Fig. 2.6).

Collecting ducts

The cortical collecting ducts are 20 mm long. They are lined with cuboidal cells that have a few projections on the luminal surface (see Fig. 2.6). Different cell types in this part of the tubule include:
- Principal cells: these contain few mitochondria and respond to antidiuretic hormone (ADH)—also known as vasopressin.
- Intercalated cells: these contain numerous mitochondria and secrete hydrogen ions (H^+).

The ducts pass through the renal cortex and medulla and, at the apices of the renal pyramids, drain the urine into the renal pelvis. The renal pelvis is lined by transitional epithelium.

In the cortex each collecting duct drains approximately six distal tubules. In the medulla the distal tubules join together and from here drain into the renal calyx.

Urine formation depends on three basic processes:
- Glomerular filtration.
- Tubular reabsorption.
- Tubular secretion.

Blood supply and vascular structure

The kidneys receive 20–25% of the total cardiac output (1.2 L/min) via the right and left renal arteries. These branch to form interlobar arteries, which further divide to form the arcuate arteries (located at the junction between the cortex and medulla). The interlobular arteries arise at 90 degrees to the arcuate arteries through the cortex, dividing up to form the afferent arterioles. These feed the glomerular capillary networks, which are then drained by the efferent arterioles.

The efferent arterioles drain blood from the glomerular capillaries and act as portal vessels (i.e., they carry blood from one capillary network to another).
- In the outer two-thirds of the cortex the efferent arterioles form a network of peritubular capillaries that supplies all cortical parts of the nephron.
- In the inner third of the cortex the efferent arterioles follow a hairpin course to form a capillary network surrounding the loops of Henle and the collecting ducts down into the medulla. These vessels are known as the vasa recta.

The vasa recta and the peritubular capillaries drain into the left and right renal veins and then into the inferior vena cava. The microcirculation of the kidney is illustrated in Fig. 2.7.

Organization of the Kidneys

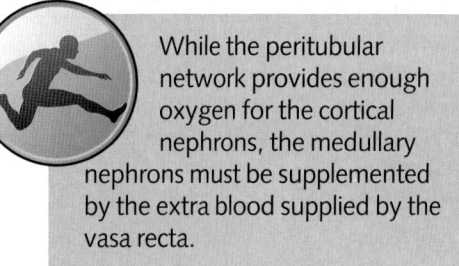

> While the peritubular network provides enough oxygen for the cortical nephrons, the medullary nephrons must be supplemented by the extra blood supplied by the vasa recta.

Function of the renal blood supply

The high rate of blood flow through the kidney is very important in maintaining the homeostatic functions of the kidney. The blood flow through the kidney determines the filtration rate. The oxygen consumption of the kidney is 18mL/min—50% of which is involved in Na^+ reabsorption in the tubules. The vasa recta helps deliver oxygen and nutrients to the nephron segments, and allows the return of reabsorbed substances into the circulation.

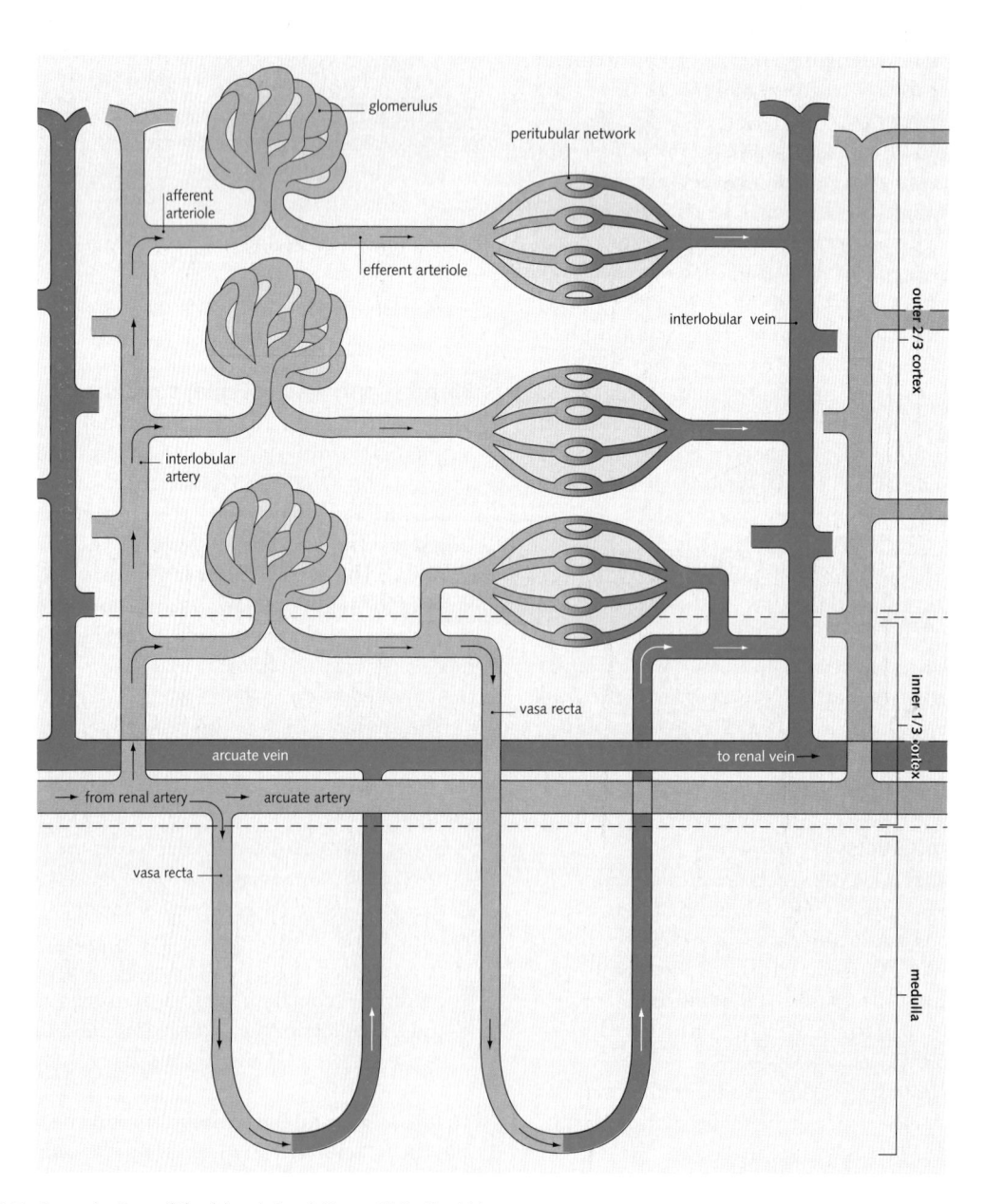

Fig. 2.7 Organization of the blood circulation within the kidney.

Although there is a very substantial blood flow, the arteriovenous oxygen difference is only about 15 mL/L, compared with 62 mL/L in the brain and 114 mL/L in the heart. This means that the oxygen extraction in the kidney is not as efficient as in other organs as a result of shunting of blood in the vasa recta through its hairpin structure.

Juxtaglomerular apparatus (JGA)
The JGA (Fig. 2.8) is located where the thick ascending loop of Henle passes back up into the cortex and lies adjacent to the renal corpuscle and arterioles of its own nephron. It is the area of distal tubule associated with arterioles. The tunica media in the wall of the afferent arteriole contains an area of specialized thickened cells (granular cells), which secrete renin. The epithelium of the distal tubule forms specialized macula densa cells that respond to changes in the composition of the tubular fluid, especially the concentration of chloride ions in the filtrate.

Hormones produced by the kidney
Renin
Renin is a protein that cleaves angiotensinogen to form angiotensin I, which in turn is converted to angiotensin II. Angiotensin II is a potent vasoconstrictor affecting blood pressure, tubular reabsorption of Na^+, and aldosterone secretion from the adrenal glands. Renin release is stimulated by sympathetic stimulation of the granular cells or a decrease in filtrate Na^+ concentration. The latter can occur following a fall in plasma volume, vasodilation of the afferent arterioles, and renal ischemia.

Erythropoietin (EPO)
The kidney is the major source (85%) of EPO production in the adult; in fetal life the liver also produces EPO. It is produced by peritubular interstitial cells of the inner cortex. EPO-sensitive cells are the erythrocyte stem cells found in the bone marrow and the effect of the hormone is to increase the production of erythrocytes, resulting in an

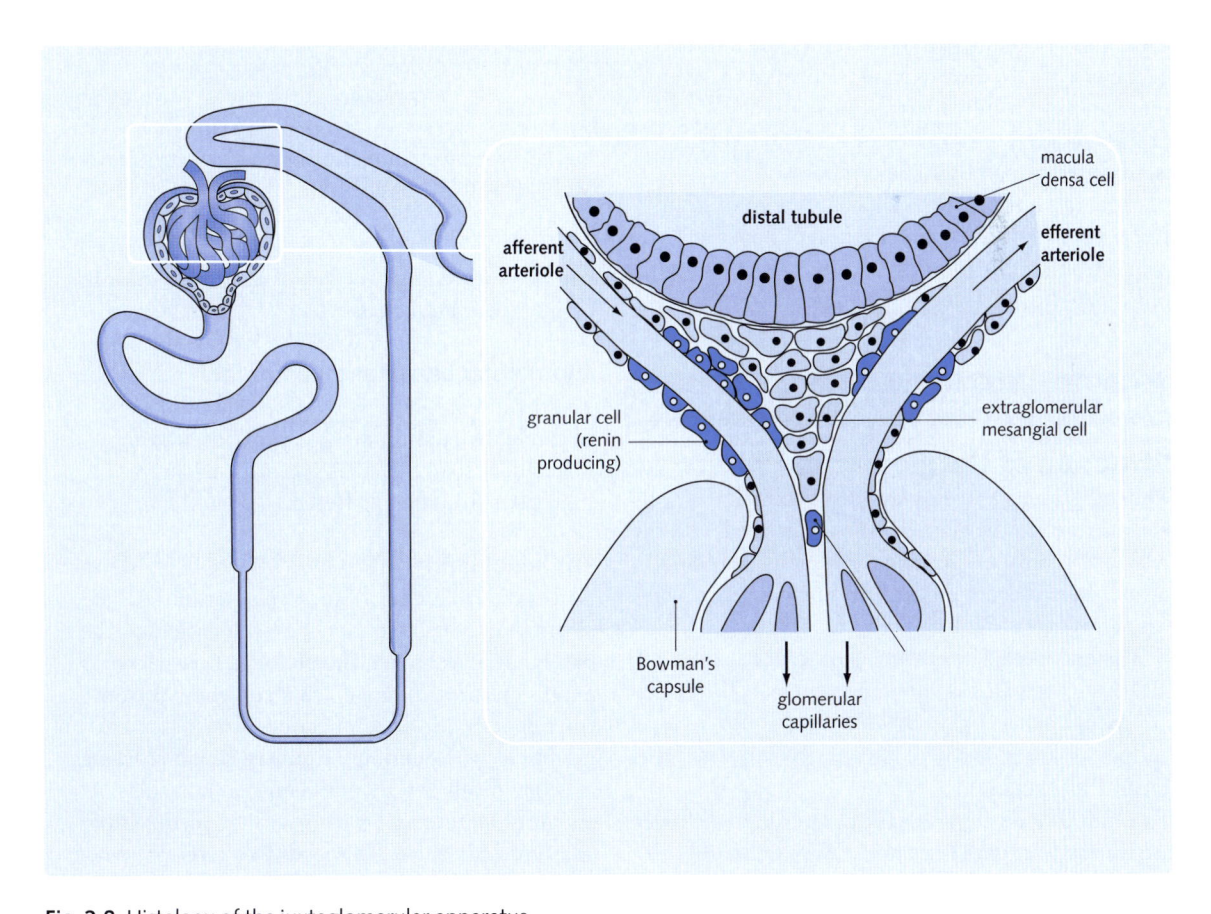

Fig. 2.8 Histology of the juxtaglomerular apparatus.

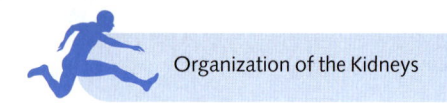

increase in the oxygen-carrying capacity of the blood. The half-life of EPO is 5hr.

Clinical use of EPO
Hypoxia, anemia, and renal ischemia stimulate EPO synthesis (this is a prostaglandin-mediated response). Increased secretion is seen in polycystic kidney disease and renal cell carcinoma, resulting in polycythemia. Patients with chronic kidney disease often have inappropriately low EPO secretion, resulting in normochromic normocytic anemia. Administration of recombinant EPO (either intravenous or subcutaneous) will correct this anemia.

Vitamin D
Vitamin D is a steroid hormone obtained in the diet and synthesized in the skin from 7-dehydrocholesterol in the presence of sunlight. This naturally occurring vitamin D (cholecalciferol) is hydroxylated in the liver to form 25-hydroxycholecalciferol ($25(OH)D_3$). It is filtered at the glomerulus, reabsorbed by the proximal tubular cells, and further hydroxylated under the influence of the enzyme 1α-hydroxylase to form the active metabolite 1,25-dihydroxycholecalciferol ($1,25(OH)_2D_3$). Production of $1,25(OH)_2D_3$ is regulated by parathyroid hormone (PTH), phosphate, and negative feedback. Active vitamin D is essential for the mineralization of bones and promotes the absorption of calcium ions (Ca^{2+}) and phosphate from the gut.

Glomerular structure and function

Structure of the glomerular filter
The first stage of urine production is the filtration of plasma through the glomerular capillary wall into the Bowman's capsule. The composition of the plasma ultrafiltrate depends on the filtration barrier, which has three layers (Fig. 2.9):
1. The endothelial cells of the glomerular capillary.
2. The glomerular basement membrane (GBM).
3. The epithelial cells of Bowman's capsule.

Endothelial cells
The endothelial cells lining the glomerular capillaries are thin and flat with large nuclei. The cells are perforated by numerous fenestrae (pores), which have a diameter of 60nm. This allows plasma

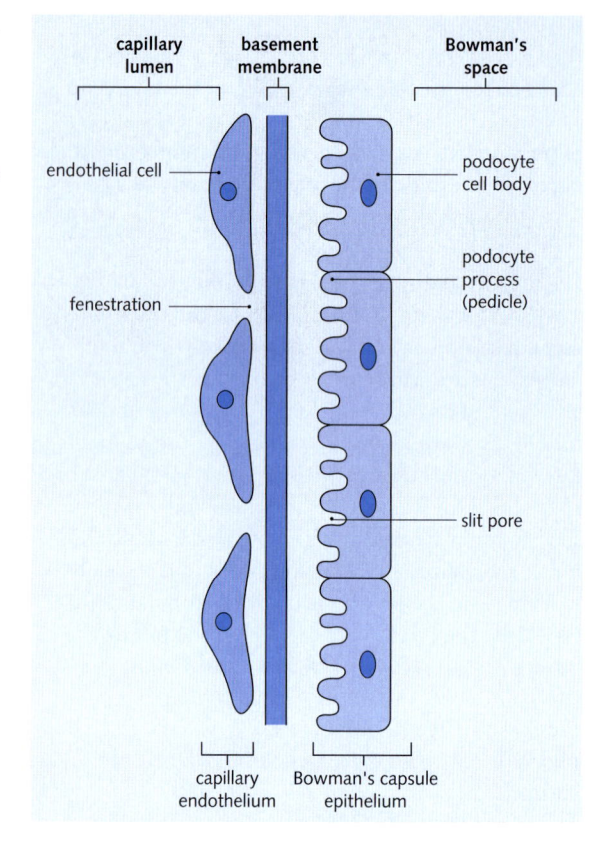

Fig. 2.9 Microscopic organization of the glomerular capillary membrane.

components to cross the vessel wall, but not blood cells or platelets.

Glomerular basement membrane
The basement membrane is a continuous layer of connective tissue and glycoproteins. It is a noncellular structure that prevents any large molecules from being filtered.

Epithelial lining
The epithelial lining of Bowman's capsule is a single layer of cells (podocytes), which rest on the basement membrane. The podocytes have large extensions or trabeculae, which extend out from the cell body and are embedded in the basement membrane surrounding a capillary. Small processes called pedicels extend out from the trabeculae and interdigitate extensively with the pedicels of adjacent trabeculae. This leads to the formation of slit pores, which control the movement of substances through the final layer of the filter. The podocytes

Glomerular structure and function

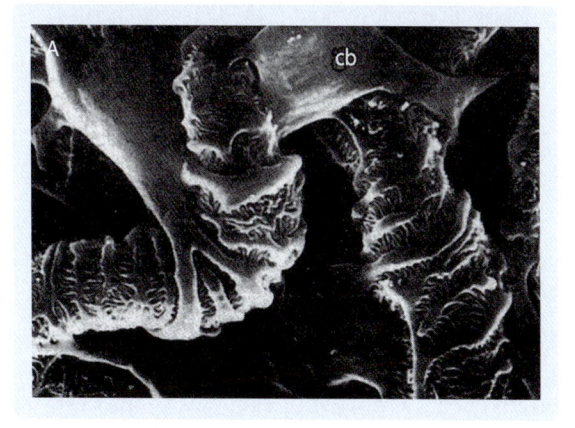

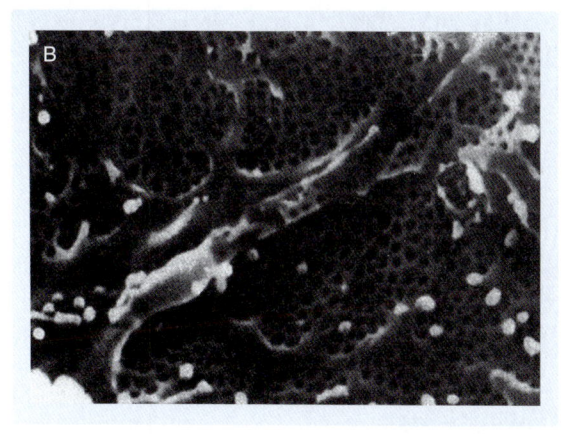

Fig. 2.10 Electron micrographs to show the arrangement of podocytes and glomerular capillaries as seen from Bowman's capsule. (A) Processes of podocytes run from the cell body (cb) toward the capillaries, where they ultimately split into foot processes (pedicles). (B) Inner surface of a glomerular capillary (from Koeppen BM, Stanton B: *Renal physiology*, 2nd ed. Mosby Year Book, 1996).

have a well-developed Golgi apparatus, used to produce and maintain the glomerular basement membrane. Podocytes can also be involved in phagocytosis of macromolecules (see Figs. 2.9 and 2.10).

Mesangium

The mesangium is also part of the renal corpuscle and consists of two components:
1. Mesangial cells.
2. Mesangial matrix.

The mesangial cells surround the glomerular capillaries and have characteristics of both monocytes and myocytes. They provide structural support for the capillaries, exhibit phagocytic activity, secrete extracellular matrix, and secrete cytokines and prostaglandins. The cells are contractile, which helps regulate the surface area of the GBM and blood flow through the glomerular capillaries.

Process of glomerular filtration

Filtration of macromolecules depends upon molecular weight, shape and electrical charge. It is a passive process that involves the flow of a solvent through a filter. Molecular weight is the main factor in determining whether a substance is filtered or remains in the capillaries. Any molecules that are small enough to pass through the filter form the filtrate. The maximum molecular weight of substances able to pass through the filter is 70kDa. Any molecule with a molecular weight of less than 70kDa passes freely through the filter (e.g., glucose, amino acids, Na, urea, K, small peptide hormones).

All three layers of the filter are coated with negatively charged glycosaminoglycans (especially heparan sulfate proteoglycan), which repel negatively charged macromolecules such as albumin. Smaller, positively charged molecules pass through the filtration barriers relatively easily, unless they are protein bound.

Serum albumin has a molecular weight of 69kDa and is a negatively charged protein. Only very tiny amounts pass through the glomerular filter because of the repelling effect of its negative charge, and all of this is normally reabsorbed in the proximal tubule. A total of 30g of protein per day enters the renal lymph vessels after reabsorption. Significant amounts of protein in the urine (proteinuria) indicate kidney disease. Proteinuria usually results from injury to one of the components of the glomerular filtration barrier.

Regulation of glomerular filtration is discussed in Chapter 3.

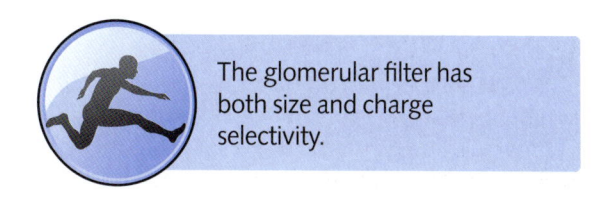

> The glomerular filter has both size and charge selectivity.

Transport processes in the renal tubule

The ultrafiltrate produced from the glomerular filter has a similar composition to plasma but is then modified by reabsorption and secretion within the tubule to produce the final urine. The general principle of this process is that bulk reabsorption of water and solutes occurs proximally; then the final urine concentration is determined by fine adjustments in the distal nephron.

Definitions

Reabsorption, secretion, and excretion are defined as follows:
- **Reabsorption:** the movement of a substance from the tubular fluid back into the circulation.
- **Secretion:** the movement of substances from the blood into the tubular fluid via tubular cells (active transport) or intercellular spaces (passive process).
- **Excretion:** the removal of waste products from the blood and the net result of filtration, secretion, and reabsorption of a substance.

Figure 2.11 illustrates the processes that occur in the nephron and result in excretion of a substance. Two types of solute transport are involved:

1. Paracellular movement (between cells) across the tight junctions that connect the cells. This is driven by concentration and the electrical and osmotic gradients.
2. Transcellular movement (through cells) via both the apical and basal membranes and the cell cytoplasm. Here, water follows the movement of solutes by osmosis.

Transport mechanisms
Diffusion

Diffusion is the movement of substances down their electrochemical gradient. It is a "passive" process, because it does not require any metabolic energy or carrier molecules.

Facilitated diffusion

Like diffusion, this is also passive movement of substances along their electrochemical gradient, but it relies on a carrier molecule to transport substances across the membrane. Consequently, it is much faster than diffusion.

Primary active transport

This is an energy-dependent process in which substances cross cell membranes against their concentration and electrochemical gradients. It involves the hydrolysis of adenosine triphosphate

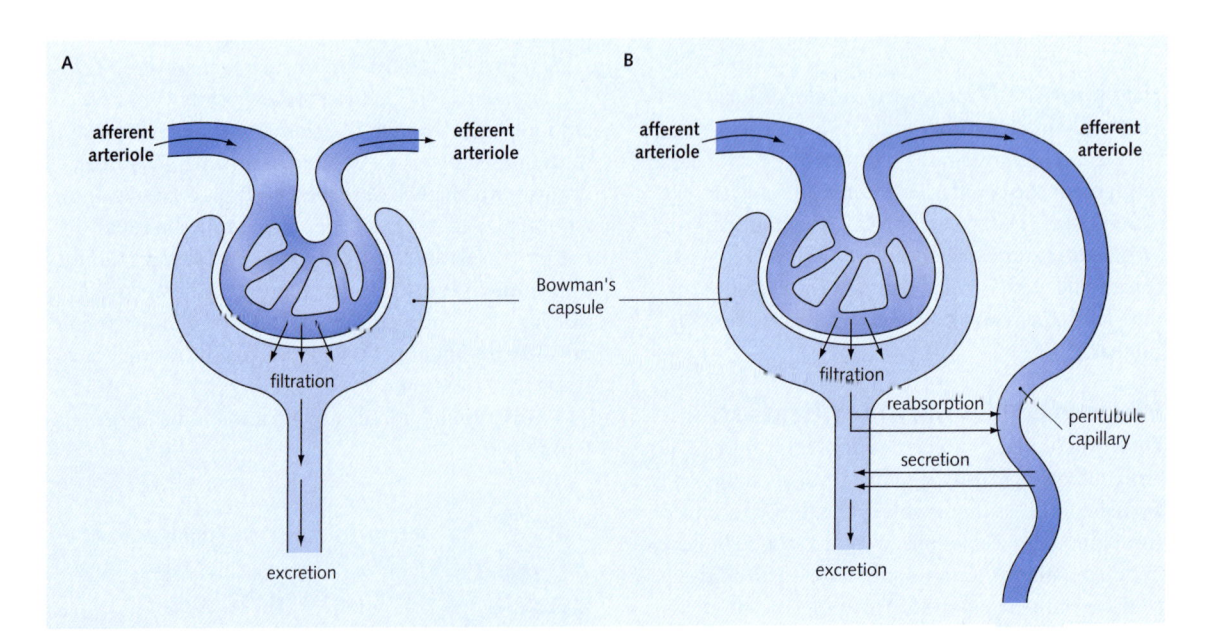

Fig. 2.11 Processes that result in the excretion of a substance in the nephron.

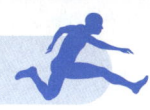

(ATP), which provides chemical energy for the transport mechanism.

The most important active transporter is the Na+/K+ ATPase pump, which is found on the basal and basolateral membranes of tubular cells. It is involved in the active transport of Na+ from intracellular to extracellular spaces, allowing the nephron to reabsorb over 99% of the filtered Na+. This maintains a low Na+ concentration and a high K+ concentration in the cell (Fig. 2.12). The other primary active transporters on the tubular cell membrane are:
- Ca^{2+} ATPase.
- H+/K+ ATPase.
- H+ ATPase.

The ATP molecule is part of the protein structure in the primary active transporters. Energy is derived from the hydrolysis of the terminal phosphate bond of the ATP molecule to form adenosine diphosphate (ADP) and phosphate (P_i) (Fig. 2.13).

Secondary active transport

This process uses the energy produced from another process to transport molecules across the cell membrane (i.e., the transport of the solutes is coupled). The most important example of this mechanism involves the Na+/K+ ATPase pump as the driving force for the secretion and reabsorption of other solutes in which the energy is provided by the Na+ gradient.

The Na+/K+ ATPase pump creates an ionic gradient across the cell membrane, which allows the energy produced from the diffusion of Na+ into the cell as it moves along its electrochemical gradient to be used for active transport (i.e., against their electrochemical gradients) of other solutes.

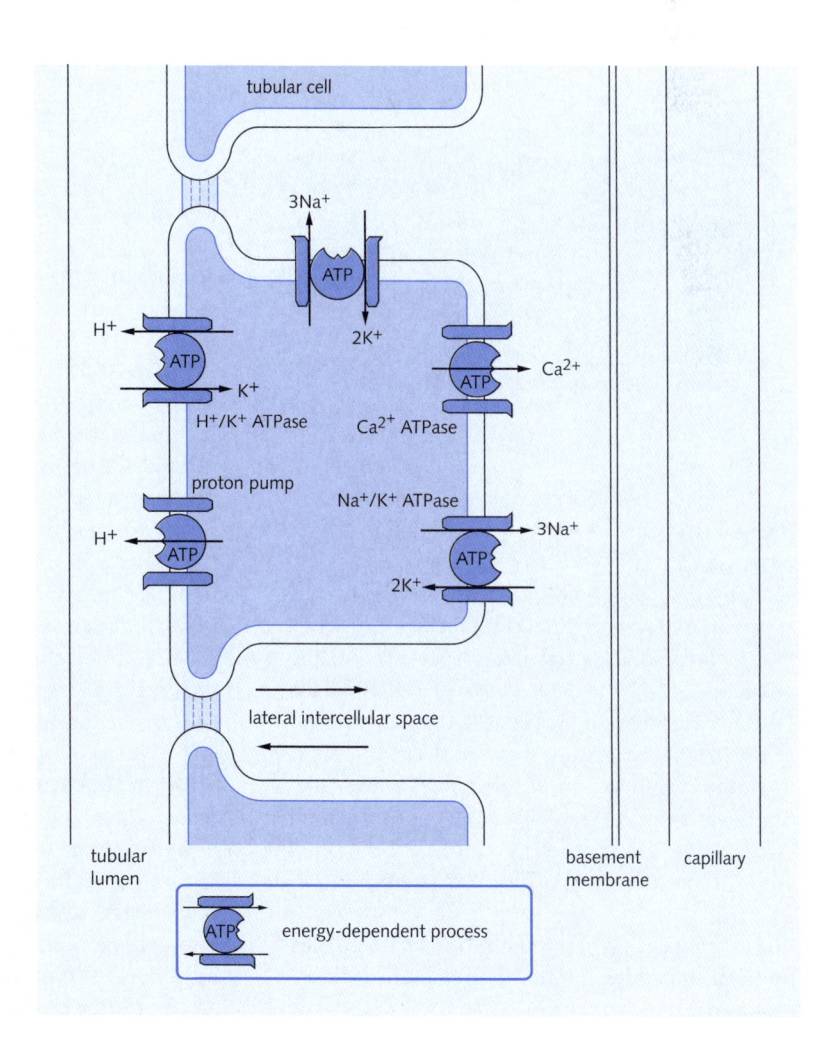

Fig. 2.12 Mechanisms of active transport in the tubules:
- H+/K+ ATPase
- proton pump
- Ca^{2+} ATPase
- Na+/K+ ATPase (sodium pump).

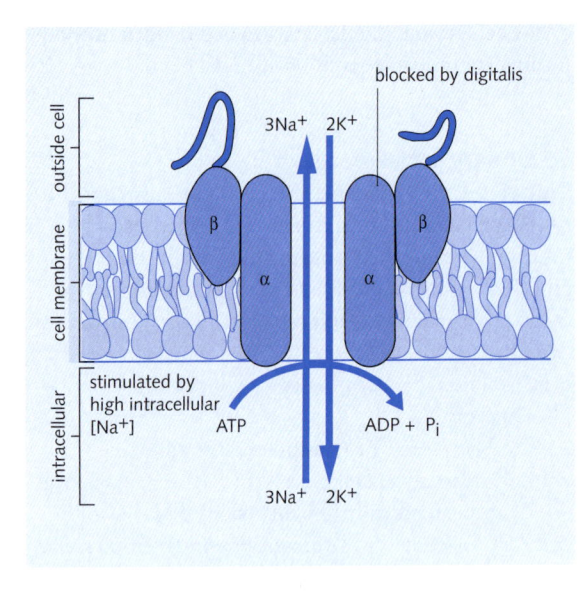

Organization of the Kidneys

Fig. 2.13 Na$^+$/K$^+$ ATPase pump found in the basal membrane of the cells. It drives secondary active transport by maintaining a low Na$^+$ concentration in the cells.

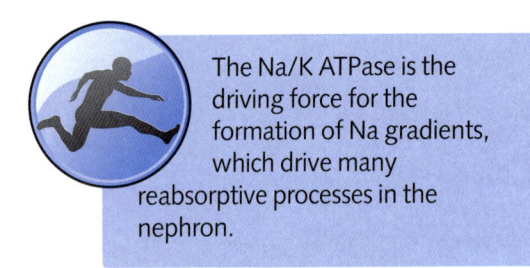

> The Na/K ATPase is the driving force for the formation of Na gradients, which drive many reabsorptive processes in the nephron.

Substances can move across the tubular cell membranes in two directions by the following processes:

- **Symport:** energy produced by the movement of Na$^+$ is used to transport other substances in the same direction across the cell membrane—i.e., into the cell (e.g., the Na$^+$/K$^+$/Cl$^-$ cotransporter in the thick ascending limb and the Na$^+$/glucose transporter in the cells of the proximal tubule cells).
- **Antiport:** movement of substances against their electrochemical gradient in the opposite direction to the Na$^+$ gradient—i.e., out of the cell (e.g., the Ca^{2+}/Na$^+$ and the H$^+$/Na$^+$ exchangers).

These processes are carried out by specific carrier proteins embedded in the cell membrane called transporters.

Ion channels

These are protein pores found on the epithelial cell membranes. They allow rapid transport of ions into the cell. Channels that are specific for Na$^+$, K$^+$, and Cl$^-$ are found on the apical membrane of all the cells lining the nephron. Although transport through these channels is very fast (10^6–10^8 ions/s) there are only about 100 channels per cell, compared with the slower (100 ions/s) but more numerous active transporters (10^7 transporters per cell).

The proximal tubule

The proximal tubule is the primary site for bulk reabsorption of water and many solutes. It also serves as an important secretory site for ammonium and protons, both important in the regulation of acid-base status.

Microstructure
The proximal tubule is made up of two parts:
1. Pars convoluta.
2. Pars recta.

The most active transport occurs in the cells of the pars convoluta. The features of a proximal tubule cell are shown in Fig. 2.14. Histology is discussed earlier (see Fig. 2.6).

Reabsorption of sodium and water
The concentration of Na$^+$ in the Bowman's capsule is equal to the plasma level because Na$^+$ is freely filtered. Virtually all the Na$^+$ that is filtered into the nephron is reabsorbed back into the circulation, with only 1% or less of the filtered Na$^+$ being excreted in the urine. This is important not only to preserve total body sodium (and extracellular volume) but also because the reabsorption processes of glucose, amino acids, water, lactate, Cl$^-$, HCO$_3^-$, and PO$_4^{3-}$ ions depend upon the movement of Na$^+$ back into the cells of the tubule.

Sodium reabsorption
Seventy per cent of the filtered Na$^+$ is reabsorbed in the proximal tubule. The Na$^+$/K$^+$ ATPase (Na$^+$ pump) on the basolateral membrane actively transports Na$^+$ out of the cell into the lateral intercellular spaces between adjacent cells. This movement of Na$^+$ out of the cell maintains a very low concentration of Na$^+$ within the proximal tubule cells

The proximal tubule

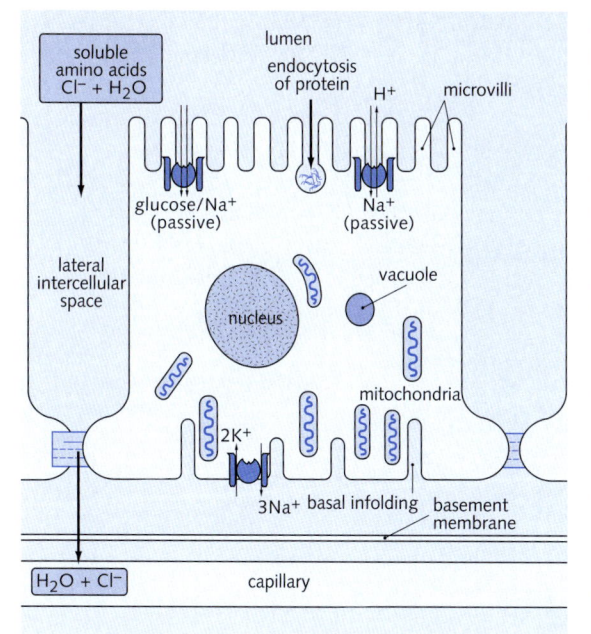

Fig. 2.14 Features of a proximal tubule cell.

(less than 30 mmol/L). This, and the fact that there is a negative transmembrane potential relative to the lumen (−70 mV), drives Na+ ions to move along their concentration and electrical gradients into the cells from the tubular fluid via carrier molecules on the apical membrane. In the early proximal tubule, movement of other substances is coupled with Na+ transport in and out of tubule cells:
- Glucose, amino acids, PO_4^{3-} and lactate are transported by symport with Na+ into the cell.
- H+ moves by antiport out of the cell and linked to the reabsorption of filtered HCO_3^-.

Much Na+ is reabsorbed in the early proximal tubule but, as the cell junctions are leaky, the concentration gradient between the lumen and the intercellular plasma is limited. Less reabsorption occurs in the late proximal tubule, but the cell junctions are tight so that a better concentration gradient is established. Here, Na+ is mainly reabsorbed with Cl− across the cells. This occurs because the cells of the late proximal tubule have different Na+ transport mechanisms and the tubular fluids have very little glucose and amino acids. The forces governing Na+ transport in the proximal tubule are shown in Fig. 2.15.

Water reabsorption

Seventy per cent of the filtered water is reabsorbed in the proximal tubule. This is driven by a transtubular osmotic gradient, created by solute reabsorption into the lateral intercellular spaces (Fig. 2.16). This fluid accumulation in the interstitium causes an increase in the hydrostatic pressure so that fluid moves by osmosis from the interstitium through the basement membrane into the peritubular capillary. This movement is also driven by the high oncotic pressure in the peritubular capillary because of the high plasma protein concentration created by the filtration process in the glomerulus.

The fluid leaving the proximal tubule is isoosmotic because both ions and water move out of the filtrate together. The proximal tubule has no concentrating capacity.

Reabsorption of other solutes in the proximal tubule
Glucose

Normal plasma glucose concentration is 50–110 mg/dl. Usually, 5–10 mg of glucose are filtered every minute. An increase in the plasma glucose concentration results in a proportional increase in the amount of glucose filtered. Virtually all filtered glucose is reabsorbed in the proximal tubule, unless

Fig. 2.15 Forces governing Na+ transport in the proximal tubule.

| Forces governing Na+ transport in the proximal tubule ||||
Part of proximal tubule	Electrical potential (mV)	Transport mechanism	Na+ concentration (mmol/L)
tubular lumen	−2	passive (carrier molecule)	150
cell	−70	active (pump)	30
extracellular fluid	0	diffusion	150

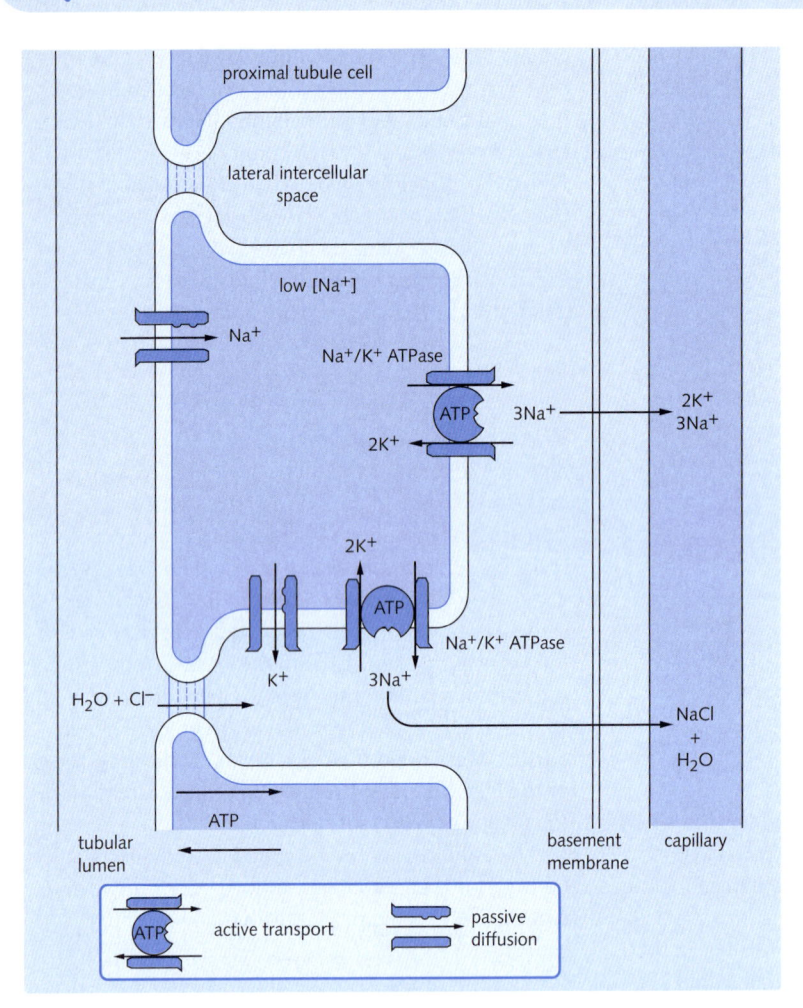

Fig. 2.16 Na⁺ transport processes in the proximal tubule.

the amount of filtered glucose exceeds the resorptive capacity of the cells. Glucose is transported into the proximal tubule cells by symport against its concentration gradient. It is driven by the energy released from the transport of Na⁺ down its electrochemical gradient because the Na⁺/K⁺ ATPase pump on the basolateral membrane maintains a low Na⁺ concentration and negative potential within the cell (Fig. 2.17). This is an example of secondary active transport.

T_m is the maximum tubular resorptive capacity for a solute (i.e., the point of saturation for the carriers), and this value can be calculated for glucose. All nephrons have different thresholds for glucose reabsorption (nephron heterogeneity). There are a limited number of Na⁺/glucose carrier molecules, so glucose reabsorption is T_m limited.

Figure 2.18 shows that the lowest renal threshold of glucose is at a plasma glucose concentration of 180mg/dl. At this level, filtered glucose will begin to be excreted in the urine (glucosuria). If the plasma glucose concentration increases further even those nephrons with highest resorptive capacity become saturated, and glucose is excreted. Urinary glucose increases in parallel with plasma glucose. The T_m for glucose is exceeded in all nephrons when the plasma glucose concentration is >360mg/dl.

Glucosuria occurs if:
- The filtered load exceeds the renal threshold.
- Tubular injury shifts the T_m for glucose lower than normal.

In diabetes, plasma glucose is elevated, so the filtered load of glucose is increased—if plasma glucose exceeds 180mg/dl, glucosuria will result.

In certain inherited tubular disorders, T_m for glucose is low and glucosuria can be found with a normal plasma glucose (renal glucosuria—the patient

Fig. 2.17 Active transport of glucose in the proximal tubule (pars convoluta). This occurs against a concentration gradient.

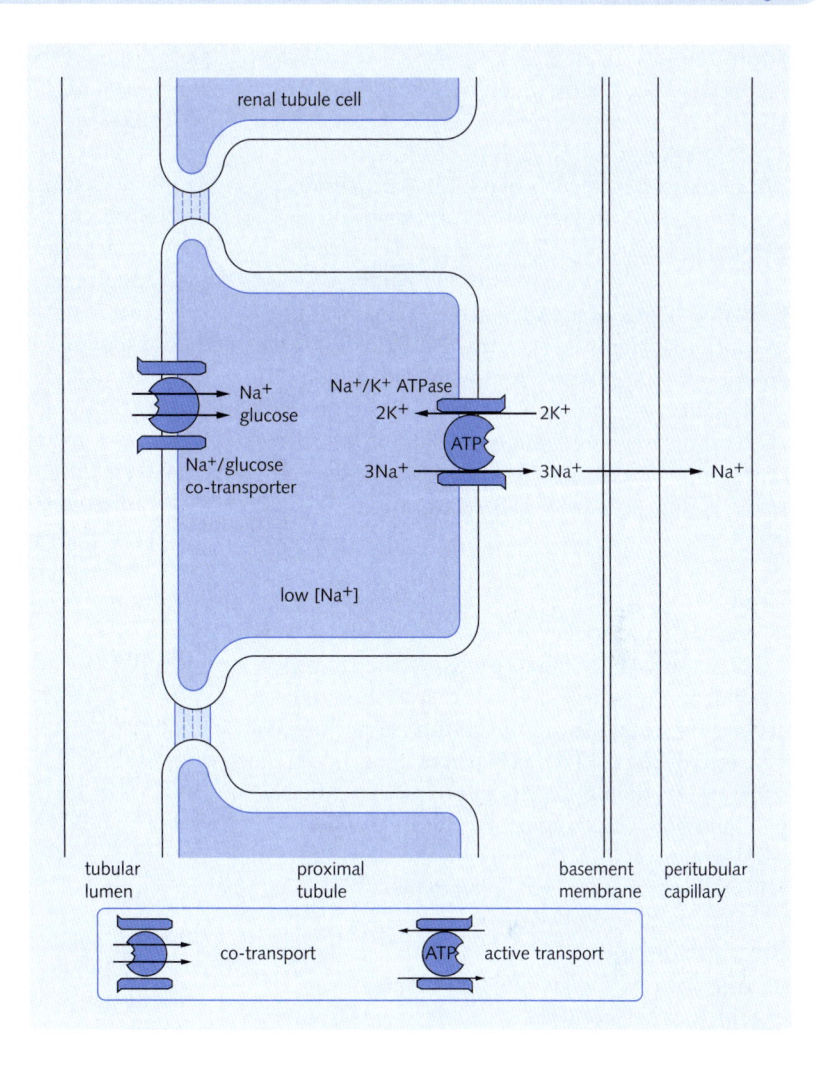

Fig. 2.18 Relationship between plasma concentration, filtration, reabsorption, and excretion of glucose (GFR = 100 mL/min). T_m is exceeded in nephrons with plasma glucose >180 mg/dl and for all nephrons when plasma glucose >360 mg/dl.

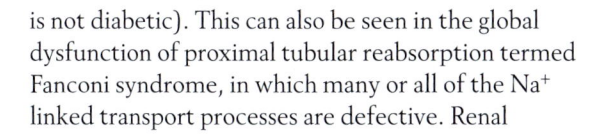

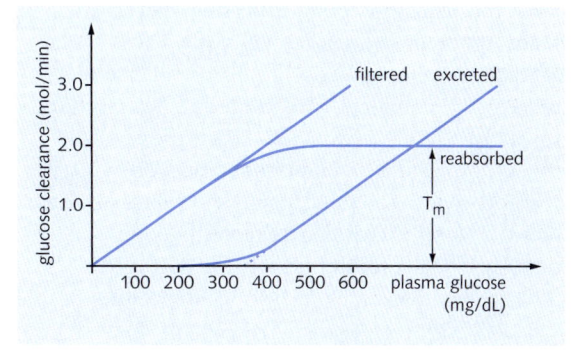

is not diabetic). This can also be seen in the global dysfunction of proximal tubular reabsorption termed Fanconi syndrome, in which many or all of the Na^+ linked transport processes are defective. Renal glucosuria can also occur in pregnancy, because T_m for glucose is reduced; however, it should be noted that true diabetes can also occur in pregnancy and cause glucosuria with hyperglycemia.

Amino acids

Amino acids are the basic unit of proteins and are absorbed constantly from the gut. The plasma concentration of amino acids is 2.5–3.5 mmol/L. They are small molecules that filter easily through the glomerulus, with most reabsorption occurring in the proximal tubule. The transport is a secondary active process (by symport with Na^+) and is driven by Na^+/K^+ ATPase, as with glucose. There are at least five different transport systems coupled with Na^+ and these are responsible for the movement of different types of amino acid residue. Because this is a T_m-limited process, amino aciduria results if the reabsorption mechanism is saturated or if the reabsorption mechanism is defective (i.e., in Fanconi syndrome).

Urea

Urea is the end-product of protein metabolism. It is made in the liver, then transported to the kidneys via the blood. It is a small molecule that is filtered freely at the glomerulus. The normal plasma concentration of urea is 8–20 mg/dl. Urea becomes concentrated along the nephron as a result of proximal tubule Na^+, Cl^- and water reabsorption. This allows passive reabsorption of 40–50% of urea in the proximal tubule along its concentration gradient.

Bicarbonate

Bicarbonate (HCO_3^-) is vital for the maintenance of acid–base balance within the body (see Chapter 3). The plasma concentration of HCO_3^- is 20–30 mEq/L. The proximal tubule reabsorbs 80% of the filtered HCO_3^-, the remaining 20% being taken up in the distal tubule and collecting ducts. Na^+ reabsorption on the apical membrane drives H^+ secretion by the tubular cells (antiport). The secreted H^+ combines with filtered HCO_3^- ions to form H_2CO_3 (carbonic acid). This is metabolized to CO_2 by luminal carbonic anhydrase. The CO_2 is reabsorbed into the tubular cell, and eventually exits into the blood as bicarbonate (see Chapter 3 for details). The net result is a reabsorption of one filtered bicarbonate for each secreted proton.

Phosphate

Phosphate (PO_4^{3-}) salts are essential for the structure of bones and teeth. Eighty per cent of the body's PO_4^{3-} content is in bone and 20% is in the intracellular fluid (ICF). The plasma concentration is 2.4–5.0 mg/dL. It is filtered easily at the glomerulus; 80% is then reabsorbed in the proximal tubule and the remaining 20% is excreted in urine.

The kidneys play an important role in the regulation of PO_4^{3-}. The amount filtered is proportional to the plasma PO_4^{3-} concentration. Therefore, any increase in plasma PO_4^{3-} concentration leads to an increase in the amount filtered and excreted, which is how plasma PO_4^{3-} levels are controlled. A fall in GFR as is seen in chronic kidney disease will result in increased plasma PO_4^{3-} concentration. Reabsorption of PO_4^{3-} occurs with Na^+ ions at the apical membrane of the tubular cells.

PO_4^{3-} is an important urinary buffer for H^+ and its overall excretion is influenced by:
- Parathyroid hormone (increases excretion).
- Vitamin D (decreases excretion).
- Acidosis (increases excretion).
- Glucocorticoids (increases excretion).

Potassium

The plasma concentration of potassium is 4–5 mmol/L. K^+ can be secreted or reabsorbed in the nephron. Excretion of the filtered K^+ can vary from 1% to 110%, depending on:
- Dietary intake of potassium.
- Acid–base status.
- Aldosterone levels.

Approximately 70% of K^+ is reabsorbed in the proximal tubule, mostly by passive paracellular reabsorption across the tight junctions between tubular cells.

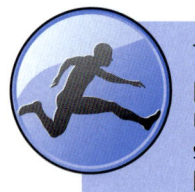

> The proximal tubule is the primary site for bulk reabsorption of water and solutes. Most of this is driven by sodium reabsorption.

Secretion by the proximal tubule

Secretion is the movement of solutes from the proximal tubule cells into the tubular fluid. It can be active (i.e., require energy) or passive. These processes are T_m limited or gradient time-limited.

Protons

As mentioned above, H^+ is secreted in the proximal tubule. This depends on the transport of Na^+ and the reabsorption of HCO_3^-. The movement of H^+ out of the cells occurs by antiport with Na^+ on the apical membrane using a specific transporter.

Ammonium
Proximal tubule cells extract glutamine from the peritubular blood and hydrolyze it to glutamate ion and ammonium (NH_4^+). This is then actively secreted to participate in net acid excretion (see Chapter 3).

Drugs and other organic substances
Numerous drugs and endogenous substances are secreted by the proximal tubule. Among the most important are:
1. Drugs: acetazolamide, furosemide, penicillin, probenecid, salicylates, sulfonamides.
2. Bile salts, oxalate, uric acid, prostaglandins.

The loop of Henle

Role of the loop of Henle
This segment continues sodium, chloride, and water reabsorption but also generates the interstitial concentrating gradient that allows regulation of water reabsorption in the distal nephron.

The loop of Henle reabsorbs 20% of the filtered Na^+ and 15% of tubular water. As filtrate flows through the loop of Henle, reabsorption of NaCl in the thick ascending limb produces a hypertonic interstitial fluid in the surrounding medulla. This creates a concentration gradient and water moves passively out of the thin descending limb.

The tubular fluid is isotonic to the plasma on entering the loop of Henle; however, by the time it leaves the loop it is hypotonic because ion reabsorption occurs within the ascending limb without water reabsorption. This mechanism generates a concentrated medullary interstitium, and this in turn allows urine to be concentrated in the distal nephron.

Structure of the loop of Henle
The different components of the loop are functionally separate units, each with its own specific properties.

Thin descending limb
The thin descending limb is permeable to water, but not to Na^+ and Cl^-. Water is reabsorbed passively down a concentration gradient caused by the hypertonic interstitium of the medulla.

- The juxtamedullary nephrons have long, thin limbs that extend deep into the inner medulla.
- The cortical nephrons only just enter the medulla and some are situated entirely in the cortex.

Thin ascending limb
The thin ascending limb has a similar structure to the thin descending limb but is impermeable to water and has some Na^+ and Cl^- transport occurring within the cells. The mechanism of ion transport in this segment remains unknown.

Thick ascending limb
The thick ascending limb consists of large cells with mitochondria, which generate energy for the active transport of Na^+ and Cl^- ions from the tubular fluid into the interstitium. 20% of filtered Na^+ is reabsorbed in the loop of Henle. As a result, the filtrate becomes progressively diluted (this part of the tubule is impermeable to water). There is cotransport (symport) of Na^+, Cl^- and K^+ (in the ratio 1:2:1—so the pump is electrochemically neutral) on the apical membrane. These pumps are inhibited by the diuretic furosemide. Overall, NaCl accumulates in the medullary interstitium. Figure 2.19 shows the transport processes in the loop of Henle; the inset shows the transport of ions in the cells in the thick ascending limb of the loop of Henle.

The distal end of the thick ascending limb contains a modified epithelial structure called the *macula densa* that functions as a sodium chloride sensor for regulation of glomerular filtration (see Chapter 3).

The distal nephron

The distal nephron has important roles in urinary dilution and concentration, sodium reabsorption, and potassium and proton excretion. It consists of the following functionally distinct segments:
1. The distal convoluted tubule.
2. The cortical collecting ducts.
3. The medullary (inner and outer) collecting ducts.

Distal convoluted tubule
The distal convoluted tubule (DCT) contains Na^+/Cl^- symporters on the apical membrane. These pumps are sensitive to thiazide diuretics. The segment is water-impermeable so that the overall process here is of urinary dilution, similar to the thick ascending limb of Henle's loop.

Organization of the Kidneys

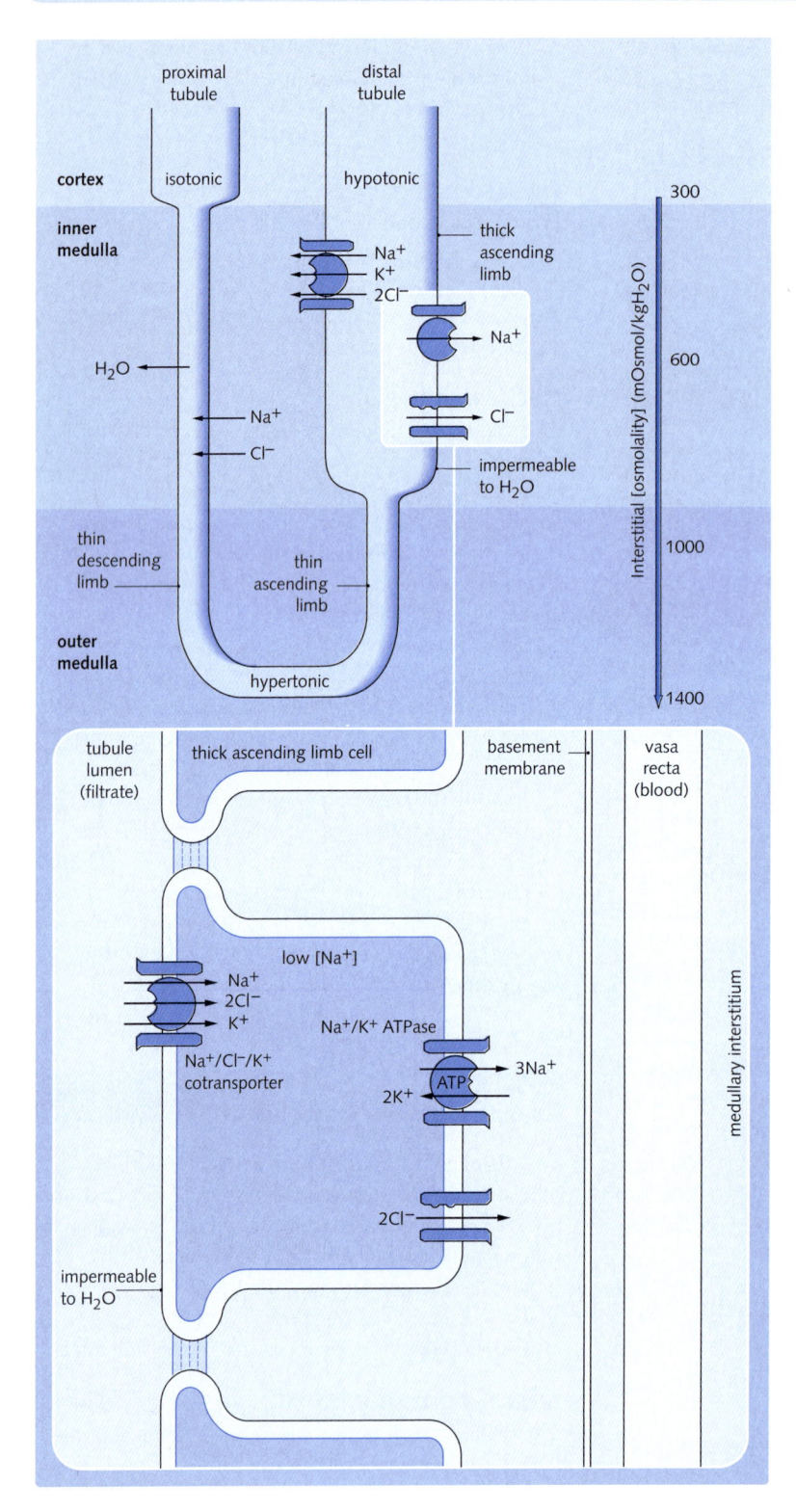

Fig. 2.19 Transport of ions in the cells of the thick ascending limb of the loop of Henle:
- $Na^+/Cl^-/K^+$ cotransporter
- Na^+/K^+ ATPase
- Cl^- channel.

The DCT also contributes to active calcium reabsorption. Calcium moves into the DCT cells via luminal calcium channels, then exits the cells via an active Ca^{2+} ATPase and a Na^+/Ca^{2+} antiporter on the basolateral membrane. This process is stimulated by parathyroid hormone. Inhibition of the luminal Na^+/Cl^- symporters with thiazide diuretics reduces intracellular Na^+, stimulates the basolateral Na^+/Ca^{2+} antiporter, and therefore increases calcium absorption and may lead to hypercalcemia.

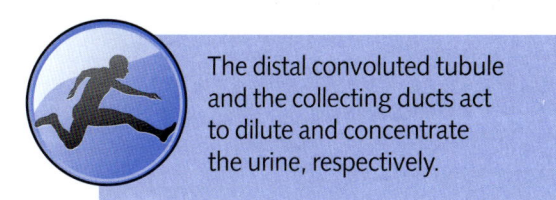

> The distal convoluted tubule and the collecting ducts act to dilute and concentrate the urine, respectively.

Cortical collecting ducts

This segment consists of three intermixed cell types:
- Principal cells.
- Type A intercalated cells.
- Type B intercalated cells.

Principal cells

Principal cells are important in sodium reabsorption, potassium excretion, and water reabsorption.

Sodium reabsorption occurs via epithelial sodium channels and a basolateral Na-K ATPase. Both are stimulated by aldosterone. The channel is inhibited by the diuretics amiloride and triamterene.

Potassium secretion occurs via apical potassium channels, and by the basolateral Na^+/K^+ ATPase. These are also stimulated by aldosterone.

Water reabsorption occurs via insertion of aquaporins in the luminal membrane under the control of the hormone ADH. When present on the basolateral side of the principal cell (Fig. 2.20), ADH causes intracellular water channels (aquaporins) to fuse with the luminal membrane. The V_2 receptors are G-protein-coupled receptors, which have a seven membrane-spanning region. Without aquaporins, the luminal membrane is water impermeable. After entering the cell, the water moves out into the concentrated interstitium through the water permeable basolateral membrane and is taken up by the capillaries.

Type A Intercalated Cells

The type A intercalated cells act to secrete protons, thus helping to excrete body acid. This is accomplished by:
- a luminal H^+/K^+ ATPase which reabsorbs potassium and excretes protons.
- a luminal H^+ ATPase.

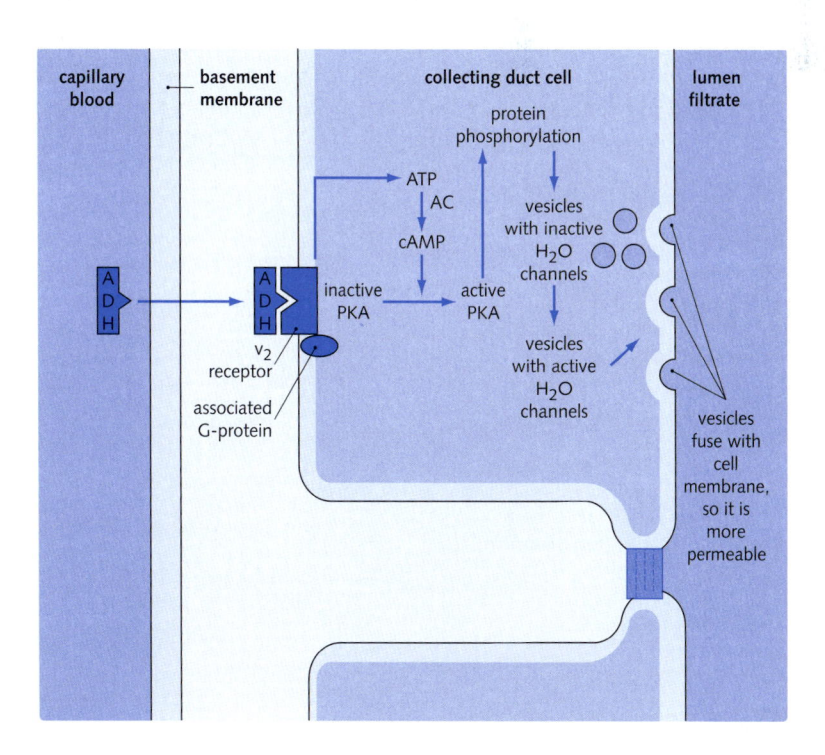

Fig. 2.20 Actions of antidiuretic hormone (ADH) in the collecting duct. AC, adenylate cyclase; cAMP, cyclic adenosine monophosphate; PKA, protein kinase.

For each proton secreted, a bicarbonate is added to the plasma via antiport with chloride on the basal membrane.

Type B intercalated cells
In contrast to the type A cells, these secrete bicarbonate, rather than reabsorb it. There are few of them in human nephrons, and their role is probably minimal in human physiology.

Medullary collecting ducts (outer and inner)
Similar to the cortical collecting duct, both of these segments have principal cells which participate in water reabsorption under the control of ADH. The outer (but not inner) segment also continues the aldosterone-sensitive reabsorption of Na^+ and secretion of K^+.

The inner medullary collecting ducts have an important function as the final determinants of sodium excretion. They are sensitive to natriuretic peptides, which inhibit sodium reabsorption by a cyclic GMP dependent mechanism. The edema seen in many glomerular diseases may occur by inducing resistance to natriuretic peptides, thus inhibiting sodium excretion.

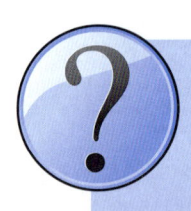

- Describe the anatomical relations of the right and left kidney.
- Describe the structure of the five anatomical regions of the nephron.
- Name the two different types of nephrons, and give three ways in which they differ.
- List four hormones that act on the kidney and four that are produced by the kidney.
- Discuss how the kidney is involved in vitamin D metabolism.
- Describe the structure of the glomerular filter.
- Explain how the molecular size and charge of particles affects filtration.
- Define reabsorption, secretion and excretion.
- Describe the difference between primary and secondary active transport.
- Outline sodium handling by the proximal tubule.
- Using a graph, explain how glucose reabsorption in the proximal tubule is T_m-limited.
- Name two other substances reabsorbed in the proximal tubule.
- Explain the reabsorption of HCO_3^- in the proximal tubule.
- Describe three functions of the principal cell.

3. Renal Function

The glomerular filtration rate (GFR): regulation and disorders

Renal blood flow (RBF) and systemic blood pressure

Autoregulation maintains a constant blood flow to the kidneys despite changes in systemic blood pressure. However, the blood flow itself is not always constant. For example, acute hemorrhage results in increased sympathetic activity to the kidney (and other parts of the body). This leads to vasoconstriction and consequently a decreased blood flow. Intrarenal vasodilator prostaglandins are produced to prevent excessive vasoconstriction and renal perfusion is thus maintained.

Glomerular filtration rate (GFR)

The GFR is the amount of filtrate that is produced from the blood flowing through the glomerulus per unit time.
- Normal GFR is 90–120 mL/min/1.73 m^2 (i.e., corrected for body surface area).
- The total amount filtered is 180 L/day, and all but 1–2 liters is later reabsorbed.

The glomerular filtrate normally:
- Contains no blood cells or platelets.
- Contains virtually no protein.
- Is composed mostly of organic solutes with a low molecular weight, and of inorganic ions.

Forces governing tissue fluid formation

The movement of fluid between plasma and tissue fluid is determined by Starling's forces (Fig. 3.1):
- Hydrostatic pressure.
- Oncotic (colloid osmotic) pressure (mainly due to serum protein).

Changes in these forces alters whether fluid leaves or enters the capillary bed.

The following factors affect tissue fluid formation in a *non*renal capillary (Fig. 3.1A):

- At the arteriole end of the capillary, hydrostatic pressure is greater than oncotic pressure as a result of resistance to flow due to the narrowing of the vessel, and fluid is forced out of the capillary—point 1 in Fig. 3.1A.
- As the fluid moves out of capillaries via the highly permeable wall, oncotic pressure increases and hydrostatic pressure decreases, so the pressure forces are reversed (most apparent at the venous end of the capillary) and there is net movement of fluid back into the capillaries—point 2 in Fig. 3.1A.

This balance allows tissue delivery of oxygen and nutrients (at the arterial end), and venous uptake of CO_2 and waste products.

Forces governing GFR

GFR is also driven by Starling forces. However, in the renal vascular bed the surface area of the glomerular capillaries is much larger than that of normal capillary beds, so there is less resistance to flow. The hydrostatic pressure falls less along the length of the capillary because the efferent arterioles, which act as secondary resistance vessels, maintain a constant hydrostatic pressure along the entire length of the glomerular capillary—see Fig. 3.1B.

The glomerular filtrate in Bowman's space is the equivalent of the interstitial fluid in a vascular bed. This fluid is produced as a result of the glomerular capillary hydrostatic pressure (50 mmHg), which exceeds the sum of the hydrostatic pressure in Bowman's capsule (12 mmHg) plus the capillary oncotic pressure (25 mmHg)—point 3 on Fig. 3.1B. As fluid leaves the glomerular capillary, the oncotic pressure rises. When these net forces are equal at the end of the glomerular capillary the filtration equilibrium is reached, with very little fluid movement (Point 4 in Fig. 3.1B).

Fluid is reabsorbed into the peritubular capillaries—point 5 in Fig. 3.1B—as a result of high oncotic pressure (35 mmHg) and low hydrostatic pressure, which fell due to efferent arteriolar

Renal Function

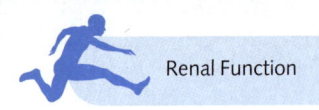

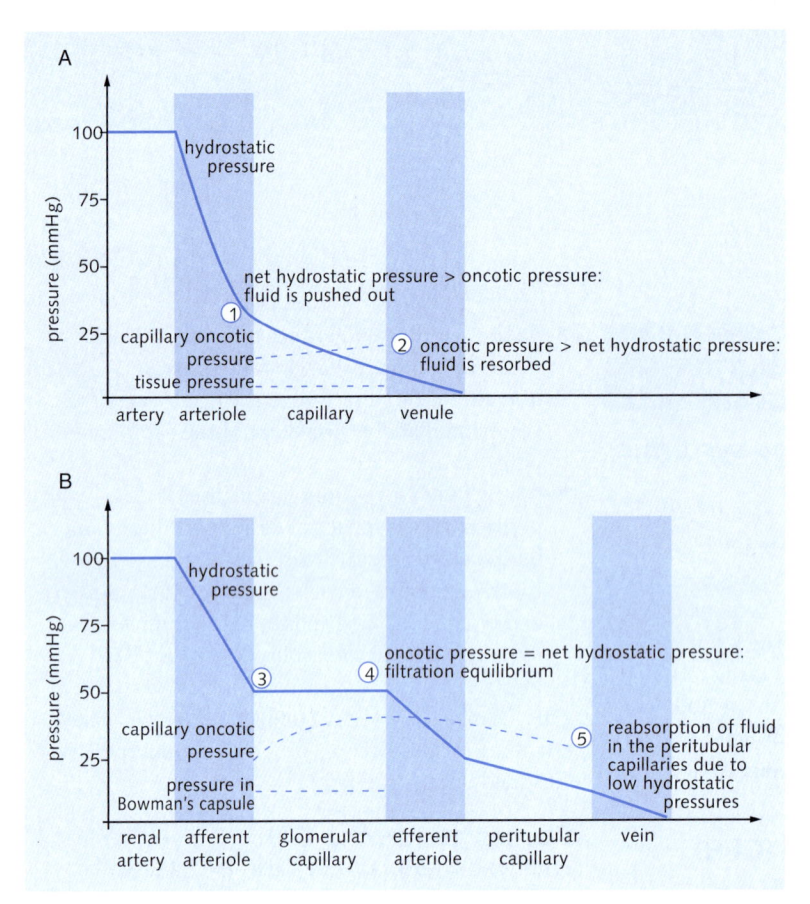

Fig. 3.1 Forces involved in tissue fluid formation in a non-renal (A) and a renal (B) vascular bed (see text for detailed explanation).

resistance. Note that this fluid reabsorption causes a fall in colloid oncotic pressure as plasma proteins become diluted.

The pressures controlling glomerular filtration into Bowman's capsule are illustrated in Fig. 3.2 and the composition of the glomerular filtrate is shown in Fig. 3.3.

Determinants of GFR

The GFR can be expressed as the following formula:

GFR = K_f × net filtration pressure

K_f is the filtration coefficient and can further be expressed as the GBM permeability (L_A) × the GBM surface area (A).

The net filtration pressure = glomerular capillary hydrostatic pressure − Bowman's capsule hydrostatic pressure − glomerular capillary oncotic pressure.
- The GBM permeability (L_A) can be increased by cytokines and angiotensin II, increasing GFR.
- The GBM surface area (A) can be reduced by mesangial cell contraction, stimulated by molecules such as angiotensin II, therefore decreasing GFR.
- The glomerular capillary hydrostatic pressure is determined mainly by the relative resistances in the afferent and efferent arteriole.
- Bowman's capsule hydrostatic pressure is normally small and can be ignored (except in urinary obstruction, where it can be significant and decrease GFR).
- The glomerular capillary oncotic pressure increases when more fluid is filtered, leaving the remaining blood more concentrated.

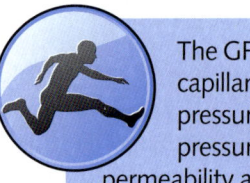

> The GFR is determined by capillary hydrostatic pressure, capillary oncotic pressure, and the permeability and surface area of the basement membrane.

The glomerular filtration rate (GFR): regulation and disorders

Fig. 3.2 Pressures controlling glomerular filtration into Bowman's capsule. A, Hydrostatic pressure of glomerular capillary = 50mmHg; B, hydrostatic pressure in Bowman's space = 12mmHg (increases fluid uptake into capillary); C, oncotic pressure of glomerular capillary = 25mmHg (increases fluid uptake into capillary).

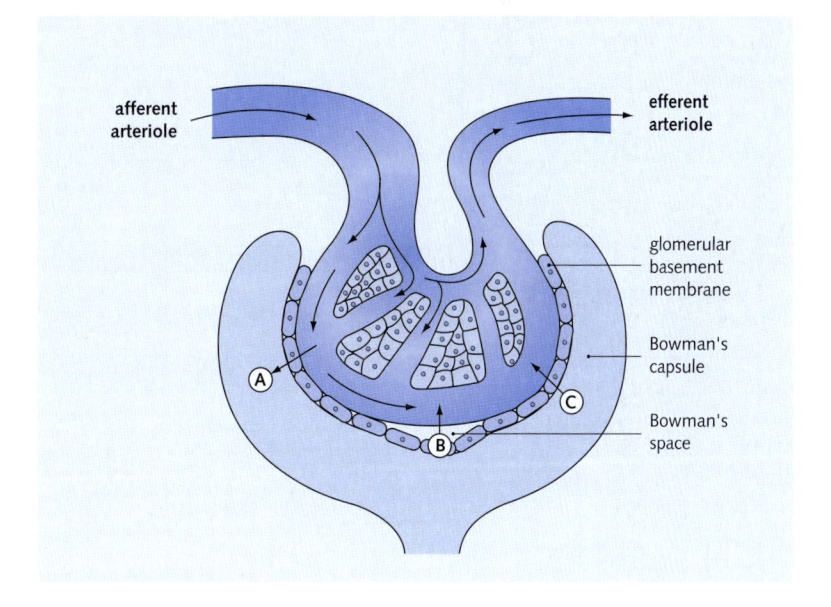

Composition of glomerular filtrate	
Component	Glomerular filtrate
Na$^+$ (mEq/L)	142
K$^+$ (mEq/L)	4.0
Cl$^-$ (mEq/L)	113
HCO$_3^-$ (mEq/L)	28–30
glucose (mmol/L)	5.9
protein (g/100mL)	0.02

Fig. 3.3 Composition of glomerular filtrate.

Regulation of RBF and GFR
- RBF is 1100mL/min (renal plasma flow is 600mL/min).
- GFR is 120mL/min.

Both remain fairly constant because of autoregulation, which involves changes in tone of the afferent and efferent arterioles (Fig. 3.4). Over the autoregulatory range of perfusion pressures (90–200mmHg), blood flow is independent of perfusion pressure so that, as the perfusion pressure increases, resistance to flow increases (Fig. 3.5). Regulation of GFR involves other vasoactive substances, which are found in the walls of blood vessels. These are summarized in Fig. 3.6.

Two principal mechanisms are involved in autoregulation:
1. Tubuloglomerular feedback mechanism.
2. Myogenic mechanism.

Tubuloglomerular feedback mechanism
The tubuloglomerular feedback mechanism controls the GFR of each nephron by sensing the NaCl concentration at the macula densa (at the distal end of the thick ascending limb of Henle's loop). When GFR increases, an increase in macula densa chloride flux is transmitted from the macula densa to cells in the juxtaglomerular apparatus (JGA), which produce vasoactive substances (e.g., angiotensin II, adenosine). These constrict the afferent arteriole, lowering glomerular hydrostatic pressure, and therefore cause the GFR to return to normal.

The system has three components:
1. A luminal component—e.g., the macula densa cells of the tubular epithelium, which detect osmolality or the rate of Na$^+$ or Cl$^-$ movement into the cells. The higher the flow of the filtrate, the higher the Na$^+$ concentration in the cells.
2. A signal, which is sent via the juxtaglomerular cells, is triggered by a change in the NaCl concentration of distal tubular fluid.
3. An effector, which acts as a vasoconstrictor to contract the smooth muscle of the adjacent afferent arterioles and therefore decreases renal plasma flow, which in turn reduces GFR.

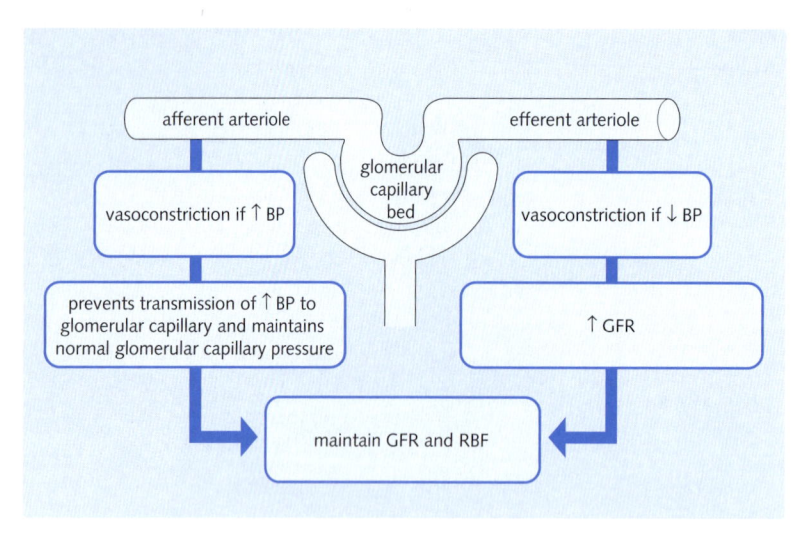

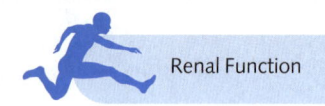

Fig. 3.4 The regulation of renal blood flow (RBF) and glomerular filtration rate (GFR) by vasoconstriction of arterioles.

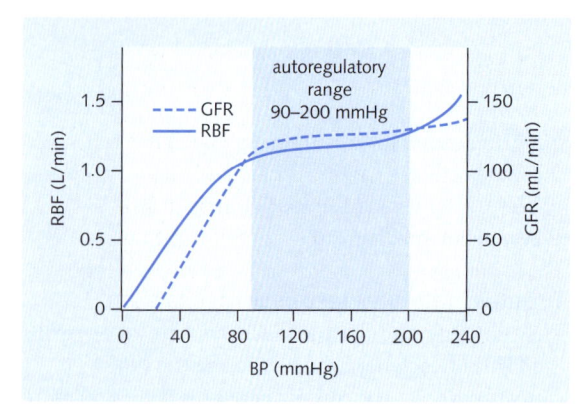

Fig. 3.5 Autoregulation of glomerular filtration rate (GFR) and renal blood flow (RBF).

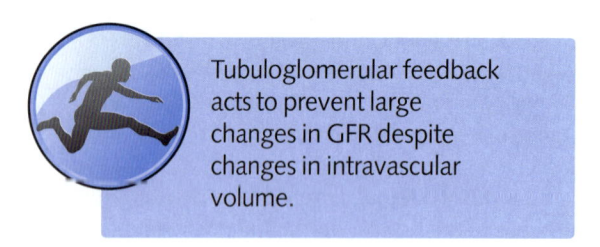

Vasoactive substances found in the blood vessel walls	
Vasodilator	**Vasoconstrictor**
prostaglandins (PGs)	adenosine
nitric oxide (NO)	angiotensin II
dopamine (DA)	antidiuretic hormone (ADH)
bradykinin	endothelin
	norepinephrine (NE)

Fig. 3.6 Vasoactive substances found in the blood vessel walls.

> Tubuloglomerular feedback acts to prevent large changes in GFR despite changes in intravascular volume.

Myogenic mechanism
This depends on the contraction of smooth muscle cells in response to stretching. Thus, when the arterial pressure rises, the renal afferent arteriole stretches and the smooth muscle cells contract. This prevents the rise in pressure being transmitted to the glomerular capillary, so that the renal blood flow and GFR remain unchanged.

Age-related changes in GFR
Age-related changes in GFR are as follows:
- Week 10 of gestation (in utero): filtration of fluid and urine production begin; this contributes to the amniotic fluid.
- Newborn: GFR <25 mL/min/1.73 m^2 body surface area; this increases progressively during the first year.
- 1 month old: progressive increase in GFR.
- By 1 year of age: GFR reaches adult values (120 mL/min).
- Old age: GFR decreases progressively.

Measurement of renal plasma flow and renal blood flow
Clearance
Clearance (C) is the volume of plasma that is cleared of a substance in a unit time. It is a measure of the

kidney's ability to remove a substance from the plasma and excrete it. The units used are volume and time—usually ml/min. If P_x = concentration of substance x in arterial plasma (mg/mL), U_x = concentration of x in the urine (mg/mL) and V = urine flow rate (mL/min), then the clearance of substance x is:

$$C_x = \frac{U_x \times V}{P_x}$$

By knowing how a substance is excreted by the kidney, its clearance can be used to quantitate various physiologic processes.

Measuring RPF and RBF

p-Aminohippuric acid (PAH) clearance provides a noninvasive estimate of the renal plasma flow. PAH is filtered at the glomerulus and secreted by the proximal tubule. If the T_m for PAH is not exceeded, 90–100% is removed from the blood as it passes through the kidney in a normal individual. Therefore the clearance of PAH can be used to measure RPF.

When the excretion of PAH is 100%, if P_{PAH} = the plasma concentration of PAH, U_{PAH} = the urine concentration of PAH and V = urinary flow rate:

$$RPF = C_{PAH} = \frac{U_{PAH} \times V}{P_{PAH}}$$

The normal RPF is 600 mL/min.

Renal blood flow (RBF) can be obtained from RPF by using the hematocrit (the percentage of total blood volume that is made of erythrocytes). The hematocrit is 45%, so 55% of blood is made up of plasma:

$$RPF = RPF \times 100/55$$
$$= 600 \times 100/55$$
$$= 1100 \, mL/min$$

Measuring GFR

Clearance of a substance will provide an accurate estimate of GFR if that substance "follows" the glomerular filtrate without being altered by the kidney (i.e., it is not reabsorbed, secreted, synthesized or metabolized by the kidney). Inulin is such a substance:
- It is a polysaccharide of molecular weight 5500.
- It is not normally found within the body; it is introduced into the body by injection or intravenous infusion.
- It passes into the glomerular filtrate but is not reabsorbed, secreted, synthesized or metabolized by the kidney—so all inulin filtered by the glomerulus is excreted in the urine. Inulin clearance can be used to assess glomerular function in disease.
- Normal inulin clearance is equal to the GFR, i.e., 120 mL/min/1.73 m² body surface area (this varies with body size).

However, measurement of inulin clearance is complicated and is rarely used to assess GFR in routine clinical practice. Instead, *creatinine clearance* is used as an estimate of GFR. Creatinine is found in the body; it is produced during muscle metabolism:

$$Phosphocreatine + ADP \xrightarrow{Creatine\ Phosphokinase} Creatine + ATP$$
$$Creatine + H_2O \rightarrow Creatinine$$

Plasma creatinine levels remain constant if renal function, muscle mass and metabolism are stable. Plasma creatinine is commonly used to follow changes in GFR. Its exact value depends upon muscle mass and therefore age, sex and size. It has a reciprocal relationship with GFR (Fig. 3.7). Note that a 25% fall in GFR would lead to a very small

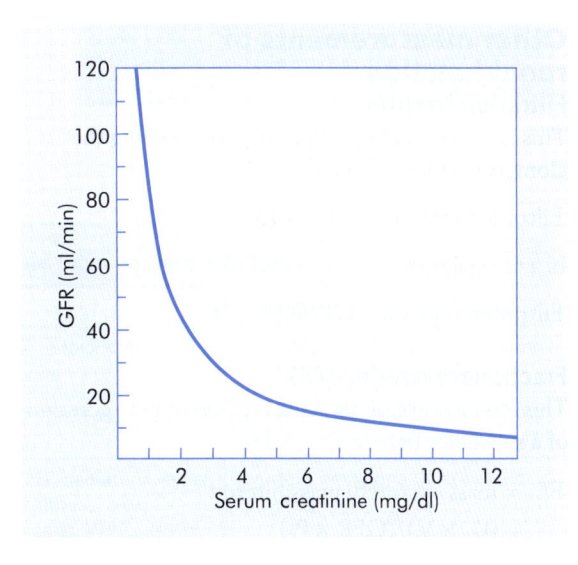

Fig. 3.7 Relationship between serum creatinine concentration and GFR.

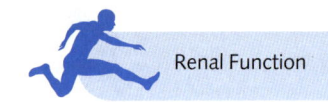

Renal Function

| Lab findings in common ARF syndromes |||||
Category	Cause	Urinalysis	FENa	Other
prerenal ARF		normal	<1%	BUN/Cr ratio >20
renal ARF	acute tubular necrosis	renal tubular epithelial cells, granular casts	>3%	
	rhabdomyolysis, myoglobinuria	heme + without RBCs		
	allergic interstitial nephritis	WBCs, WBC casts, eosinophils		
	rapidly progressive GN	protein, dysmorphic RBCs, RBC casts	<1% (often)	
postrenal ARF		crystals, hematuria (variable)	variable	ultrasound shows hydronephrosis

Fig. 3.9 Lab findings in common ARF syndromes.

Complications of ARF
- Hyperkalemia.
- Metabolic acidosis and an increased anion gap.
- Increased plasma phosphate and decreased plasma calcium (less marked than in CKD).
- Volume overload.
- Uremic symptoms (confusion, weakness, itching, nausea).

Treatment
- Treatment of the specific cause should begin immediately.
- Oliguric patients should have fluids restricted.
- Potassium and phosphorus should be restricted while maintaining adequate caloric intake.
- Hemodialysis may be required if electrolyte or fluid problems are not correctable, or if uremic symptoms ensue (see next section).

Chronic kidney disease (CKD)
Unlike ARF, which is generally reversible with early treatment, chronic kidney disease may lead to chronic renal failure (CRF), in which there is irreversible impaired renal function. It can result from intrinsic renal disease or be secondary to other systemic diseases.

Causes
Causes of CKD (also see Chapter 4) are:
- **Renal:** glomerulonephritis, chronic pyelonephritis, bladder or urethral obstruction, polycystic kidneys, interstitial nephritis, amyloid, myeloma, renal vascular disease, Alport's syndrome.
- **Extrarenal:** diabetes mellitus, hypertension (especially if accelerated—malignant), heart failure, SLE, gout, hypercalcemia, renovascular disease (atheroma), vasculitis.
- **Drugs:** cyclosporine, analgesics.

Diagnostic approach
The diagnostic approach to CKD can involve:
- **Urine:** urinalysis (hematuria, glucosuria, proteinuria), microscopy (white cells, eosinophilia, granular casts, red cell casts, red cells), biochemistry (24-hr creatinine clearance, 24-hr protein excretion, urine protein electrophoresis).
- **Blood:** urea and creatinine, electrolytes, glucose, calcium (decreased), phosphate (increased), urate (increased), protein, osmolality, full blood count, protein electrophoresis, autoantibody screen, complement components, test for sickle-cell disease.
- **Radiology:** ultrasound (to assess kidney size), CT, plain radiography of the abdomen. Hand radiographs can show evidence of osteodystrophy.
- **Renal biopsy:** consider if kidneys are of normal size and the cause of CKD is not clear from other investigations.

Complications
- **Hematologic:** anemia (due to lack of erythropoietin), bleeding (platelet dysfunction).
- **Cardiac:** pericarditis, hypertension, increased atherosclerosis.
- **Bone:** hyperparathyroidism, hyperphosphatemia, osteodystrophy.

Fig. 3.10 Comparison of two different methods of dialysis. (A) hemodialysis; (B) peritoneal dialysis (adapted from O'Callaghan CA, Brenner BM: *The kidney at a glance*, Blackwell Science, 2001 p. 96, 98).

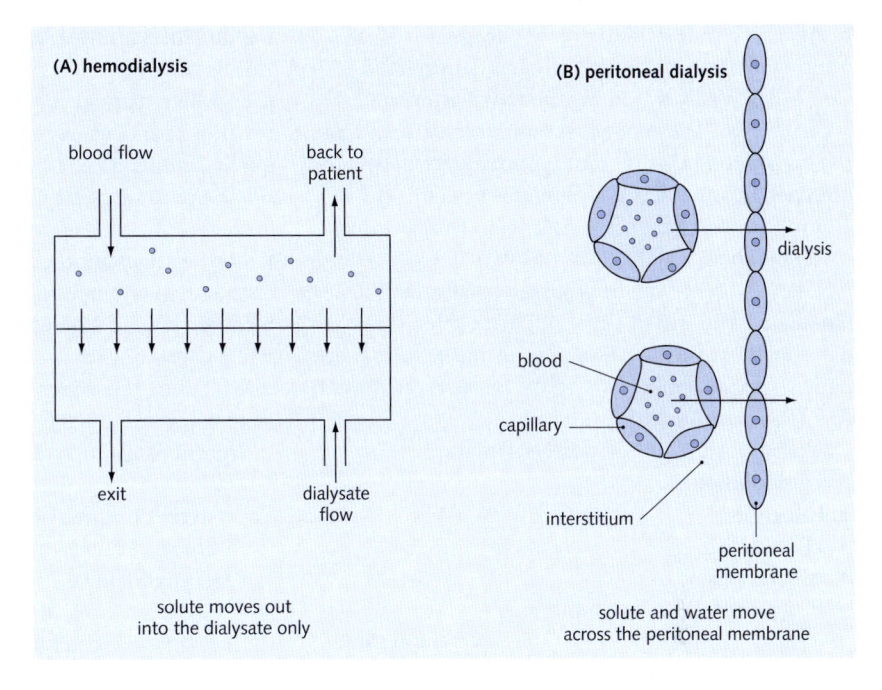

- Infectious: high risk.
- Electrolyte: acidosis, hyponatremia, hyperkalemia.
- Neurologic: confusion, asterixis, peripheral neuropathy.

Treatment: medical
All the measures suggested for ARF above should be done. In addition, the following have been demonstrated to slow progression in many cases:
- Hypertension control to <130/90mmHg.
- ACE inhibitors or angiotensin receptor blockers have separate protective effect.
- Tight glucose control in diabetic nephropathy.
- Reduced protein diets (0.6–0.8gm/kg/day) may be effective in some glomerular diseases.
- Phosphate binders and 1,25-dihydroxy Vitimin D for bone disease.
- Erythropoietin for anemia.

Treatment: dialysis
Dialysis imitates the kidney by temporarily removing waste products and excess fluids that accumulate in renal failure. It is used to treat renal failure in patients with acute or chronic renal failure. Dialysis is indicated when there is:
- GFR <10 ml/min.
- Hyperkalemia.
- Acidosis.
- Pulmonary edema.
- Pericarditis.
- Mental status changes.
- Malnutrition.

There are two main forms of dialysis: hemodialysis and continuous ambulatory peritoneal dialysis (Fig. 3.10). At best, they provide an equivalent average clearance of approximately 10mL/min (normal GFR, 125mL/min).

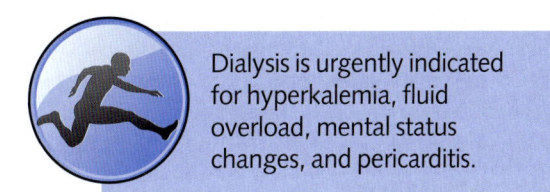

> Dialysis is urgently indicated for hyperkalemia, fluid overload, mental status changes, and pericarditis.

Hemodialysis
This involves pumping the blood through an artificial kidney, called a dialysis machine. Blood flows on one side of a semi-permeable membrane, with dialysis fluid being passed in the opposite direction on the other side. Dialysis occurs across the semipermeable membrane removing toxins from the blood down a concentration gradient.

The dialysate is made of purified water with a solute composition similar to plasma, but without any of the waste products, so that solutes move along their concentration gradient out of the blood.

Renal Function

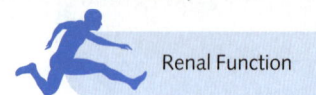

Access to the circulation is ideally gained by an arteriovenous (AV) fistula, which is constructed surgically, usually by joining the radial artery and cephalic vein. The venous system "arterializes," and the high blood flows required for dialysis can be obtained by cannulating the venous system. Complications of the AV fistula include infection and thrombosis.

Dialysis "dose" can be adjusted by altering the blood flow, the area of the semipermeable membrane, or the duration of treatment. On average, patients require approximately 4 hours of treatment 3 times/week.

Complications of hemodialysis include:
- Hypotension.
- Infection.
- Hemolysis.
- Air embolism.
- Reactions to dialysis membrane.

Continuous ambulatory peritoneal dialysis (CAPD)

This procedure uses the peritoneal membrane as the semipermeable membrane. Unlike hemodialysis, peritoneal dialysis does not require an AV fistula for circulatory access. Instead, it requires the insertion of a permanent Tenchkoff catheter through the anterior abdominal wall into the peritoneal cavity. Dialysate solution is introduced into the peritoneum and exchanged regularly for fresh fluid—up to 5 times/day is necessary to maintain the efficiency of dialysis. Waste products pass into the dialysate along their concentration gradients, and water is removed by osmosis. Dialysis solutions with high osmolarity (usually dextrose) will remove more water. CAPD is used in the maintenance dialysis of end-stage renal failure, but technique survival declines to 50% after 5 years due to loss of peritoneal membrane function.

Complications of peritoneal dialysis include:
- Peritonitis (50% of cases are caused by *Staphylococcus epidermidis*). Treatment is with intraperitoneal or intravenous antibiotics.
- Mechanical problems with fluid drainage.
- Infections or blockage around the site of the catheter.

Contraindications to CAPD are:
- Peritoneal adhesions as a result of peritonitis.
- Abdominal hernia.
- Colostomy.

Renal transplantation

This is the most successful organ transplant and is the ideal treatment for irreversible renal failure. It restores near-normal renal function and improves quality of life. The kidney comes from a cadaver or a related or unrelated live donor and is usually placed in the iliac fossa. The renal vessels from the donated kidney are anastomosed onto the iliac blood vessels of the recipient, and the ureter is inserted into the bladder (Fig. 3.11). Success depends upon:
- ABO group.
- Matching the donor and the recipient for human leukocyte antigen (HLA) types.
- Immunosuppressive treatment.

Short-term complications include:
- Acute rejection (within 3 months).
- Operative failure.

Rejection is reduced by immunosuppression therapy, which is started after the transplant and continued indefinitely. However, patients are at risk of opportunistic infection (e.g., with cytomegalovirus).

Long-term complications include:
- Infection.
- Recurrence of original disease.
- Obstruction at the ureteric anastomoses.
- Malignancy, especially lymphomas.

Currently, the 5-year graft survival rate is about 70% for both cadaveric and living transplants.

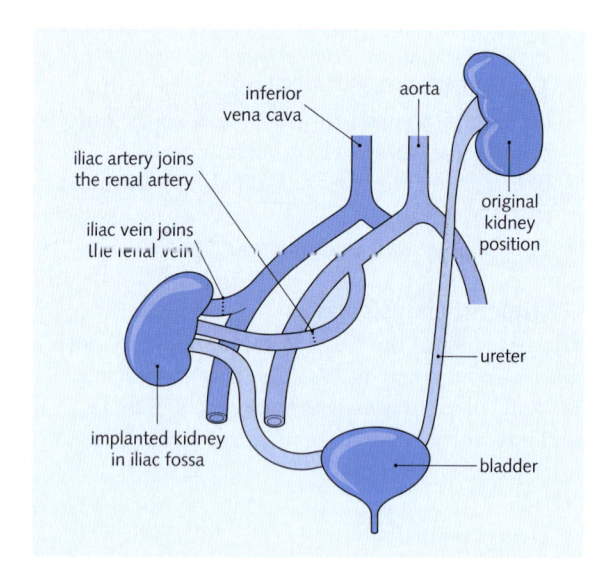

Fig 3.11 Implantation of a transplanted kidney.

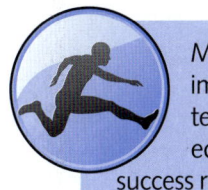

> Modern immunosuppressive techniques have led to near-equivalent transplant success rates for cadaveric, living related, and living unrelated donors.

Body fluids: regulation and clinical disorders

Effective circulating volume and extracellular volume

The volume of fluid that effectively perfuses tissues is the effective circulating volume; this needs to be kept constant. Its determinents include the extracellular volume (which determines the intravascular volume), the blood pressure, and the cardiac output. It cannot be measured directly, but is estimated by noting the body's physiological responses to it.

The main determinant of the extracellular volume is the total body sodium. Since Na^+ is the major extracellular ion, a rise in the amount of extracellular Na^+ results in increased serum osmolality, which leads to renal water retention and thirst (increased drinking of water). This increases extracellular volume. Thus, the extracellular volume can be regulated by controlling the total body sodium.

If effective circulating volume decreases sufficiently, multiple renal and nonrenal mechanisms can act to return it to normal (Fig. 3.12).

Regulation of total body sodium and extracellular volume

The extracellular volume can be expanded by either increasing total body sodium or by increasing total

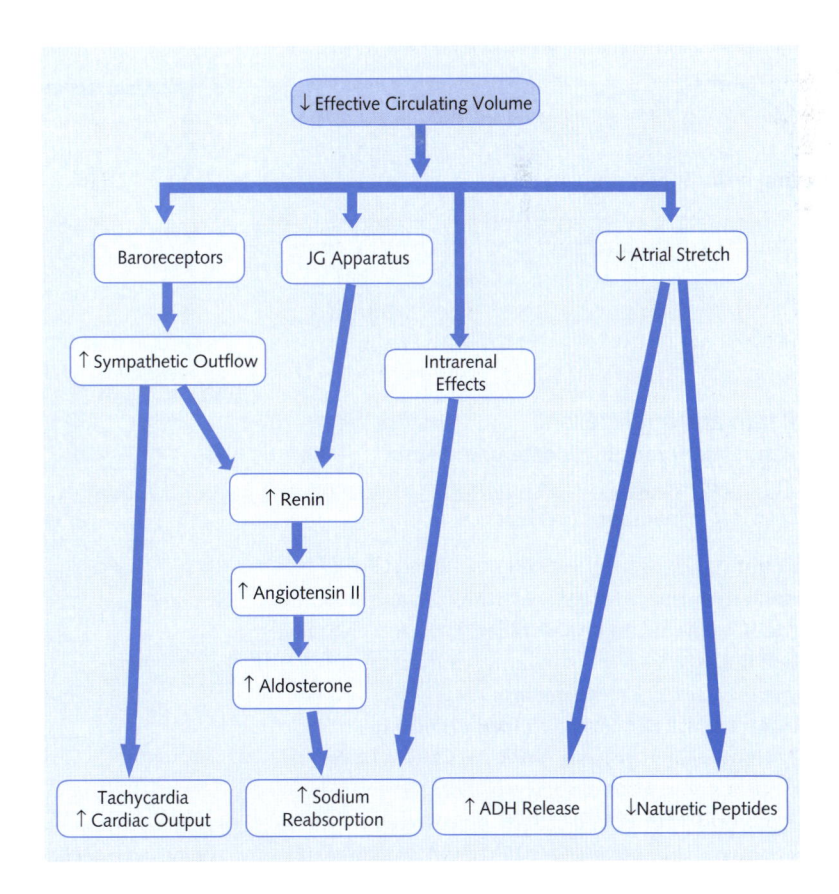

Fig 3.12 Response to decreased effective circulating volume. JGA, juxtaglomerular apparatus.

Na⁺ transport along the nephron			
Part of nephron	Percentage of filtered Na⁺ reabsorbed	Method of entry into the cell	Regulatory hormones
proximal tubule	65–70	Na⁺ co-transport, paracellular	angiotensin II
loop of Henle	20–25	Na⁺/Cl⁻/K⁺ pump (1:2:1)	aldosterone
early distal tubule	5	Na⁺/Cl⁻ symport	aldosterone
late distal tubule and collecting ducts	5	Na⁺ channels	aldosterone, natriuretic peptides

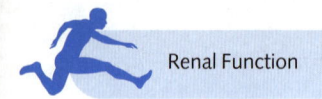

Fig 3.13 Na⁺ transport along the nephron.

body water. The former is more effective, since sodium is confined to the extracellular space, while water distributes in both the extracellular and intracellular spaces. The kidney is the main determinant of total body sodium, since it can tightly regulate sodium reabsorption or excretion. Multiple mechanisms exist to increase renal sodium reabsorption. Na⁺ reabsorption along the nephron is shown in Fig. 3.13.

> The kidney has multiple mechanisms to respond to a fall in effective circulating volume. Sodium and water reabsorption help to correct the deficit.

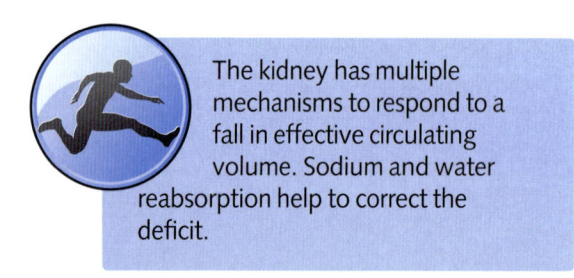

Renin and angiotensin
Renin–angiotensin–aldosterone system
The renin–angiotensin–aldosterone (RAA) system (Fig. 3.14) maintains Na⁺ balance.

Renin
Renin is an enzyme that is synthesized and stored in the JGA in the kidneys. A fall in total body Na⁺ leads to a fall in extracellular volume, causing the release of renin via several mechanisms:
- Increased sympathetic innervation: a fall in extracellular volume results in a fall in blood pressure. This is detected by baroreceptors in carotid arteries and causes increased sympathetic activity. Granular cells of the JGA are innervated by the sympathetic system, so an increase in sympathetic activity leads to an increase in renin release. The process is mediated by beta-adrenergic receptors.
- The wall tension in afferent arterioles falls: decreased extracellular volume reduces perfusion pressure to the kidneys. Changes in the blood

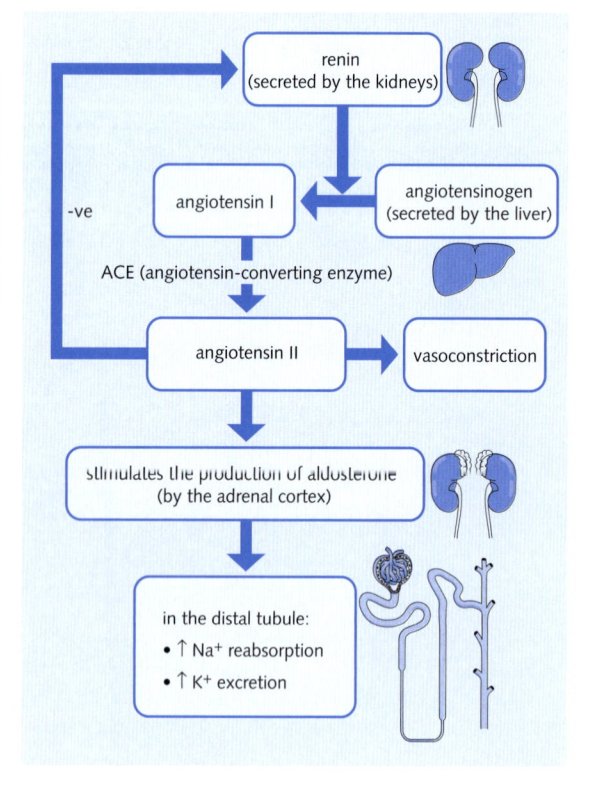

Fig. 3.14 The renin–angiotensin–aldosterone system. -ve, negative feedback.

pressure decrease wall tension at granular cells, which stimulates renin release.
- Decreased Na^+ or Cl^- delivery to the macula densa: if less NaCl reaches the macula densa, the macula densa is stimulated to secrete the prostaglandin PGI_2. This acts on the granular cells to cause renin release.

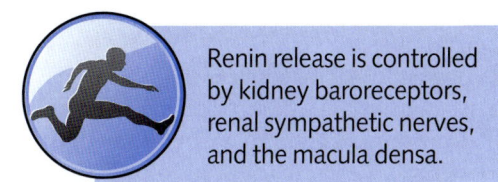

> Renin release is controlled by kidney baroreceptors, renal sympathetic nerves, and the macula densa.

Conversion of angiotensinogen to angiotensin
Renin cleaves angiotensinogen, converting it to angiotensin I (a decapeptide). Angiotensin-converting enzyme (ACE) in the lungs then removes two amino acids to produce angiotensin II (an octapeptide). Angiotensin II:
- Stimulates the zona glomerulosa of the adrenal cortex to release aldosterone.
- Directly vasoconstricts arterioles within the kidney (efferent > afferent).
- Directly increases Na^+ reabsorption from the proximal tubule.
- Releases ADH.
- Stimulates thirst.

- Provides negative feedback to the JGA cells, and therefore reduces renin release (see Fig. 3.14).

In addition to the generation of circulating angiotensin II, the local generation of angiotensin II by ACE (within the tissues) might have an important pathogenic role. ACE inhibitors are used to treat high blood pressure. They decrease the production of angiotensin II and consequently:
- Decrease vasoconstriction.
- Decrease aldosterone (and prevent an increase in extracellular volume).

Aldosterone
Aldosterone is synthesized by zona glomerulosa cells in the adrenal cortex. Its release (Fig. 3.15) is stimulated by:
- Angiotensin II
- Extracellular volume: indirectly, via renin–angiotensin II.
- ↑ serum K^+ concentration: stimulates direct release of aldosterone from the adrenal cortex. This returns K^+ to normal by increasing distal tubular secretion of K^+.
- ACTH: not normally a major mediator of volume regulation.

Aldosterone primarily regulates total body sodium content. It acts within cells to:
- Promote Na^+ reabsorption in the kidney, colon, gastric glands and sweat and salivary gland ducts.
- Promote K^+ and H^+ secretion by the kidney.

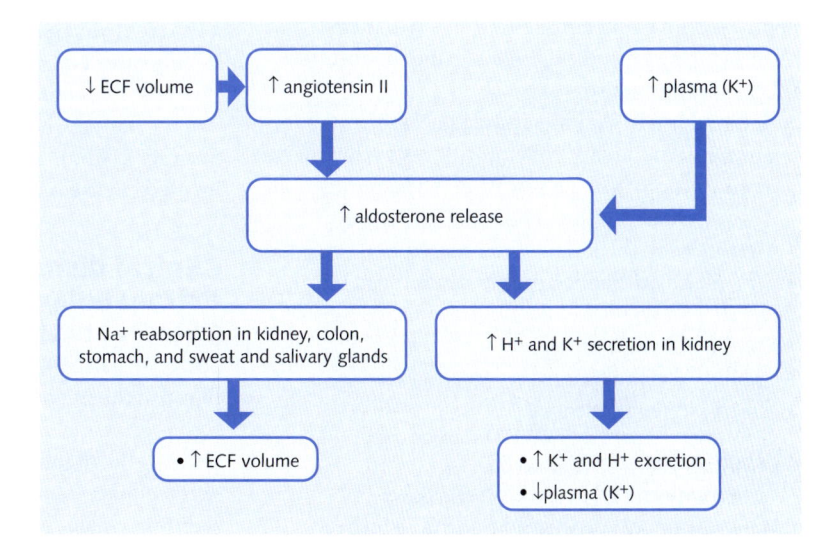

Fig. 3.15 Factors causing aldosterone release and the effects of aldosterone. ECF, extracellular fluid.

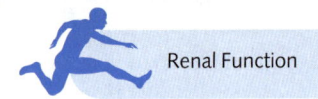

Other factors affecting renal Na⁺ reabsorption
Starling forces in the proximal tubule
The amount of Na⁺ and water reabsorbed into the peritubular capillaries from the proximal tubule depends on the rate and amount of uptake from the lateral intercellular spaces into the capillaries.

Changes in the body fluid volume alters plasma hydrostatic and oncotic pressure. For example, increased NaCl intake is mirrored by a rise in extracellular volume, which in turn increases hydrostatic pressure and decreases tubular capillary oncotic pressure. As a result, NaCl and water reabsorption by the proximal tubule cells decreases.

Sympathetic drive from the renal nerves
The arterial baroreceptors regulate renal sympathetic nerve activity. For example, a fall in extracellular volume decreases blood pressure, which is sensed by baroreceptors and results in an increase in sympathetic activity. This stimulates Na⁺ retention and an increase in peripheral resistance, thus restoring extracellular volume and blood pressure.

A rise in sympathetic nerve activity to the kidney stimulates renin release directly (this activates the JGA). Catecholamines from sympathetic nerve endings also stimulate Na⁺ reabsorption by the proximal tubule, but it is unclear if this is a direct effect or secondary to altered peritubular forces.

Natriuretic peptides
Natriuretic peptides are produced by cardiac atrial cells (and others) in response to an increase in extracellular volume. Their general action is to increase sodium excretion by the kidney. Natriuretic peptides bind to specific cell surface receptors, resulting in increased cyclic guanosine monosulfate (cGMP). They act to:
- Inhibit Na⁺/K⁺ ATPase and close Na⁺ channels of the inner medullary collecting ducts, reducing Na⁺ reabsorption. Na⁺ reabsorption is also reduced in the proximal tubules. Thus, Na⁺ and water excretion by the kidney is increased.
- Vasodilate afferent arterioles, thereby increasing GFR.
- Inhibit aldosterone secretion.
- Inhibit ADH release.
- Decrease renin release.

Prostaglandins
A decrease in the effective circulating volume stimulates cortical prostaglandin (PG) synthesis.

In the kidney, PG synthesis occurs in the:
- Cortex (arterioles and glomeruli).
- Medullary interstitial cells.
- Collecting duct epithelial cells.

Several renal prostaglandins exist: PGE_2 (medullary), PGI_2 (cortical), $PGF_2\alpha$, PGD_2, and TXA_2 (thromboxane). The main functions of each are as follows:
- PGE_2, PGI_2: vasodilators, preventing excessive vasoconstriction.
- PGI_2 (prostacyclin): renin release.
- PGE_2 (medullary): promotes water and sodium excretion within the collecting tubules and thus overrides the water retaining action of ADH. PGE_2 protects the medullary tubule cells from excessive hypoxia when the extracellular volume decreases.
- TXA_2: a vasoconstrictor, which is synthesized after repeated kidney damage (e.g., ureteral obstruction). It reduces the amount of blood available for filtration by a poorly functioning kidney.

Kinins
Kininogens are cleaved by the enzyme kallikrein to form kinins. The effects of kinins are similar to those of PGs and include:
- Vasodilation.
- Inhibition of ADH release.
- Increased Na⁺ excretion.

Dopamine
This is synthesized by the proximal tubule cells and:
- Inhibits Na⁺/K⁺ ATPase and Na⁺/H⁺ antiport, thereby decreasing tubular Na⁺ transport.
- Increases Na⁺ excretion (natriuresis).
- Causes vasodilation.

See Fig. 3.12 for a summary of the mechanisms involved in the regulation of body fluid

Clinical disorders of extracellular volume
Overview: total body sodium vs. serum sodium concentration
Because the main ECF solute is sodium, "total body sodium *content*" is nearly synonymous with "extracellular volume" (i.e., most decreases in extracellular volume also show decreased total body sodium). Since sodium is confined to the

extracellular space, and since the extracellular volume is only about one-third of total body water, a gain (or loss) of isotonic saline will result in a threefold more potent change in the extracellular volume than an equivalent volume of pure water alone.

In contrast, the serum sodium *concentration*, tightly controlled by ADH, *does not* predict total body sodium or extracellular volume status. It is mainly a function of the amount of water present in the circulation *relative* to sodium. Therefore, a patient with hyponatremia (low sodium concentration) may not have a low total body sodium content.

- The extracellular volume status reflects total body sodium content and is assessed by clinical criteria, *not* by serum sodium concentration.
- The serum sodium *concentration* reflects serum osmolality and is determined by total body water, not by sodium intake.

Extracellular volume depletion (hypovolemia)

Mechanism: loss of salt and water from ECF.
   Causes include:
- Gastrointestinal loss: vomiting, diarrhea, bleeding, suction.
- Renal loss: diuretics, salt wasting, osmotic diuresis (including DKA).
- Skin: burns, sweat.
- Lungs: insensible loss.
- Hemorrhage.

Symptoms: thirst, dizziness, confusion.

Signs: dry skin and mucous membranes, flat jugular venous pulse, orthostasis, hypotension, tachycardia.
   Lab tests include:
- Urine Na < 10mEq/L, which reflects avid renal Na reabsorption.
- Urine osmolality >450mosm/kg-, which reflects ↑ ADH in response to ↓ effective circulating volume.
- BUN/Cr ratio >20:1, which reflects avid urea reabsorption in proximal tubule.
- Elevated hematocrit, which reflects concentration of plasma volume.

Therapy includes the following:
   Sodium and water repletion is critical in initial management. Rapid IV administration of at least 2L/hr is essential for patients in shock. Monitor fluid status frequently, especially in elderly patients or patients with suspected heart disease. Overtreatment can precipitate congestive heart failure.
   Which fluid is best to use?
- Blood is an excellent volume expander but expensive and in short supply; it stays in intravascular space. Use for hemorrhage and severe hypoalbuminemia.
- Colloid solutions (e.g., albumin) have theoretical advantages over salt solutions, since they are confined to intravascular space. However, they are expensive, and clinical studies have *failed* to confirm this advantage.
- Salt solutions have a varying extracellular/intracellular distribution, depending on Na concentration (Fig. 3.16). Note that hypertonic saline pulls water from the ICF into the ECF.

Expanded extracellular volume

Disorders of expanded ECF are normally caused by excessive renal sodium reabsorption. This can be secondary to decreased effective circulating volume, or due to primary renal sodium retention due to aberrant hormonal or renal responses.

Expanded ECF due to decreased effective circulating volume

Overall mechanism: renal salt and water retention in response to ↓ effective circulating volume.
   Mechanisms for reduced effective circulating volume:
- Congestive heart failure: reduced cardiac output.
- Hepatic cirrhosis: systemic vasodilation and pooling of blood in splanchnic beds.
- Drugs: vasodilators (minoxidil, hydralazine, nitroprusside).
- Nephrotic syndrome with <u>severe</u> hypoalbuminemia (<1.0mg/dl) and decreased low plasma oncotic pressure, causing reduced intravascular volume.
- Sepsis/shock: capillary leak reduces intravascular volume.

Renal Function

Composition and volume of distribution of 1 liter of common IV fluids		
Solution	Volume of distribution (liters, approx.)	
	ECF	ICF
0.9% normal saline (150mM Na)	1	0
0.45% normal saline (75mM) "half normal"	0.65	0.35
D_5W (0 Na, 5gm/L glucose)	0.35	0.65
lactate ringer's (130mM Na, 28mM HCO_3, 4mM K, 2mM Ca)	1	0
3% saline (500mM Na)	+2.6	−1.6

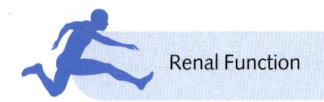

Fig. 3.16 Composition and volume of distribution of 1 liter of common IV fluids.

Consequences include the following:
- Edema: pulmonary in left heart failure, peripheral in other causes.
- Ascites.
- Variable hypertension.
- Other symptoms specific to disease.

Lab tests: The urine is concentrated (high osmolality) due to high ADH and has a Na concentration of <10mEq/L.

Expanded ECF: due to primary renal salt and water retention

Mechanism: primary renal sodium retention despite normal initial volume status and normal effective circulating volume.

Key causes include:
- Glomerulonephritis: probably due to resistance to natriuretic peptides.
- Severe renal failure: reduced GFR and reduced Na excretion.
- Primary hyperaldosteronism: increased Na reabsorption.

Consequences include the following:
- Edema (GN and renal failure only). Edema is unusual in ↑ aldosterone states, due to the action of natriuretic peptides to counteract the Na retaining action of aldosterone. There is hypertension, however, from unknown mechanisms. Renal diseases, in contrast, often manifest resistance to natriuretic peptides; thus edema results.
- Hypertension (seen in all the above).

Lab tests: the urine Na is < 10mEq/L due to the avid sodium reabsorption by the disordered kidney. Major causes of edematous disorders are listed in Fig. 3.17.

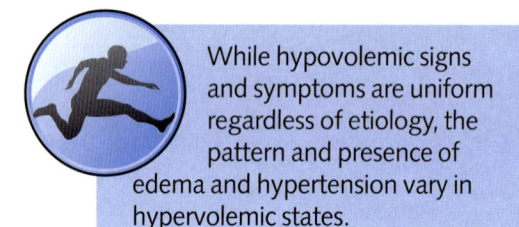

While hypovolemic signs and symptoms are uniform regardless of etiology, the pattern and presence of edema and hypertension vary in hypervolemic states.

Treatment of expanded extracellular volume
- Evaluate cause of edema and optimize treatment of underlying cause.
- Restrict sodium intake.
- Mobilize edema—bed rest, support stockings.
- Diuretics.

Diuretics
Diuretics increase the volume of urine produced by increasing renal sodium excretion (natriuresis), which is followed passively by water. Each type of diuretic inhibits Na reabsorption in a particular segment (Fig. 3.18). All can cause volume depletion and hypokalemia (except potassium-sparing diuretics). They should be used judiciously.

Osmotic diuretics
Osmotic diuresis can be induced by an inert substance that is not reabsorbed in the tubule. The proximal tubule and the descending limb of the loop of Henle allow free movement of water molecules. If an agent such as mannitol is introduced into the tubular fluid, it is not absorbed and thus reduces water reabsorption. There is increased urine flow through the nephrons, resulting in reduced sodium reabsorption.

Body fluids: regulation and clinical disorders

Selected causes of edema			
Cause	Why?	Intravascular volume	Effective circulating volume
CHF, cirrhosis	low effective circulating volume	↑	↓
glomerular disease	renal ANF resistance	↑	↑
vasodilators (minoxidil)	precapillary vasodilation	↓	↓
sepsis, shock	capillary leak	↓	↓

Fig. 3.17 Selected causes of edema.

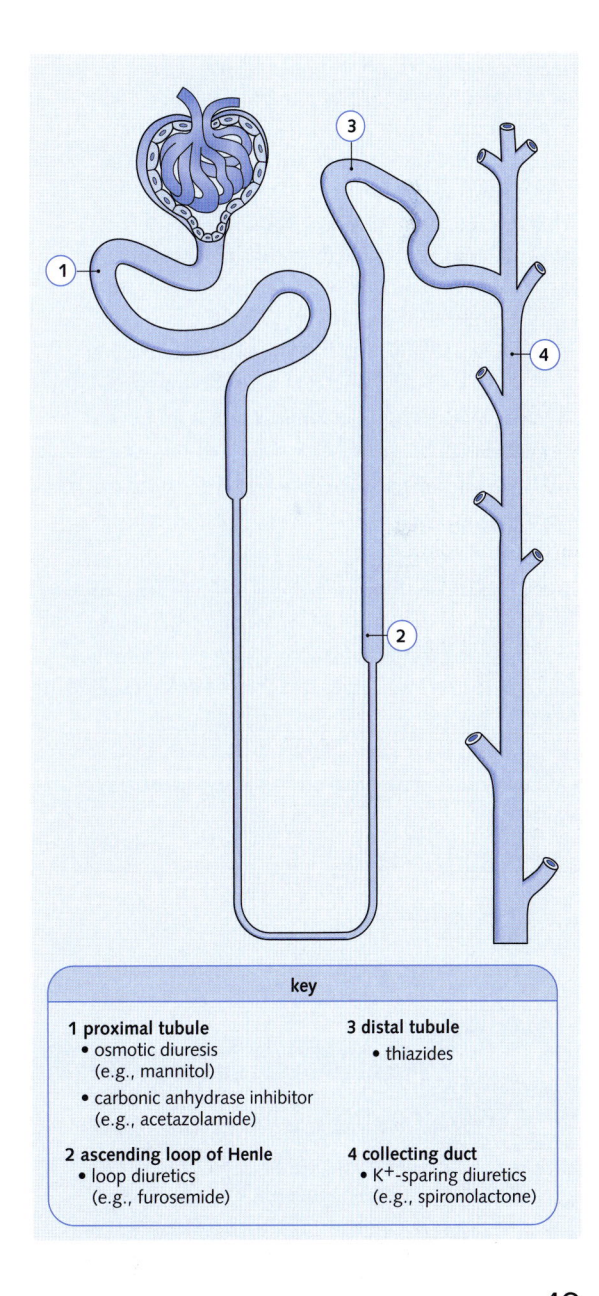

key

1 proximal tubule
- osmotic diuresis (e.g., mannitol)
- carbonic anhydrase inhibitor (e.g., acetazolamide)

2 ascending loop of Henle
- loop diuretics (e.g., furosemide)

3 distal tubule
- thiazides

4 collecting duct
- K$^+$-sparing diuretics (e.g., spironolactone)

Fig. 3.18 Sites of diuretic action.

49

Osmotic diuretics are used to:
- Increase urine volume.
- Reduce intracranial pressures in neurological conditions.
- Reduce intraocular pressures before ophthalmic surgery.

Excessive use of osmotic diuretics without adequate fluid replacement can cause dehydration and hypernatremia.

Loop diuretics

These are the most potent diuretics, causing up to 20% of filtered Na^+ to be excreted. They inhibit sodium transport out of the thick ascending limb of the loop of Henle into the medullary interstitium. Examples include furosemide and bumetanide. Loop diuretics act by inhibiting the $Na^+/K^+/2Cl^-$ cotransporter on the luminal membrane of the cells. This inhibits Na^+ reabsorption, thereby diluting the osmotic gradient in the medulla. This results in increased Na^+ and water excretion.

Loop diuretics are used to:
- Treat acute pulmonary and peripheral edema.
- Reduce end-diastolic ventricular filling pressure.
- Treat acute hypercalcemia.
- Avoid complications in acute renal failure (increase urine output and K^+ excretion).

Thiazide diuretics

These reduce active Na^+ reabsorption in the early distal tubule by inhibiting the Na^+/Cl^- cotransporter. As there is more reabsorption of Na^+ in the loop of Henle, the loop diuretics are more potent than thiazide diuretics. Thiazides reduce peripheral vascular resistance and consequently are used to manage hypertension. They are also used to treat calcium containing renal stones and nephrogenic diabetes insipidus. They can cause:
- hyponatremia (they limit the ability of the kidney to dilute the urine maximally).
- hypercalcemia

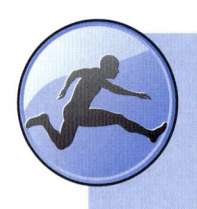

Side effects of thiazide diuretics are summarized in the mnemonic HyperGLUC (increased levels of glucose, lipid, uric acid, and calcium).

Potassium-sparing diuretics

These diuretics are K^+-sparing and act in the principal cells of the collecting ducts. They inhibit the uptake of Na^+ in the cells of the principal cells by one of two mechanisms:
- Inhibiting the luminal sodium channel (e.g., amiloride and triamterene).
- Competing with aldosterone for the aldo receptor sites (spironolactone).

They therefore reduce sodium reabsorption in the distal nephron making the cells more electronegative and therefore decreasing K^+ secretion (potassium-sparing activity).

Potassium-sparing diuretics are used if there is mineralocorticoid excess such as primary aldosteronism (Conn's syndrome) or ectopic ACTH production. They are also used in secondary aldosteronism with salt and water retention (esp. liver disease). They are fairly weak and often used with loop diuretics or thiazides to prevent K^+ loss.

The side effects include:
- Hyperkalemia: this results from renal K^+ retention as Na^+ absorption falls and ranges from mild to life-threatening.
- Endocrine effects with spironolactone (e.g., gynecomastia).

Potassium-sparing diuretics are contraindicated in patients with hyperkalemia or chronic renal failure.

Carbonic anhydrase (CA) inhibitors

CA inhibitors such as acetazolamide interfere with the action of proximal tubule luminal carbonic anhydrase and inhibit HCO_3^- reabsorption (see Chapter 2). The presence of HCO_3^- in the lumen reduces Na^+ reabsorption.

CA inhibitors such as acetazolamide are weak diuretics, which cause the excretion of only about 5–10% of the filtered Na^+ and water. Their main clinical use is to treat acute and chronic glaucoma by reducing intraocular pressure (the production of aqueous humor in the eye involves secretion of HCO_3^- by the ciliary body in a process similar to that in the proximal tubule).

The side-effects of CA inhibitors include:
- Metabolic acidosis (from HCO_3^- loss).
- Renal stones.
- Nervous system effects—paresthesias and drowsiness.

Summary of diuretic action

Diuretic	Specific indications	Side effects
loop diuretics (furosemide, bumetanide)	severe CHF: most potent diuretics available	↓K ototoxicity
thiazides (hydrochlorothiazide, metolazone)	essential hypertension diabetes insipidus only metolazone is useful in chronic renal failure	↓K, ↓Na, ↑Ca inhibits urinary dilution
potassium-sparing diuretics (spironolactone, triamterene, amiloride)	cirrhosis mild diuretic; added to thiazides to avoid ↓K	↑K if GFR reduced! gynecomastia (spironolactone)
osmotic agents (mannitol)	cerebral edema	vascular space expansion with volume overload
acetazolamide	glaucoma altitude sickness weak diuretic	metabolic acidosis ↓K

Fig. 3.19 Summary of diuretic action.

CA inhibitors should be avoided in patients with liver disease or advanced chronic renal failure.

A summary of the main classes of diuretics is shown in Fig. 3.19.

Regulation and clinical disorders of serum osmolality

Regulation of serum osmolality

Body weight remains relatively constant from day to day because total body water remains constant. The normal intake and output of water are discussed in Chapter 1. At least 400mL/day of urine must be produced for the kidney to maintain homeostasis.

The normal serum osmolality is 285–295 mOsmol/kg H_2O. Na^+ and other associated anions are the main constituents that determine plasma osmolality. Water loss or gain alters the Na^+ concentration. Changes in other solutes without the addition or loss of water can also change the osmolality.

The serum osmolality is strictly regulated by water ingestion and renal water reabsorption. An increase or decrease of 3mosm/kg will stimulate the body's osmolality regulation mechanism.

Osmoreceptors

Osmoreceptors detect changes in the plasma osmolality and are located in the supraoptic and paraventricular areas of the anterior hypothalamus. Their blood supply is the internal carotid artery. They have two functions:
1. To regulate the release of antidiuretic hormone (ADH, also known as vasopressin).
2. To regulate thirst (this also depends on other osmoreceptors in the lateral preoptic area of the hypothalamus).

Figure 3.20 illustrates the roles of thirst and ADH in maintaining osmolality.

Not all solutes stimulate the osmoreceptors to the same degree—this depends on how easily they can cross the cell membrane (i.e., their ability to cause cellular dehydration).

> Total body water balance depends upon:
> - Regulation of water excretion by the kidneys.
> - Water intake via the thirst mechanism.
>
> Both are controlled by the osmoreceptors.

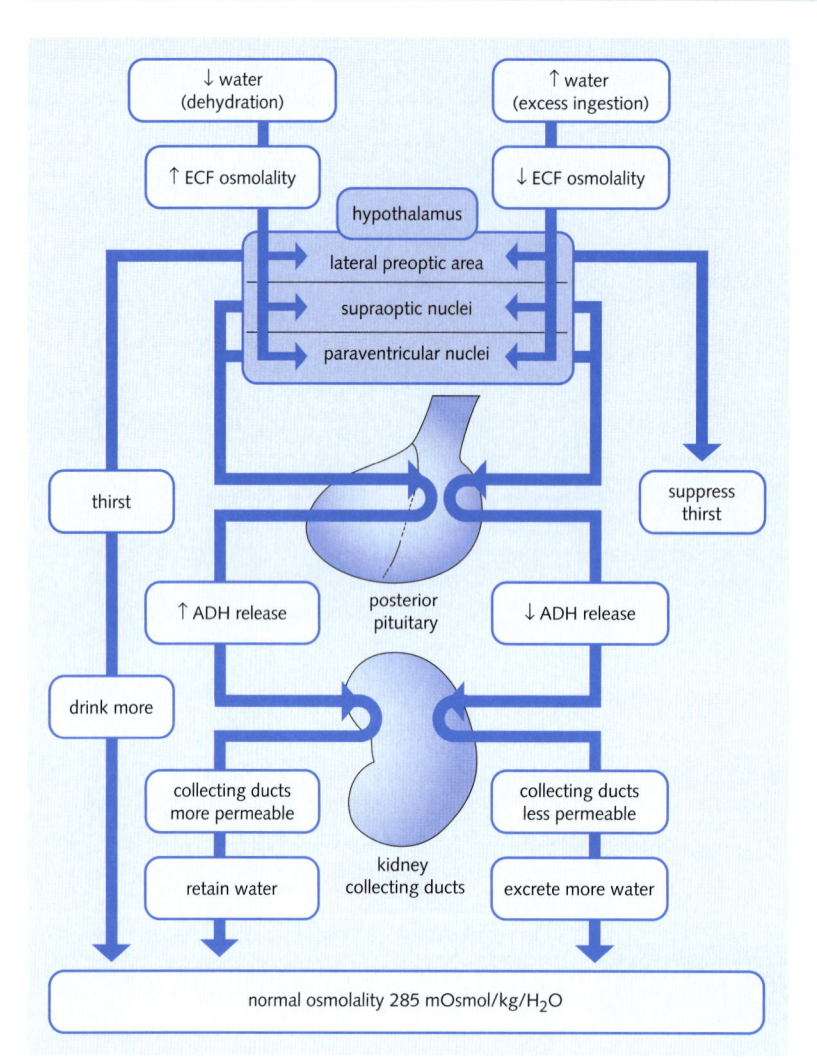

Fig. 3.20 Role of antidiuretic hormone (ADH) in maintaining osmolality. ECF, extracellular fluid.

Renal water reabsorption

Although about 20% of the initial glomerular filtrate enters the distal nephron, only 5% enters the medullary collecting ducts. This is mainly due to water reabsorption in the cortical collecting duct. In order to reabsorb water, the kidneys must have the following present:
- Circulating ADH.
- A concentrated medullary interstitium.

In the presence of these factors, water moves through the aquaporins into the principal cells, then through the water permeable basolateral membrane into the concentrated medullary interstitium. The water reabsorbed is then taken up by the capillaries and returned to the circulation.

ADH (antidiuretic hormone/vasopressin)

ADH levels within the body determine the concentration and volume of urine:
- Average daily urine volume is 1.0–1.5 L (normal range: 400 mL to 2–3 L).
- Average urine osmolality is 450 mosm/kg (normal range: 60–1400 mosm/kg).

Synthesis and storage

ADH is a peptide hormone synthesized in the supraoptic nucleus of the hypothalamus as a large precursor molecule. It is transported to the posterior pituitary gland, where its synthesis is completed and it is stored until release (Fig. 3.21).

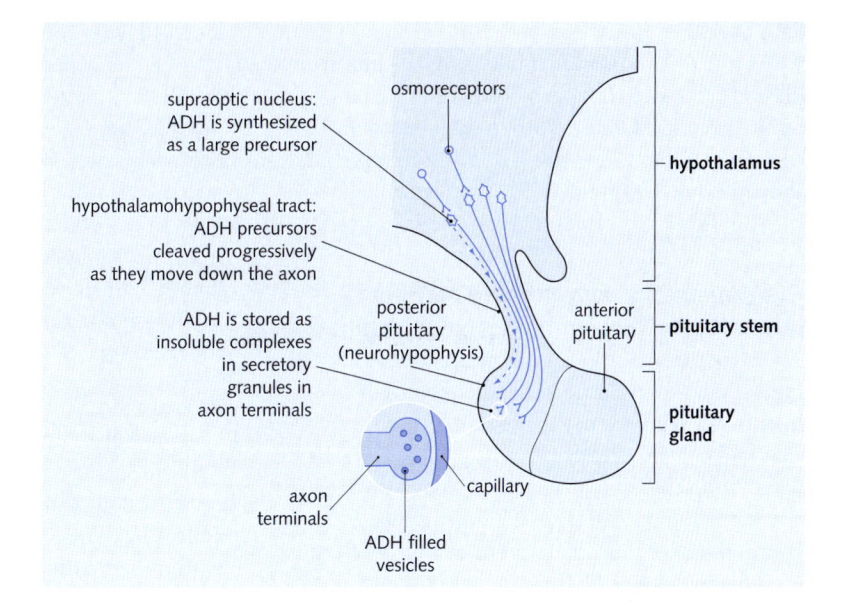

Fig. 3.21 Synthesis and storage of antidiuretic hormone (ADH).

Release

ADH secretion is controlled by:
- Osmoreceptors (which detect changes in the body fluid osmolarity).
- Baroreceptors (which detect changes in blood volume, i.e., blood vessel wall "stretch").

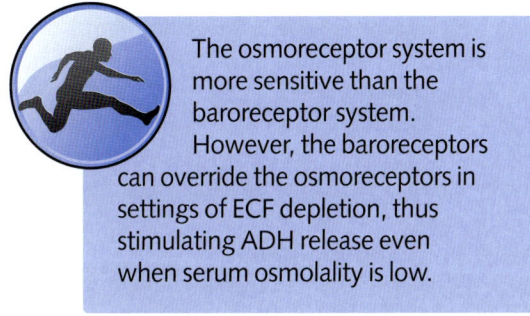

> The osmoreceptor system is more sensitive than the baroreceptor system. However, the baroreceptors can override the osmoreceptors in settings of ECF depletion, thus stimulating ADH release even when serum osmolality is low.

A rise in plasma osmolality is sensed by osmoreceptors and triggers ADH release. Action potentials in the neurons from the hypothalamus (which contains ADH) depolarize the axon membrane, resulting in Ca^{2+} influx, fusion of secretory granules with the axon membrane, and the release of ADH and neurophysin into the bloodstream.

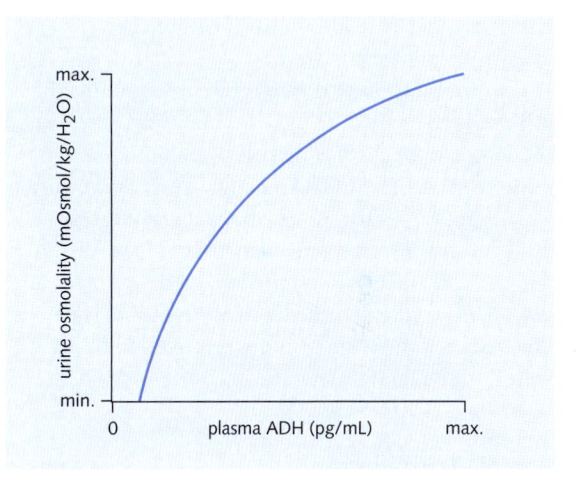

Cellular actions

ADH has several functions:
1. To increase renal water reabsorption (V_2 receptor-mediated). This is accomplished by insertion of aquaporins into the luminal membrane of collecting duct principal cells (see Chapter 2). In the presence of a concentrated medullary interstitium, water leaves the collecting duct and the urine osmolality rises (Fig. 3.22).
2. To stimulate blood vessel vasoconstriction (V_1 receptor mediated).
3. To increase collecting duct urea reabsorption, increasing interstitial osmolality.

Fig. 3.22 Urine osmolality in relation to plasma antidiuretic hormone (ADH) concentration (from Berne RM, Levy MN: *Physiology*, 3rd ed. Mosby Year Book, 1996).

The presence of cortisol is vital for the action of ADH.

Fate of ADH

ADH must be removed rapidly from the blood once plasma osmolality has been corrected. This is done by the liver and kidneys (50%), with less than 10% appearing in the urine; the rest is metabolized. Its short plasma half-life (10–15min) also ensures that the duration of its effect in the blood is limited.

Generation of a concentrated medullary interstitium: the countercurrent multiplier

The structure, location and function of the loop of Henle has a central role in the development of a hypertonic gradient in the medulla. Any mechanism that will concentrate urine must be able to reabsorb water from the tubular fluid as it passes through the collecting ducts. The loop of Henle, which acts as a countercurrent multiplier, produces a hypertonic medulla by pooling NaCl in the interstitium, which favors the subsequent reabsorption of water out of the collecting ducts (under the regulation of ADH). Each portion of the loop contributes to the effectiveness of this system.

The mechanism of the countercurrent multiplier is illustrated in Fig 3.23. The tubular fluid entering the loop has the normal plasma osmolality of 300mosm/kg. The thick ascending limb can maintain a difference of 200mosm/kg between the tubular fluid and the interstitium at any point along its length. The maximum osmolality of the interstitium is 1400mosm/kg is at the tip of the loop. As the fluid ascends the loop, solute is removed without water, so the fluid leaving the loop of Henle is hypotonic (100mosm/kg).

Role of the vasa recta

The countercurrent mechanism requires an environment in which the waste products and water are cleared without disturbing the solutes that maintain the medullary hypertonicity. This exchange is provided by the vasa recta capillary system derived from the efferent arterioles of the longer juxtaglomerular nephrons.

The capillaries have a hairpin arrangement surrounding the loop of Henle and are permeable to water and solutes. As the descending vessels pass through the medulla they absorb solutes such as Na^+, urea and Cl^-. Water moves along its osmotic gradient out of the capillaries. At the tip of the loop the capillary blood has the same osmolality as the interstitium, and an osmotic equilibrium is reached. The capillaries that ascend with the corresponding loop of Henle contain very viscous concentrated blood as a result of the earlier loss of water from the capillaries. There is a consequent increase in oncotic pressure because of the concentration of plasma proteins, which favors the movement of water back into the blood vessel from the interstitium. However, most of the NaCl is retained in the interstitium to maintain the hypertonic medullary environment. Figure 3.24 shows the vasa recta and countercurrent exchanger and the collecting duct as it passes through the medulla.

Role of urea

The medullary interstitial osmolality of 1400mosm/kg consists of about half NaCl and half urea. Although urea is impermeable in the cortical collecting ducts, ADH stimulates uptake of urea within the medullary collecting ducts. Urea, along with NaCl, helps maintain medullary hypertonicity as follows:

- 50% of the filtered urea is reabsorbed in the proximal tubule with Na^+.
- In the ascending loop, the tubular concentration of urea increases as it diffuses out of the medullary interstitium into the lumen down its concentration gradient.
- The remaining urea becomes further concentrated within the tubular lumen as water and other solutes are reabsorbed into the cells of the distal tubule and the cortical collecting tubules, which are impermeable to urea.
- Urea diffuses out of the lumen into the interstitium (facilitated diffusion when ADH is present), thus increasing the concentration of urea in the medulla and recycling it.

Low protein intake decreases the amount of urea in the blood for excretion. Consequently, there is less urea in the medullary interstitium, resulting in a lower maximal urine osmolality (see Nephrogenic diabetes insipidus below).

Clinical disorders of osmolality: hyponatremia

The serum sodium concentration is a quickly measured convenient surrogate for the more laborious measurement of serum osmolality. In most cases hyponatremia = hypoosmolality. For example, in hyponatremia serum $[Na^-]$ is <130mEq/L, and there is a decreased solute:water ratio in the extracellular fluid. This is usually due to excess

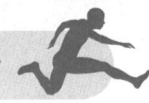

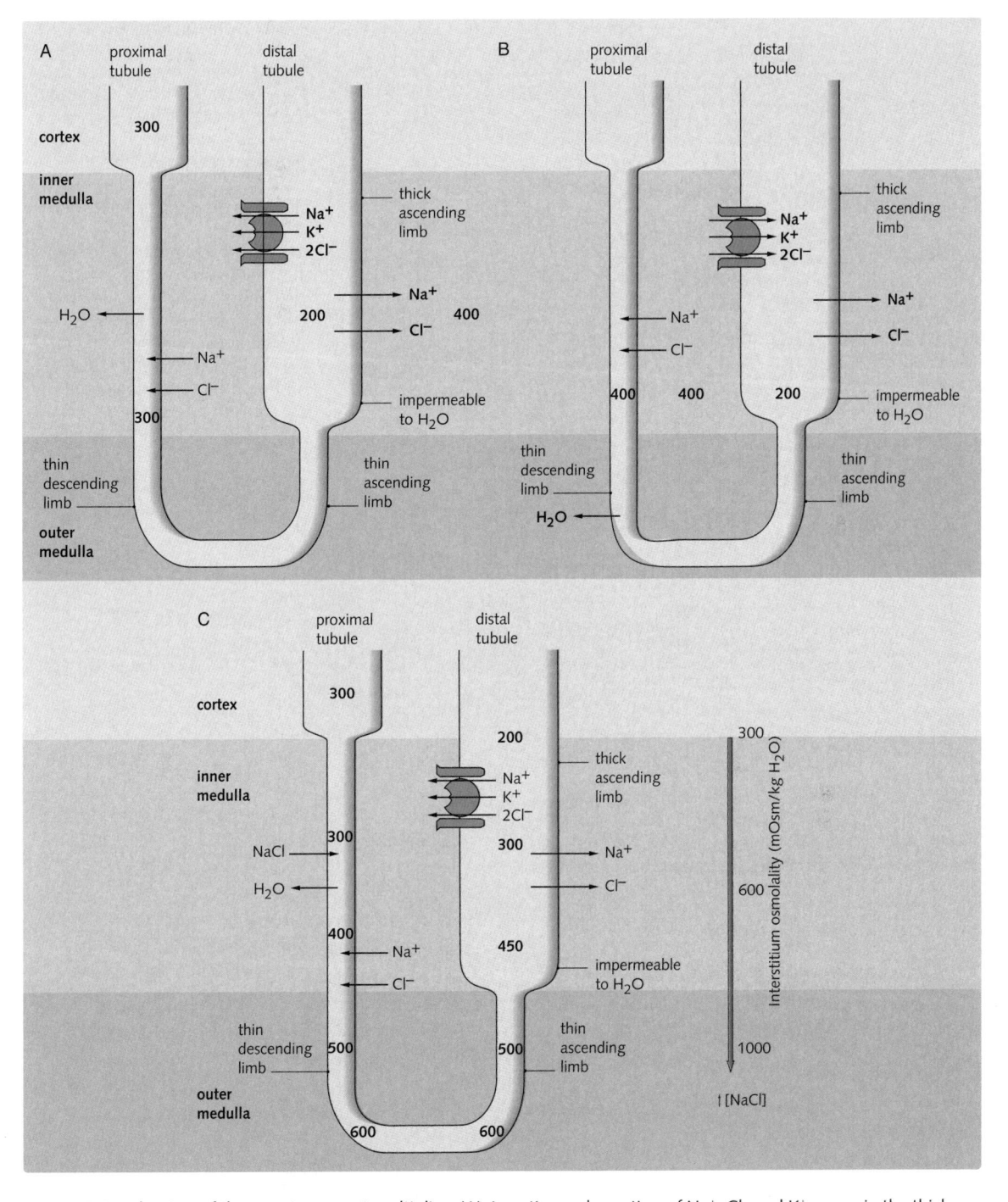

Fig. 3.23 Mechanism of the countercurrent multiplier: (A) As active reabsorption of Na⁺, Cl⁻ and K⁺ occurs in the thick ascending limb, the concentration of solutes in the medulla increases. Because there is no movement of water in the thick ascending limb, the osmolality of the tubular fluid decreases (200 mosm/kg) and the osmolality of the interstitium increases (400 mosm/kg). (B) The increase in the interstitial osmolality stimulates passive movement of water out of the thin descending limb into the medullary interstitium. It also causes NaCl to move into the filtrate. This occurs until an equilibrium is reached (400 mosm/kg) between the thin descending limb and the interstitium. (C) The constant removal of NaCl will continue to decrease the osmolality of the tubular fluid in the thick ascending limb, with maximal reabsorption occurring at the tip of the loop (600 mosm/kg). This will further increase the osmolality of the fluid in the thin descending limb as it comes into equilibrium with its surroundings. In this way, a longitudinal gradient of osmolality is created in the medulla.

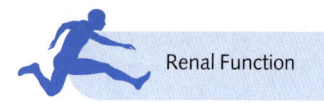

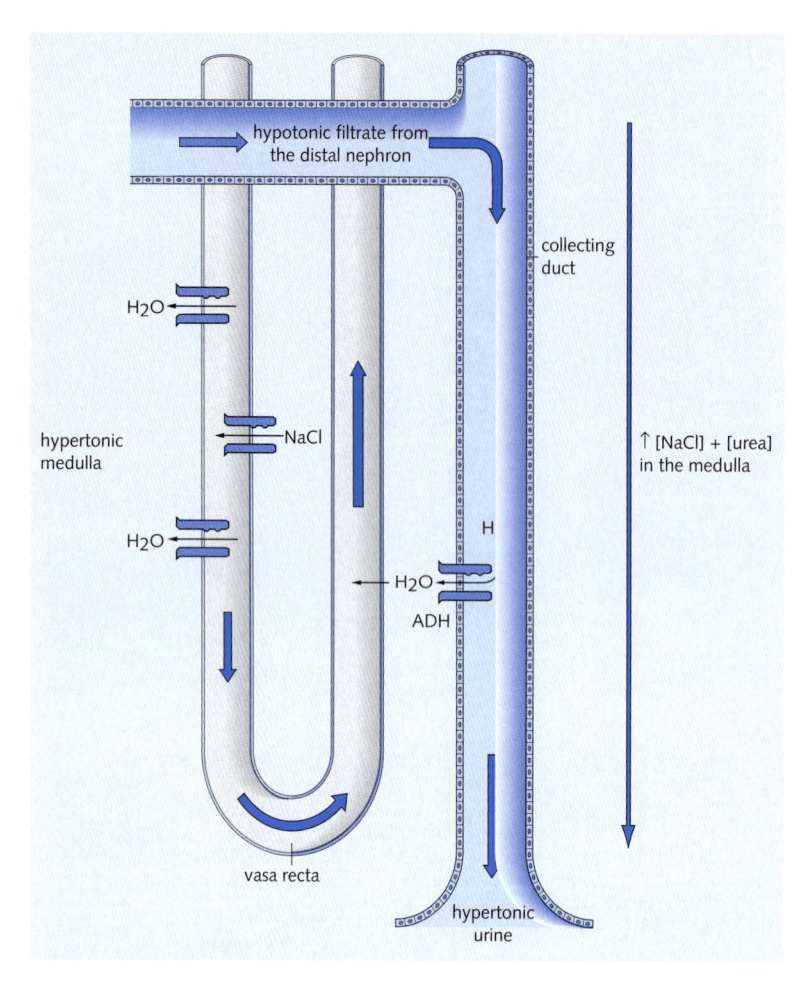

Fig 3.24 Countercurrent exchanger as it passes through the medulla. The descending vessels of the vasa recta lose water as they pass through the hypertonic medulla. As a result of increasing oncotic pressure in the ascending vessels, water is reabsorbed passively back into the blood vessels from the interstitium as water uptake occurs in the collecting ducts under the influence of ADH. Because of this uptake of water by the vasa recta, the high osmolality of the medullary interstitium is maintained and this hypertonic environment allows continued concentration of the tubular fluid in the collecting duct.

water. The clinical consequences of hyponatremia reflect the low serum osmolality, not low sodium *per se*.

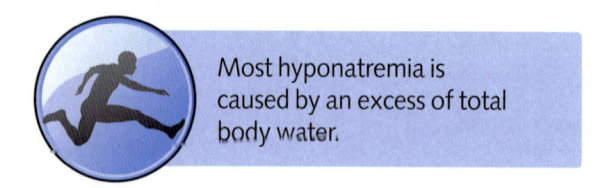

> Most hyponatremia is caused by an excess of total body water.

Symptoms
When hyponatremia is due to hypoosmolality, symptoms may develop due to brain swelling in the low osmotic environment. As the hyponatremia worsens, the symptoms worsen:
- Headache.
- Anorexia.
- Nausea and vomiting.
- Stupor.
- Seizures.
- Coma, death.

Classifying hyponatremia
A general diagnostic approach to hyponatremia is shown in Figure 3.25.
1. First exclude *pseudohyponatremia*, in which serum osmolality is normal. This is an artifact of lab measurement seen in some clinical labs. Causes are hyperlipidemia or paraproteinemia. No specific treatment of the hyponatremia is required.
2. Then exclude *hyponatremia with hyperosmolality*, caused by shifting of water from the intra- to the extracellular space in response to intravascular hypertonicity from a nonsodium osmole. Hyperglycemia is the most common cause. No specific treatment of the hyponatremia is required, but hyperglycemia should be treated.
3. Most remaining cases of hyponatremia reflect true hypoosmolality and therefore represent an excess

Regulation and clinical disorders of serum osmolality

Fig. 3.25 Diagnostic approach to hyponatremia. ECF, extracellular fluid; SIADH, syndrome of inappropriate ADH secretion; TURP, transurethral resection of the prostate.

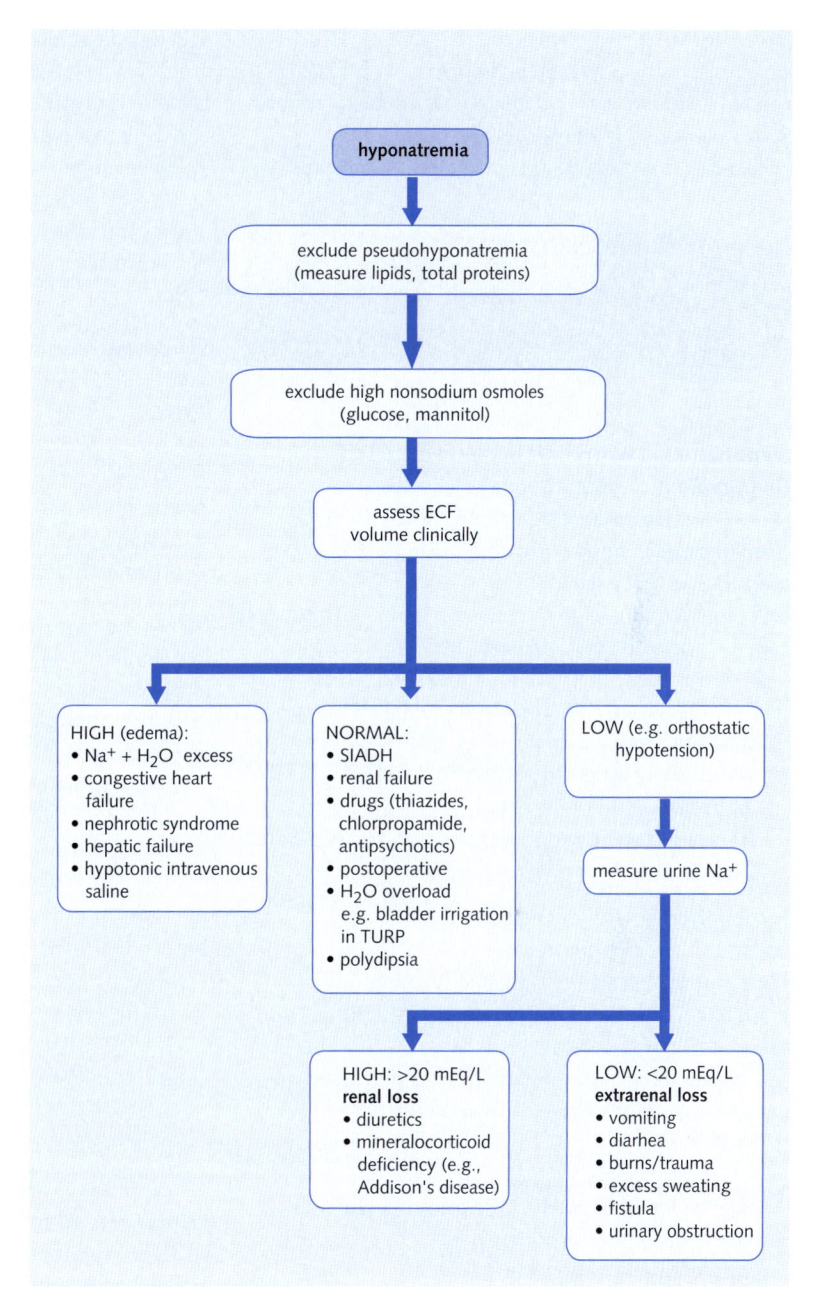

```
                    hyponatremia
                         ↓
           exclude pseudohyponatremia
           (measure lipids, total proteins)
                         ↓
           exclude high nonsodium osmoles
               (glucose, mannitol)
                         ↓
                  assess ECF
                volume clinically
          ↙              ↓              ↘
   HIGH (edema):    NORMAL:         LOW (e.g. orthostatic
   • Na⁺ + H₂O      • SIADH           hypotension)
     excess         • renal failure         ↓
   • congestive     • drugs (thiazides,  measure urine Na⁺
     heart failure    chlorpropamide,
   • nephrotic        antipsychotics)
     syndrome       • postoperative
   • hepatic        • H₂O overload
     failure          e.g. bladder
   • hypotonic        irrigation in TURP
     intravenous    • polydipsia
     saline
                      ↙              ↘
              HIGH: >20 mEq/L    LOW: <20 mEq/L
              renal loss        extrarenal loss
              • diuretics       • vomiting
              • mineralocorticoid • diarrhea
                deficiency (e.g., • burns/trauma
                Addison's disease) • excess sweating
                                  • fistula
                                  • urinary obstruction
```

of water. This is usually due to an inability of the kidneys to excrete a water load. This may be due to an elevated level of ADH or a primary renal disorder. Many of these causes can be differentiated by clinical assessment of the extracellular volume status.

Before assessing volume status, a good history should exclude pathologic water drinking (*psychogenic polydipsia*). This can also be identified by the appropriately dilute urine osmolality (<100 mosm/kg), unlike all other causes in which the urine is more concentrated.

The remaining causes of hyponatremia reflect hypoosmolality due to inadequate water excretion by the kidney. *Most* have higher ADH levels and urine osmolality than would be normal in the setting of low serum osmolality (most show urine osmolality

57

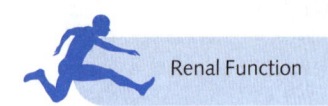

>200mosm/kg, sometimes much greater). The difference between them is the stimulus for ADH release. Evaluating the patient's *extracellular volume status* clinically provides the best clue to this. Measuring the urine [Na] is often helpful as well.

> The clinical extracellular volume status is the key to diagnosing hyponatremia.

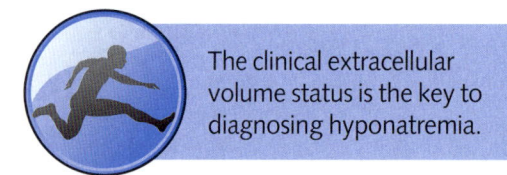

Hyponatremia with clinically increased ECF (hypervolemic hyponatremia)

Here effective circulating volume drops due to a drop in cardiac output or vasodilation (cirrhosis), stimulating ADH release.

- Hypervolemic hyponatremia presents with the usual signs of CHF, cirrhosis, etc., including sodium retention (with low urine Na).
- Patients have excess total body NaCl and water but have more water than NaCl.
- Serum [Na] usually does not drop below 120mEq/L.
- Treatment: treat underlying disease, restrict water intake to 1 liter per day.

Hyponatremia with decreased ECF (hypovolemic hyponatremia)

Here low ECF leads to low effective circulating volume and increased ADH release, overriding the effect of hypoosmolality to suppress ADH. This is due to the same causes of low ECF as discussed earlier (e.g., hemorrhage, GI loss, diuretics).

- Patients lack both NaCl and water but have more water than NaCl.
- Hypovolemic hyponatremia presents with the usual signs of extracellular volume loss (e.g., tachycardia, hypotension).
- Urine [Na] is usually <20mEq/L, due to avid renal Na retention. The exception to this will occur in ongoing diuretic use, where urine [Na] is often >20.
- Serum [Na] usually does not drop below 120mEq/L.
- Treatment: correct effective circulating volume with isotonic saline (0.9% normal saline).

Hyponatremia with clinically normal ECF

In general, these disorders are characterized by marked elevations in total body water, with mild, subclinical increases in ECF (i.e., the patient does not develop severe peripheral or pulmonary edema). Despite this mild ECF increase, the patient *appears* clinically to have a normal ECF.

- The total body sodium is near-normal, and urine Na > 20 reflects salt balance on a normal sodium diet (i.e., Na input = output).
- Serum [Na] can drop to symptomatic or even fatal levels (<110mEq/L).

Syndrome of inappropriate ADH (SIADH)
Ectopic ADH production leads to elevated ADH levels.
  Causes include:
- Oat cell carcinoma of the lung.
- Bronchogenic cancer.
- Granulomatous disease of lung (i.e., TB) and other pulmonary diseases.

Increased hypothalamic ADH release   Increased hypothalamic ADH release leads to elevated ADH levels.
  Causes include:
- Psychosis.
- Drugs: nicotine, morphine, oxytocin, chlorpropamide, carbamazepine, tolbutamide, antipsychotic medications.
- Hypothyroidism (severe only; ADH release occurs via decreased cardiac output and/or peripheral vasodilation).
- Glucocorticoid deficiency–two possible mechanisms:
  1. Decreased cardiac output or vasodilation.
  2. Low cortisol level disinhibits CRH. CRH stimulates ADH release.
- Postoperative: stress or anesthesia-mediated ADH release

Primary renal inability to excrete water   ADH levels are variable here. The problem is the kidney's inability to excrete a dilute urine despite low ADH levels.
- Chronic kidney disease: decreased GFR, with decreased water excretion (note: CKD can also present with *increased* extracellular volume).
- Thiazide diuretics: hyponatremia is usually seen in conjunction with poor intake of protein, increased intake of water, and/or decreases in GFR. The drugs inhibit the distal convoluted tubule Na transport, inhibiting urinary dilution; the minimum urinary osmolality may then be

150–200 mosm/kg rather than 50, limiting ability to excrete a water load.

Treatment
Acute hyponatremia
- Always treat the underlying problem (e.g., low T4, malignancy, thiazide).
- Hypotonic IV solutions are contraindicated (e.g., D_5 0.5 NS)
- If volume depleted clinically, give 0.9 normal saline)
- Water restriction (1 liter per day if possible).
- If symptoms are severe (seizures, coma, usually Na < 120 mEq/L) add:
  1. Hypertonic saline: raise the serum sodium by giving patient a fluid with higher osmolality than *urine* osmolality.
  2. Furosemide: lowers urine osmolality in SIADH and edematous states.
- Monitor serum sodium frequently (every 2–4 hours!).
- Aim for no more than 1 mEq/hr increase in serum Na, and back off when symptoms resolve, usually when [Na] > 120 mEq/L.
- Overcorrection can lead to *central pontine myelinolysis*, a potentially fatal CNS lesion.

Chronic hyponatremia
Treatments usually needed in SIADH:
- Water restriction.
- High-salt, high-protein diet—increases total body osmoles.
- Loop diuretic—reduces urine osmolality (see above).
- Demeclocycline—reduces urinary osmolality by blocking ADH receptors in collecting duct.

Clinical disorders of osmolality: hypernatremia
Hypernatremia results from a deficiency of water relative to solutes and almost always involves an absolute water deficit. Unlike hyponatremia, in which the kidneys' ability to excrete water is the only defense, hypernatremia is prevented by both the kidneys' generation of a concentrated urine and by the thirst mechanism.

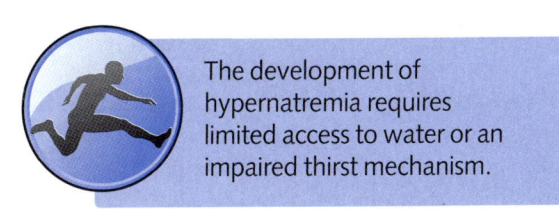

Symptoms/Signs
- Polydipsia;
- Polyuria (in diabetes insipidus only).
- Neurologic changes: lethargy, irritability and weakness, then seizures, coma, death.
- Death in 60–75% of cases if [Na] > 160 mEq/L.

Etiology
Hypernatremia is virtually always caused by lack of water intake, usually in association with one of the following:
1. Increased water loss:
   - Insensible loss (sweating, fever, exercise)—most common cause.
   - Renal loss (central diabetes insipidus [DI], nephrogenic DI).
   - GI loss (osmotic diarrhea).
2. Excessive sodium ingestion (rare):
   - Infants given salt instead of sugar by error in their feeding formulas.
   - Hypertonic saline or sodium bicarbonate.

Excess renal water loss: diabetes insipidus (DI)
DI is due to the lack of ADH or unresponsiveness to ADH. It is classified as either central or nephrogenic.
A. Central DI: decrease in ADH secretion by hypothalamus; this corrects with administration of ADH. Causes include:
   - Idiopathic (most common, 50% of cases).
   - Post-intracranial surgery.
   - Head trauma.
   - Intracranial malignancy (primary or metastatic).
   - Autoimmune disorders.
   - Drugs (caffeine, ethanol): short-acting.
2. Nephrogenic DI: decrease in kidney response to ADH. Causes include:

A. Interference with the ADH-receptor interaction in the collecting duct:
   - Drugs (lithium, demeclocycline)—lithium is the most common cause of DI overall.
   - Interstitial disease: polycystic kidneys, pyelonephritis.
   - Hypercalcemia.
   - Hypokalemia.
   - Congenital ADH receptor defects.
   - Amyloidosis.

> The development of hypernatremia requires limited access to water or an impaired thirst mechanism.

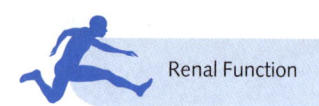

B. Interference with countercurrent multiplier mechanism, with reduced medullary interstitial osmolality:
- Renal failure.
- Hypercalcemia.
- Hypokalemia.
- Sickle cell anemia (sickling in the vasa recta vessels that supply Henle's loop cause ischemic damage to the loop and loss of transport function).
- Prolonged diuresis from other causes (washes out concentrating gradient).
- Protein malnutrition (decreases urea in interstitium)

Evaluation of hypernatremia
1. A good physical exam, especially assessing extracellular volume status.
2. Urine chemistry.
   - Urine osm <150 mosm/kg = **renal water loss**; patients with diabetes insipidus (central or nephrogenic) are generally volume-depleted and have urine sodium <20 mEq/L; central DI corrects with dosed ADH (vasopressin).
   - Urine osm >300 mosm/kg with Na <10 mEq/L = **nonrenal water loss** (sweat, GI loss, osmotic diuresis); these patients usually have signs of extracellular volume depletion (e.g., orthostatic hypotension).
   - Urine osm >300 mosm/kg with Na >20 mEq/L = **osmotic diuresis**, due to hyperglycemia, mannitol, etc.

Treatment of hypernatremia
First, always treat the underlying problem (e.g., stop lithium, correct hypokalemia, remove pituitary mass). Then in all patients:
- First correct any effective circulating volume deficit, using 0.9% normal saline.
- Then give water—orally, by nasogastric tube, or as D_5W IV. The amount may be calculated by determining the free water deficit:

$$\text{Free water deficit} = 0.6\,[\text{body weight (kg)}] \times \left(\frac{[Na]_s}{140} - 1\right)$$

where $[Na]_s$ = the patient's current Na serum level

Note: In a 70-kg person, a sodium serum level of 150 represents a water deficit of 3 liters.

- In symptomatic patients, replace water deficit at no more than 1 mEq/L/hr. until symptoms resolve, then the rest over 24–48 hours—too rapid a correction may cause *cerebral edema*. The more chronic the hypernatremia, the slower you should go.
- Concurrently, reduce renal water excretion:
  ○ For central DI, give ADH in the form of desamino-8-D-arginine (ddAVP) nasal spray or other vasopressin formulation.
  ○ For nephrogenic DI, consider:
    i Thiazide diuretics: decrease urine osmolality and urine volume (remember: they are a *cause* of the "opposite" clinical condition, hyponatremia).
    ii ↓ Protein and sodium intake → ↓ renal solute load and urea delivery to kidney → ↓ obligatory water excretion.
    iii Prostaglandins inhibitors may reduce urine water loss by unknown mechanisms.

Regulation and clinical disorders of body fluid pH

Body fluid pH is tightly controlled because most enzyme reactions are sensitive to pH changes.
- Normal pH range is 7.35–7.45.
- Normal serum H^+ concentration is 35–45 nmol/L.

Basic principles
Buffers
A buffer is a mixture of a weak acid (HA) and a conjugate base. It undergoes minimal pH change when either an acid or a base is added to it:

$$HA \leftrightarrow H^+ \text{ (acid)} + A^- \text{ (conjugate base)}$$

It can also be a mixture of a weak base (BH) and conjugate acid:

$$BH \leftrightarrow H^+ \text{ (conjugate acid)} + B^- \text{ (base)}$$

For example, if there is an increase in H^+, the equations above shift to the left so that the extra H^+ combines with the buffer and the H^+ concentration in the body falls.

The kidneys act together with the lungs and buffer systems to minimize any changes in plasma [H].

pK values and equilibrium constants
The equations below demonstrate the equilibrium constants in terms of conjugate acids and bases, proton donators, and acceptors.

Regulation and clinical disorders of body fluid pH

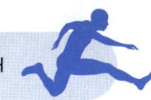

$$HA \leftrightarrow H^+ + A^-$$

Equation 1. At equilibrium:

$$K = \frac{[H^+][A^-]}{[HA]}$$

$$\therefore [H^+] = \frac{K[HA]}{[A^-]}$$

Equation 2:

$$pH = -\log[H^+]$$
$$= \log(1/[H^+])$$

$$pK = -\log K$$
$$= \log(1/K)$$

Combining equations 1 and 2 gives the Henderson-Hasselbach equation:

$$pH = pK + \log\frac{[HA]}{[A^-]}$$

Physiologic buffers

There are several buffer systems in the different body compartments (Fig. 3.26), of which the most important is the bicarbonate buffer system.

Bicarbonate buffer system

The bicarbonate buffer system is important in all body fluids. Carbon dioxide (CO_2) and water (H_2O) are combined to form carbonic acid (H_2CO_3) by the enzyme carbonic anhydrase (CA). The H_2CO_3 dissociates spontaneously to form bicarbonate ions (HCO_3^-) and H^+. This is summarized in the equation below:

$$CO_2 + H_2O \xrightarrow{\text{Carbonic anhydrase}} H_2CO_3 \leftrightarrow H^+ + HCO_3^-$$

CO_2 concentration is regulated by the lungs and HCO_3^- concentration is regulated by the kidneys. Therefore, pH regulation depends equally on both these organs. Substituting this equation in the Henderson–Hasselbach equation, we get:

$$pH = pK + \log[HCO_3^-]/[H_2CO_3]$$

$[H_2CO_3]$ is determined by dissolved CO_2: $[H_2CO_3]$ = $0.23 \times pCO_2$ (0.23 is the CO_2 solubility coefficient at 37°C; pCO_2 is the pressure of CO_2 in the lungs). Therefore,

$$pH = pK + \log\frac{[HCO_3^-]}{0.3 \times pCO_2}$$

Normal values are:
- $[HCO_3^-]$: 20–30 mmol/L.
- pCO_2: 36–44 mmHg.
- pK of HCO_3^-/pCO_2 system: 6.1.

Therefore, pH = 7.4.

In summary: $pH \propto \dfrac{HCO_3^-}{pCO_2}$

Renal regulation of acid-base status

H^+ is produced during metabolism, and significant amounts are produced from catabolism of protein ingested in a normal diet. Cellular metabolism stimulates CO_2 production:

$$H^+ + HCO_3^- \leftrightarrow H_2CO_3 \leftrightarrow H_2O + CO_2$$

The CO_2 is exhaled by the lungs. The kidneys retain HCO_3^- and make more HCO_3^-.

The kidney has two major functions in acid-base physiology:
- It reabsorbs filtered bicarbonate buffer so it can continue to participate in serum buffering.
- It excretes the excess acid produced from dietary protein and cellular metabolism, generating one HCO_3^- for each proton excreted.

Buffer systems in different body compartments			
Buffer systems	**Blood**	**ECF and CSF**	**ICF**
HCO_3^-/CO_2	X	X	X
hemoglobin	X		
plasma proteins	X		
phosphate	X	X	X
organic phosphate			X
proteins		X	X

Fig. 3.26 Buffer systems in different body compartments. CSF, cerebrospinal fluid; ECF, extracellular fluid; ICF, intracellular fluid.

The kidney reclaims filtered bicarbonate and excretes excess acid generated from diet and metabolism.

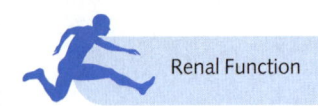

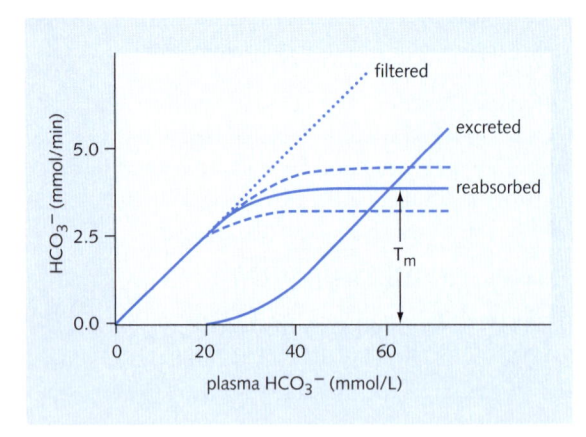

Fig. 3.27 How HCO_3^- ions are handled by the kidney. HCO_3^- absorption is dependent on H^+ secretion into the tubule. This dependency causes the T_m for HCO_3^- absorption to vary. The limits of the T_m variability are illustrated by the dotted lines on the graph above.

Renal HCO_3^- reabsorption

The concentration of HCO_3^- in the plasma filtered by the kidney is 24 mmol/L. Ninety percent of HCO_3^- is absorbed in the proximal tubule. HCO_3^- is reabsorbed by the kidney using a T_m-dependent mechanism (Fig. 3.27). The T_m is similar to the amount of HCO_3^- filtered at a normal plasma concentration. If plasma HCO_3^- increases, T_m is exceeded and HCO_3^- is excreted until the plasma level returns to normal.

Mechanism of HCO_3^- reabsorption (Fig. 3.28)

Na^+ reabsorption on the apical membrane drives H^+ secretion by the tubular cells (antiport). The secreted H^+ combines with filtered HCO_3^- ions to form H_2CO_3 (carbonic acid). Carbonic anhydrase on the brush border of the cells catalyses the dissociation of H_2CO_3 to H_2O + CO_2 within the tubular lumen. Both H_2O and CO_2 diffuse freely into the cell, where they reform H_2CO_3, this process being catalyzed by intracellular carbonic anhydrase. H_2CO_3 again dissociates into:
- H^+, which is secreted into the lumen.
- HCO_3^-, which enters the plasma via the peritubular fluid.

HCO_3^- and Na^+ are actively transported out of the cell across the basolateral membrane. H^+ is secreted out of the cell into the tubular lumen and recycled to allow continuation of this cycle.

The net result is reclamation of the filtered bicarbonate. However, no new bicarbonate is generated, so this process cannot excrete extra acid generated by diet or metabolism (see Fig. 3.28 for summary of this process). This process is stimulated by both systemic acidemia and increased systemic pCO2. Carbonic anhydrase inhibitors (e.g., acetazolamide) block this pathway for HCO_3^- reabsorption, leading to a bicarbonate diuresis (with accompanying sodium), and thus act as weak diuretics.

Renal acid excretion

The protons that are secreted in the tubules cannot be effectively excreted as free protons, since the minimum urine pH is 4.5, limiting proton solubility. Therefore, *net acid excretion* relies on the presence of luminal buffers to buffer the secreted protons.

The kidney excretes excess acid (and generates bicarbonate) via two pathways, titratable acid and ammoniagenesis.

Titratable acid

This is an noninducible process using filtered serum buffers, mainly phosphate and sulfate. Alkaline phosphate Na_2HPO_4 and acid phosphate NaH_2PO_4 are present in the plasma in the ratio of 4:1. Both are filtered at the glomerulus. Alkaline phosphate traps a secreted proton and is converted to acid phosphate, mainly in the distal tubule but also in the proximal tubule (Fig. 3.29). This allows the secreted proton to be excreted in the urine. The process also generates HCO_3^- for the plasma. A similar process exists for sulfates. Because the phosphate buffers appear in the urine via passive glomerular filtration, there is an upper limit on the ability of the kidney to generate titratable acid, and it may not be able to fully buffer a large acid load solely with this mechanism.

Ammonia secretion

This is the main inducible means of net acid excretion. Deamination of glutamine in the proximal tubule produces urinary ammonium ions (NH_4^+) and generates bicarbonate for the serum, helping to excrete an acid load (Fig. 3.30). Although the liver can metabolize NH_4^+ to urea, it is only by secretion of NH_4^+ in the kidney that HCO_3^- can be regenerated to act as a buffer in the plasma. The ammonium ions are reabsorbed in the thick ascending limb of Henle's loop and eventually reappear as NH_3 in the cortical collecting duct, now

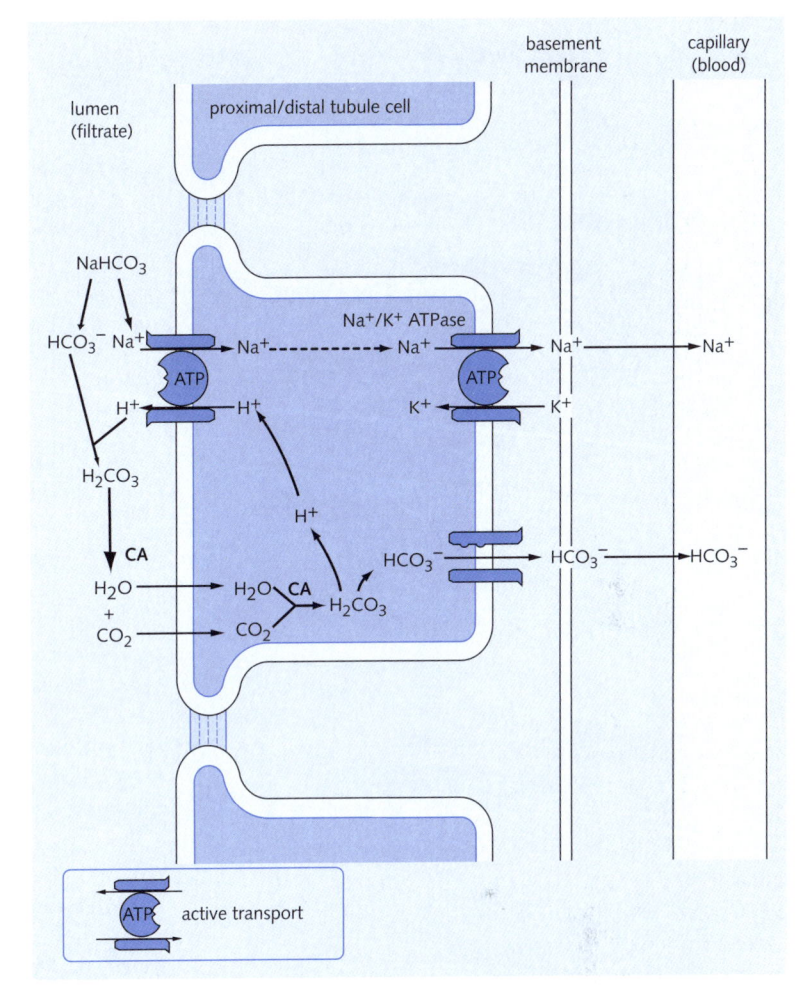

Fig. 3.28 HCO_3^- reabsorption in the proximal tubule cells. Secreted H^+ combines with HCO_3^- to form carbonic acid. This is broken down by carbonic anhydrase (CA) in the brush border to CO_2 and H_2O, which diffuse freely into the cell. The process is reversed inside the cell to re-form HCO_3^-.

available to buffer secreted protons. Figure 3.30 illustrates the secretion of ammonia (NH_3) and Fig. 3.31 shows NH_4^+ handling by the nephrons.

Acidosis and hypokalemia increase NH_4^+ excretion (and net acid excretion) because they stimulate enzymes that deaminate glutamine, thereby increasing NH_4^+ synthesis by the proximal tubule. Hyperkalemia inhibits the same enzymes, limiting ammoniagenesis. Clinically, a hyperkalemic (type IV) renal tubular acidosis results when chronic hyperkalemia inhibits proximal tubule ammoniagenesis, limiting the ability of the kidney to excrete an acid load.

> Titratable acid and ammonium secretion allow excretion of an acid load.

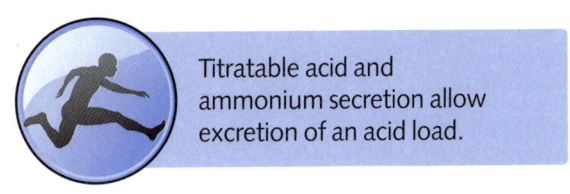

Acid–base disturbances

There are four types of disorders, which can exist singly or with other disorders:
1. Respiratory acidosis.
2. Respiratory alkalosis.
3. Metabolic acidosis.
4. Metabolic alkalosis.

Metabolic disturbances result from changes in cellular metabolism or diet, leading to a gain or loss of H^+. In contrast, respiratory disturbances arise from changes in ventilation, ledding to a gain or loss of CO_2. If the body fluid pH alters, the buffering system mechanism is activated. Thus, overall, there might be very little change in arterial pH despite acid–base imbalance. A change in the arterial pH results in a change in the pH of body cells, which adversely affects many cellular processes.

Renal Function

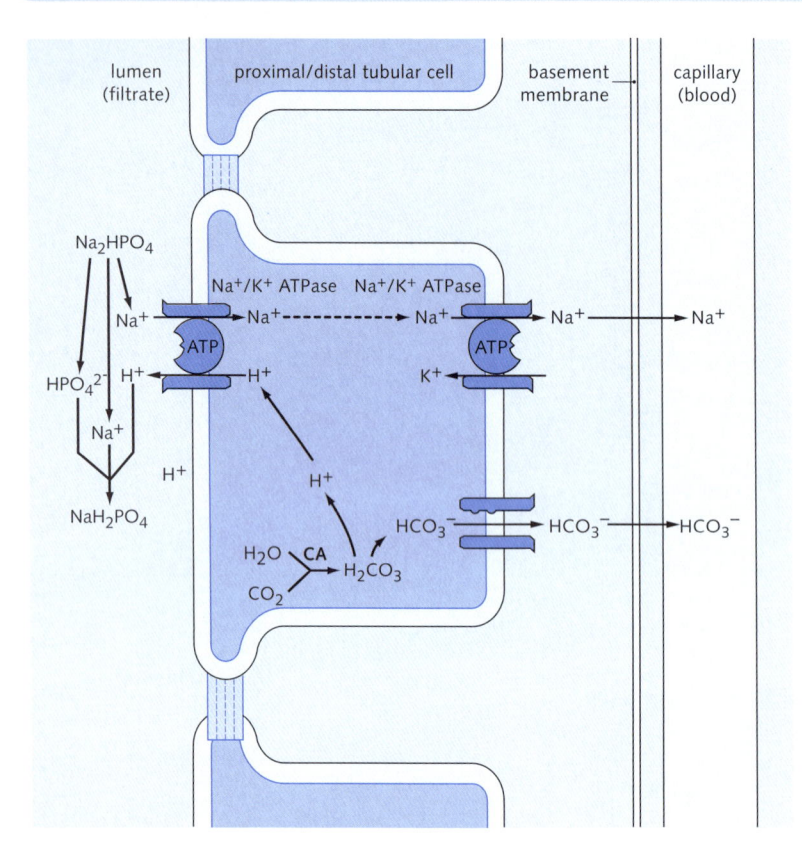

Fig. 3.29 Conversion of alkaline phosphate to acid phosphate in the tubule lumen. Sodium is transported into the tubule cell by an Na^+/H^+ antiporter, causing H^+ secretion into the lumen and the generation of a bicarbonate by the tubule cells. CA, carbonic anhydrase.

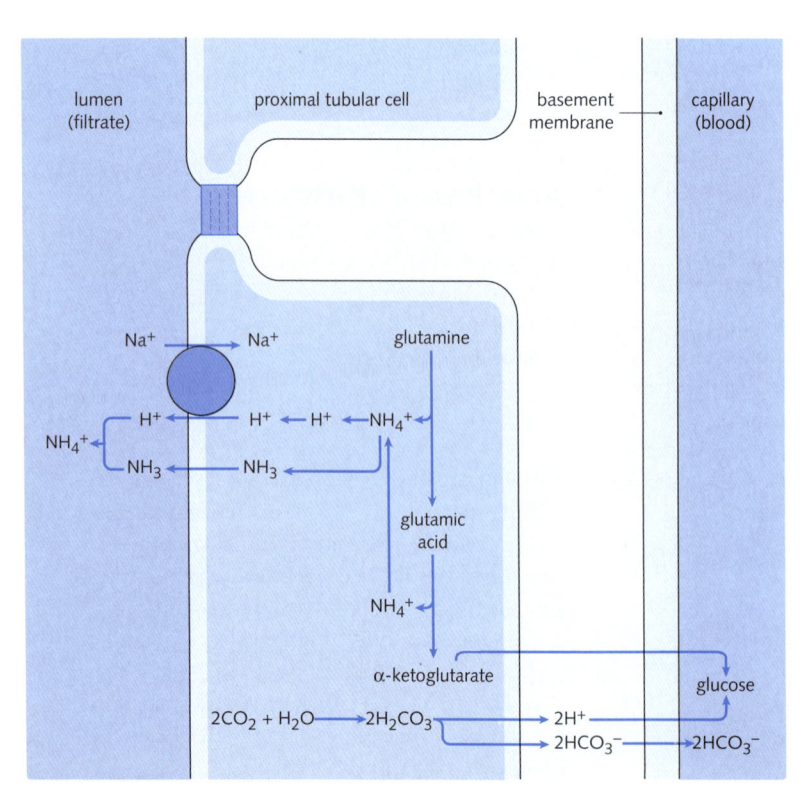

Fig. 3.30 Renal secretion and handling of NH_3.

Fig. 3.31 Handling of NH_3 and NH_4^+ by nephrons.

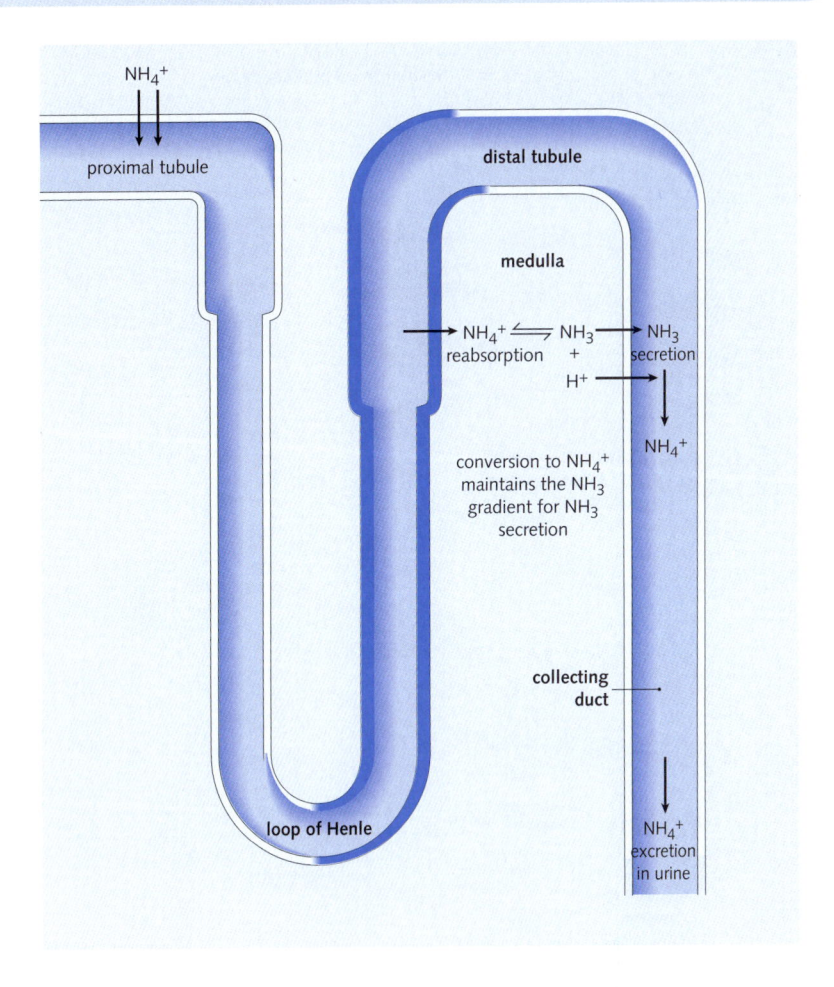

Compensation for acid-base abnormalities

Compensation is the normalization (but not complete correction) of systemic pH even when an acid–base imbalance is still present.
- The kidney compensates for respiratory abnormalities by retaining or excreting bicarbonate.
- The lungs compensate for metabolic abnormalities by hyper- or hypoventilating, changing the pCO_2.

Identifying acid-base abnormalities

Arterial blood gases (ABGs) measure the pH, pO_2, and pCO_2 in an arterial blood sample. An arterial blood gas is required to correctly identify acid base abnormalities. The ABG pattern seen in each disturbance is shown in Fig. 3.32.

Routinely follow three steps to identify acid base disorders:
1. Identify the primary disorder (Figure 3.32).
2. Determine whether compensation is appropriate (Figure 3.33) and if not, identify the additional acid base disorder.
3. Calculate the anion gap. If elevated, the patient has an elevated anion gap metabolic acidosis.

Examine Fig. 3.33. The shaded area of the nomogram shows the normal physiologic compensations for each of the acid base disorders.

Classification of acid-base disturbances by ABG pattern			
Disturbance	pH	pCO_2	HCO_3
metabolic acidosis	↓	↓	↓
metabolic alkalosis	↑	↑	↑
respiratory acidosis	↓	↑	↑
respiratory alkalosis	↑	↓	↓

Fig. 3.32 Classification of acid-base disturbances by ABG pattern.

Renal Function

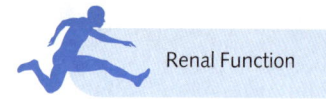

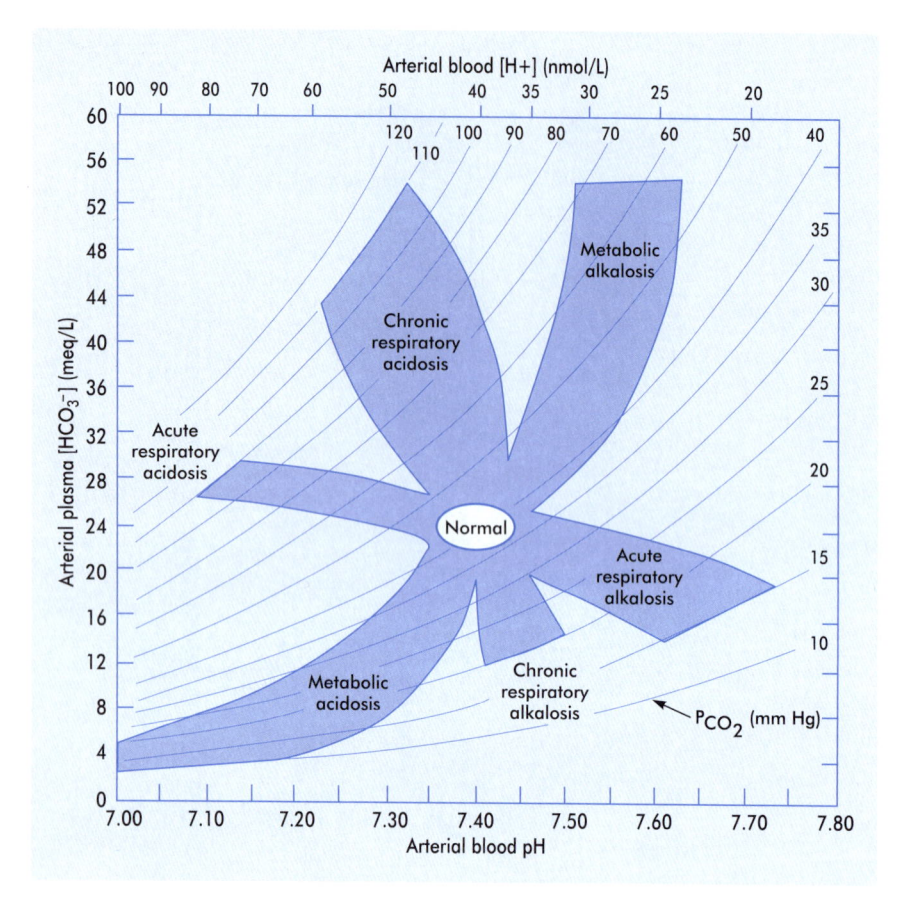

Fig. 3.33 Acid and base disturbances with compensatory changes demonstrated on the acid-base nomogram.

Note that if any two variables (e.g., pH and pCO$_2$) are known, the third [HCO$_3^-$] can be calculated and that any two variables can identify the acid base abnormality. For example, if pH = 7.30 and pCO$_2$ is 25 mmHg, by looking at Fig. 3.33 it can be seen that [HCO$_3^-$] will be reduced to 12 mEq/L and that the disturbance is a compensated metabolic acidosis. The normal compensations for the primary disorders are based on experimental data. If the patient's blood gases show a pattern outside the shaded regions, then the disturbance is not a compensated single disorder, and a multiple acid base disorder is present. For example, a patient with a pH 7.20, pCO$_2$ 40, and HCO$_3^-$ 14 has a metabolic acidosis and respiratory acidosis.

Examples of acid–base disturbances
Respiratory acidosis

The causes of respiratory acidosis are:
- Chronic bronchitis.
- Emphysema.
- Obstruction of the airway (e.g., tumor, foreign body).
- Mechanical chest injuries.
- Severe asthma.
- Drugs: general anesthetic, morphine, barbiturates (respiratory center depressant).
- Injuries and infections to the respiratory center in the brainstem.

ABG results show pCO$_2$ > 45 mmHg and decreased pH. Clinically, the respiratory system cannot remove enough CO$_2$, so CO$_2$ increases together with pCO$_2$. Therefore, the following equation is shifted to the right:

$$CO_2 + H_2O \leftrightarrow H_2CO_3 \leftrightarrow H^+ + HCO_3^-$$

This results in elevated [H$^+$] and [HCO$_3^-$]. The reduced serum pH and increased pCO$_2$ lead to increased proximal H$^+$ secretion and increased HCO$_3^-$ reabsorption (renal compensation for respiratory acidosis). This restores pH, acting as a compensatory response. In general, compensations do not return the pH to 7.40, but do moderate the problem.

Respiratory alkalosis
The causes of respiratory alkalosis are:
- Hypoxia, detected by chemoreceptors in the carotid body, resulting in hyperventilation and decreased pCO_2.
- High altitude.
- Fever.
- Brainstem damage resulting in hyperventilation.
- Anxiety with hyperventilation.

The ABG results show a $pCO_2 < 36\,mmHg$ and an elevated pH. Clinically, too much CO_2 is removed by the respiratory system. Therefore the following equation is shifted to the left:

$$CO_2 + H_2O \leftrightarrow H_2CO_3 \leftrightarrow H^+ + HCO_3^-$$

This causes $[H^+]$ to fall and leads to an increased pH and a slight decrease in $[HCO_3^-]$. The compensatory renal response involves reduced H^+ secretion, increased HCO_3^- excretion, and decreased HCO_3^- reabsorption, thus restoring pH. Correction requires rectification of the underlying respiratory defect.

Metabolic acidosis
The causes of metabolic acidosis are:
- Ingestion of acids (H^+).
- Excess metabolic production of H^+ (e.g. lactate acidosis, diabetic ketoacidosis).
- Extrarenal loss of HCO_3^- (e.g. severe diarrhea, drainage from fistulae).
- Renal disease (renal tubular acidosis = failure to excrete H^+).

There is an increase in $[H^+]$. Therefore, the following equation is shifted to the left:

$$CO_2 + H_2O \leftrightarrow H_2CO_3 \leftrightarrow H^+ + HCO_3^-$$

Consequently, $[HCO_3^-]$ falls to under $23\,mEq/L$ as it is used to "mop up" the excess H^+ ions. The decreased pH stimulates respiration to cause hyperventilation. This respiratory compensation decreases pCO_2 and returns the pH towards normal. For this compensation, the $\Delta pCO_2 = 1.2 \pm 0.2 \times \Delta HCO_3^-$ The low serum HCO_3^- leads to low filtered load of bicarbonate, which hinders the normal response of the kidneys to acidemia, which would be to increase HCO_3^- reabsorption.

Anion gap vs. non-anion gap metabolic acidosis
The *anion gap* represents the net difference between plasma anions and cations not measured on the normal electrolyte panel.

Serum anion gap = $[Na^+] - [Cl^-] - [HCO_3^-]$

The normal value is $8 \pm 3\,mEq/L$ (a recent change in the normal value, based on changed autoanalyzer chloride determination). The excess of anions represents largely anionic albumin, phosphates, and sulfates. Since metabolic acidosis may be associated with an elevated anion gap, it should be calculated on all patients with acid base abnormalities.

Elevations in the anion gap help define the cause of a metabolic acidosis, and elevations above 15–16 mEq/L are usually clinically significant. For example, when an excess of an exogenous (aspirin) or endogenous acid (e.g., ketones) is present, the anion gap is elevated and the pH falls.

Elevations can be due to retained endogenous acids (lactic, ketoacids, renal failure) or ingestions (ethylene glycol [metabolized to oxalate], methanol [formate], and aspirin [both the drug itself and secondary lactic acidosis]).

> The causes of elevated gap are remembered as **MUDPALES**: **M**ethanol, **U**remia, **D**KA, **P**araldehyde, **A**lcoholic ketoacidosis, **L**actic, **E**thylene glycol, **S**alicylates.

In uremia (renal failure) the anion gap is raised due to failure to filter titratable acid, increasing the serum phosphates and sulfates and preventing buffering of secreted acids in the collecting duct.

In contrast to the above situations, metabolic acidosis due to diarrhea or renal tubular acidosis does not alter the anion gap (a *nongap* metabolic acidosis). In diarrhea, bicarbonate is lost in the stool, lowering serum pH. In the renal tubular acidoses, various tubular abnormalities lead to either an inability to excrete an acid load or a loss of filtered bicarbonate. Figure 3.34 characterizes the renal tubular acidoses. The hyperkalemic (type IV) RTA is the most common and is commonly seen in diabetic patients, often due to hyporeninemic hypoaldosteronism from a failure of renin secretion by the juxtaglomerular apparatus.

Metabolic alkalosis
In this disorder the pH is elevated and the serum bicarbonate is $>28\,mEq/L$, due to loss of acid or gain of bicarbonate.

In all these situations there is a rise in plasma $[HCO_3^-]$. Respiratory compensation occurs via

Renal Function

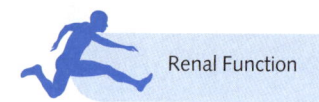

Types of renal tubular acidosis			
Type	Mechanism	Causes	Diagnostic clues
I (distal)	failure of type A intercalated cell H+ secretion	interstitial renal disease, obstruction, amphotericin, Sjögren's syndrome	urine pH > 5.5 renal stones
II (proximal)	proximal tubule dysfunction with inability to reabsorb HCO_3^-	Fanconi syndrome, multiple myeloma, acetazolamide	elevated urine bicarbonate hypokalemia glucosuria
IV (hyperkalemic)	hyperkalemia suppresses proximal ammoniagenesis and net acid excretion	diabetes mellitus (hyporeninemic hypoaldosteronism), interstitial disease (tubular resistance to aldosterone), primary hypoaldosteronism	hyperkalemia

Fig. 3.34 Types of renal tubular acidosis.

hypoventilation and increased pCO_2. For this compensation, $\Delta pCO_2 = 0.7 \pm 0.2 \times \Delta HCO_3^-$. The increase in pH acts on chemoreceptors, which reduce the ventilatory rate and so increase pCO_2. pH returns towards normal. The kidney cannot excrete the excess bicarbonate because of proximal reabsorption driven by volume depletion that is common with this abnormality (esp. in diuretics, vomiting). The causes of metabolic alkalosis can be classified as saline responsive or non-saline responsive.

The saline responsive metabolic alkaloses (most common) are:
- Vomiting (loss of HCl).
- Diuretics (renin-AT-aldosterone mediated H+ losses).
- "Contraction alkalosis" from depleted extracellular volume (e.g., hemorrhage, burns). This stimulates renal bicarbonate reabsorption because of its linkage to sodium reabsorption.

The most helpful diagnostic test is the urine chloride, which is low (<25mEq/L) in saline responsive alkaloses. A caveat is that ongoing diuretic use will keep the urine Cl (and Na and K) high, due to continued inhibition of reabsorption of NaCl.

Saline unresponsive alkaloses include: ingestion of alkali (e.g., antacid ingestion), hyperaldosteronism (increases distal H+ secretion), and other mineralocorticoid excess states. It is also seen when a severe respiratory acidosis drives renal bicarbonate reabsorption. If the respiratory problem quickly resolves (for example, by tracheal intubation), the patient is left with a markedly elevated serum bicarbonate and alkalemia. All these disorders usually lead to an elevated urine chloride (>40 mEq/L), distinguishing them from the disorders listed above.

Metabolic alkalosis is commonly associated with hypokalemia due to:
- Shifting of K+ to the intracellular space.
- Urinary K+ losses due to diuretics.
- Urinary K+ losses seen with the bicarbonate diuresis early in vomiting.
- Urinary K+ losses driven by renin-AT-aldosterone in the setting of volume depletion.

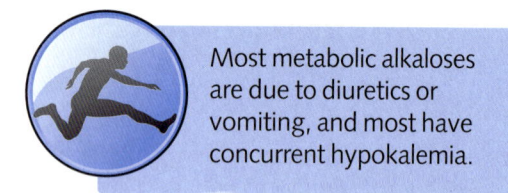

> Most metabolic alkaloses are due to diuretics or vomiting, and most have concurrent hypokalemia.

Potassium: regulation and clinical disorders

Introduction
K+ is the main intracellular cation. The intracellular and extracellular [K+] is very important in the function of excitable tissues (e.g. nerves and muscles) as it determines the resting potentials of cell membranes. Therefore, a constant [K+] is critical for survival. Concentration is as follows:
- Intracellular fluid (ICF) K+: 98%; 150–160mEq/L.

Fig. 3.35 Potassium transport in the kidney.

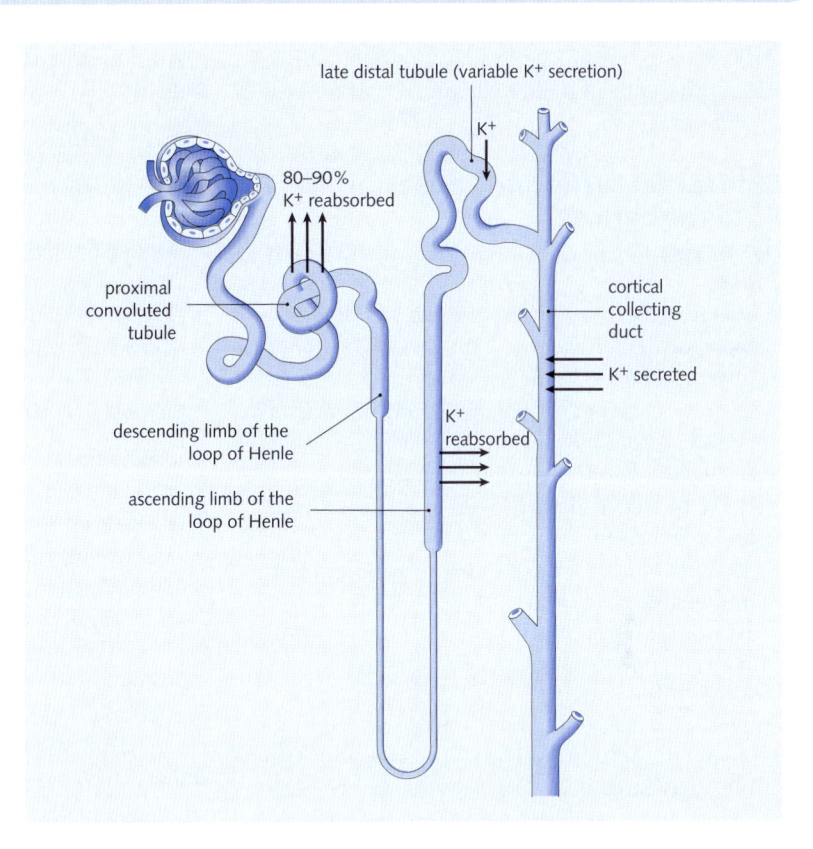

Diagram labels: late distal tubule (variable K⁺ secretion); 80–90% K⁺ reabsorbed; proximal convoluted tubule; descending limb of the loop of Henle; ascending limb of the loop of Henle; cortical collecting duct; K⁺ secreted; K⁺ reabsorbed.

- Extracellular fluid (ECF) K⁺: 2%; 4–5 mEq/L.
- If extracellular [K⁺] rises, the resting membrane potential is increased (less negative), bringing it closer to the threshold potential (i.e., depolarizing the membrane). Cardiac membranes become excitable, leading to dysrhythmias.
- If extracellular [K⁺] falls, the resting membrane potential is decreased (i.e., hyperpolarized).

Extracellular—intracellular shifting of K⁺

The high intracellular K⁺ concentration is maintained by the Na⁺ K⁺ ATPase, found on virtually all cells. Several factors can induce K⁺ to shift into cells by stimulating the ATPase, lowering serum K⁺ concentration:

- Beta adrenergic stimulation.
- Alkalemia.
- Insulin.

Conversely, these factors can shift K⁺ out of cells, causing hyperkalemia:

- Alpha adrenergic stimulation.
- Acidemia.
- Hyperglycemia (via solvent drag or water shifts).

K⁺ handling by the kidney

K⁺ is filtered freely in the glomerulus. The proximal tubule reabsorbs 80–90%. In the distal tubule the collecting ducts secrete K⁺ into the urinary filtrate (passively via an electrochemical gradient) according to the body's needs. Increased principal cell intracellular K⁺ concentration or increased K⁺ channels result in increased tubular secretion. This secretion is increased by:

- Aldosterone.
- Increased urine flow (such as with diuretics).
- Increased luminal negative charge (nonreabsorbable anions, such as some penicillins).

Figure 3.35 illustrates K⁺ transport in the kidney.

Increased plasma K⁺ concentration and angiotensin II stimulate aldosterone production by the adrenal cortex, so plasma aldosterone concentration rises. This in turn increases K⁺ secretion and therefore K⁺ excretion. Aldosterone increases K⁺ collecting duct secretion by increasing the activity of the basolateral Na⁺ K⁺ ATPase and by increasing insertion of potassium and sodium channels in the luminal membrane. These factors increase intracellular K^+ concentration and increase the positive voltage gradient driving K^+ out of the cell and into the urine.

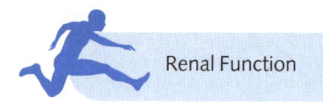

Clinical features and causes of K^+ disturbances

Hypokalemia
Causes
- Vomiting: K^+ is lost in the urine as part of a bicarbonate diuresis.
- Diarrhea: K^+ lost in the stool.
- Diuretics (except potassium-sparing diuretics like spironolactone): K^+ lost in the urine.
- Excess insulin: K^+ shifts intracellularly.
- Renal tubular acidosis (proximal and distal): K^+ lost in the urine.
- Metabolic alkalosis: K^+ lost in the urine and shifts intracellularly.
- Hyperaldosteronism.

Consequences
Hypokalemia is asymptomatic until K^+ concentration falls below 2–2.5 meq/L. The low K^+ concentration results in a decreased resting potential (more negative) so the nerve and muscle cells become hyperpolarized. This means that cells are less sensitive to depolarizing stimuli and therefore less excitable, so fewer action potentials are generated and paralysis ensues.

Clinical effects of hypokalemia are:
- Muscle weakness, cramps and tetany, which starts in the lower extremities and progresses upward (death is usually by paralysis of respiratory muscles).
- Cardiac arrhythmias.
- Impaired ADH action, causing thirst and polyuria and inability to concentrate the urine.
- Metabolic alkalosis due to an increase in intracellular H^+ concentration.

Treatment
Treatment involves treating the underlying cause and administration of oral or intravenous administration of potassium salts.

Figure 3.36 shows the diagnostic approach to hypokalemia.

Hyperkalemia
Causes
- Renal failure (usu. GFR <20 mL/min).
- Drugs that limit K excretion: ACE inhibitors, angiotensin receptor blockers, spironolactone.
- Ingestion of K^+.
- Metabolic acidosis (diabetes mellitus).
- Type 4 RTA.
- Insulin deficiency, hyperglycemia.
- Excess cell breakdown (e.g., tumor lysis after cytotoxic cancer therapy).
- Hypoaldosteronism.

Consequences
Hyperkalemia is asymptomatic until $K^+ > 6.5$ mEq/L. The increased K^+ concentration results in cell depolarization and increased excitability. The resting potential might be above the threshold potential, so cells cannot repolarize after an action potential, leading to paralysis. Death results from cardiac arrest due to the effects of hyperkalemia on cardiac conduction. The EKG initially shows peaked T waves, then prolonged PR and QT intervals. Fatal arrhythmias can occur when $K^+ > 7$ mEq/L.

Treatment
Treatment involves:
- Calcium salts to raise the activation potential and protect excitable tissues (of heart) against toxic effects of K^+.
- Dextrose and insulin to drive K^+ into cells.
- HCO_3^- to correct acidosis by stimulating K^+ entry into cells.
- Beta agonists to drive K^+ into cells.
- K^+ removal from body using loop diuretics, gut exchange resins (e.g., Kayexalate), and dialysis.

Figure 3.37 shows the diagnostic approach to hyperkalemia.

> Hyperkalemia with EKG changes is a medical emergency and requires urgent treatment to stabilize the cardiac membranes, shift K^+ into cells, and remove K^+ from the body.

Calcium, phosphate, and magnesium: regulation and clinical disorders

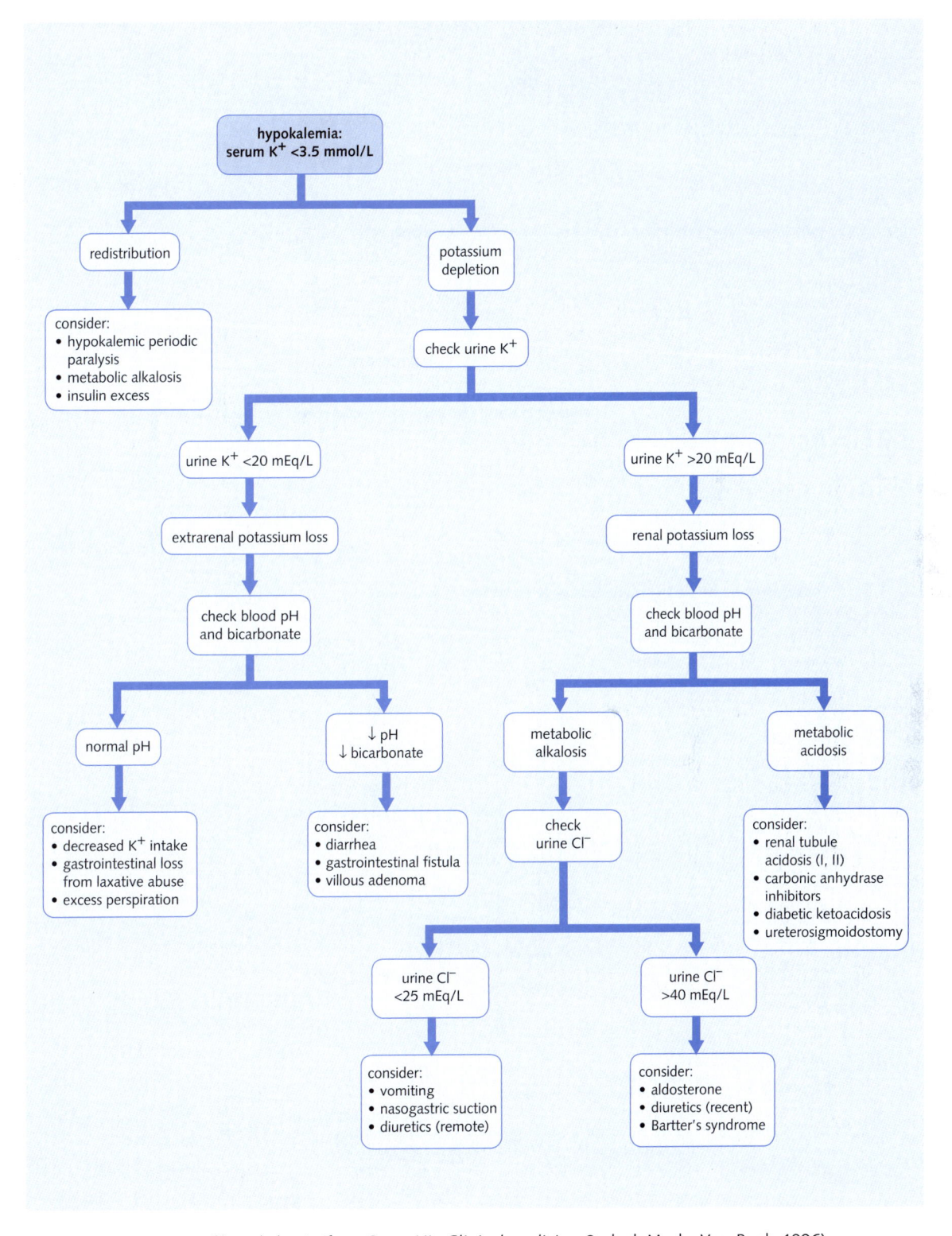

Fig. 3.36 Investigation of hypokalemia (from Green HL: *Clinical medicine*, 2nd ed. Mosby Year Book, 1996).

Renal Function

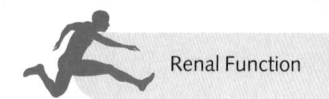

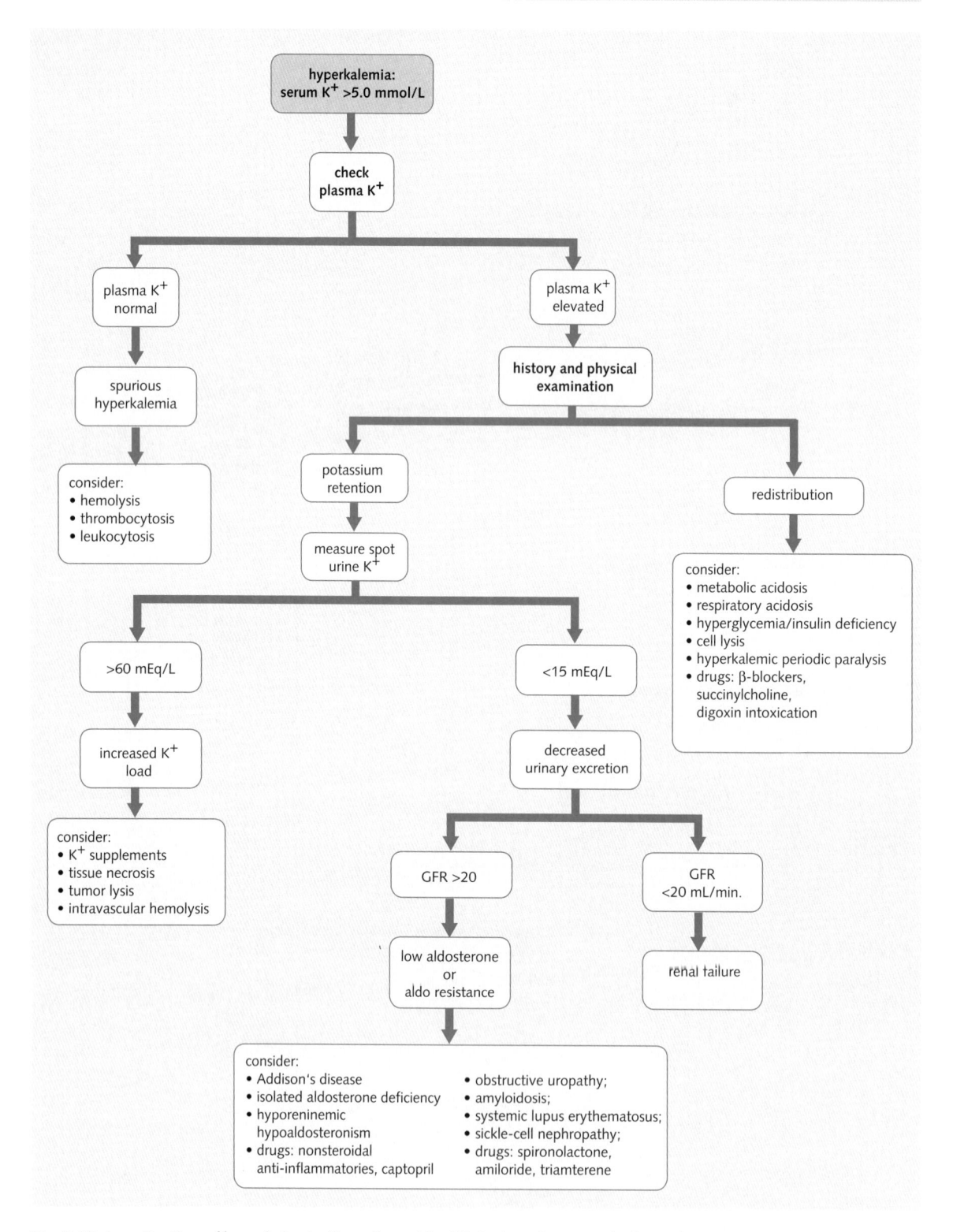

Fig. 3.37 Investigation of hyperkalemia (from Green HL: *Clinical medicine*, 2nd ed. Mosby Year Book, 1996).

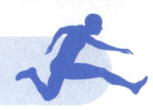

Calcium, phosphate, and magnesium: regulation and clinical disorders

Calcium (Ca^{2+})

Ca^{2+} is present mainly in bone but has an important extraskeletal function. The threshold potential of cell membranes of nerve and muscle for action potentials varies inversely with plasma calcium concentration. Thus it is important to keep calcium levels constant.

Calcium exists in two forms in the plasma, each with about half the total calcium (normal total serum calcium is 9–10.5mg/dl):
1. Ionized Ca^{2+}, which is physiologically more important (normal concentration: 1–1.25 mmol/L).
2. Ca^{2+} bound to protein—mainly albumin.

Calcium and phosphate homeostasis

Ca^{2+} and PO_4^{3-} concentrations are inversely proportional.

$$[Ca^{2+}] \times [PO_4^{3-}] = constant$$

Therefore, a rise in Ca^{2+} leads to a decrease in PO_4^{3-}, whereas a fall in Ca^{2+} stimulates an increase in PO_4^{3-} concentration, and vice versa.

Ca^{2+} and PO_4^{3-} enter the ECF via the intestine (diet) and bone stores. They leave the ECF via the kidneys (urine) and move into the bone.

Parathyroid hormone, vitamin D, and calcitonin regulate Ca^{2+} and PO_4^{3-}.

Ca^{2+} transport by the kidney

Only ionized Ca^{2+} is filtered through the glomerulus (approximately 50% of plasma Ca^{2+}). Reabsorption proceeds as follows:
- Proximal tubule: 70% is reabsorbed by diffusion, Ca^{2+}-activated ATPase and the Ca^{2+}/Na^{+} countertransport system.
- Thick ascending loop of Henle: 20–25% is reabsorbed passively.
- Distal convoluted tubule: 5–10% is reabsorbed against an electrochemical gradient. Sodium reabsorption inhibits calcium reabsorption in this segment while thiazide diuretics stimulate it.
- Collecting tubule: less than 0.5% is reabsorbed against an electrochemical gradient.

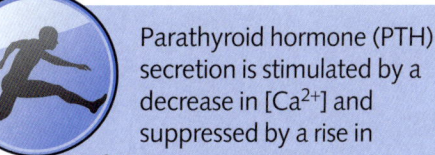

> Parathyroid hormone (PTH) secretion is stimulated by a decrease in $[Ca^{2+}]$ and suppressed by a rise in $[Ca^{2+}]$. Patients with chronic kidney disease have elevated PTH secondary to both hyperphosphatemia and low vitamin D.

Parathyroid hormone (PTH)

PTH is a polypeptide secreted by the parathyroid gland when there is a fall in plasma Ca^{2+}. PO_4^{3-} also affects PTH release, both directly and secondary to changes in Ca^{2+} levels. Figure 3.38 illustrates mechanisms of Ca^{2+} and PO_4^{3-} homeostasis. Vitamin D can also affect PTH release because it alters sensitivity of the parathyroid gland to Ca^{2+}.

Vitamin D

Vitamin D refers to a group of closely related sterols obtained from the diet or by the action of ultraviolet light on certain provitamins. It is metabolized to 25-hydroxycholecalciferol in the liver, then to 1,25-dihydroxycholecalciferol by the kidney. This metabolically active form causes an increase in Ca^{2+} and PO_4^{3-} by:
- Enhancing intestinal absorption of Ca^{2+}.
- Increasing Ca^{2+} release from bone.
- Decreasing Ca^{2+} and PO_4^{3-} excretion.

Patients with chronic kidney disease cannot form metabolically active 1,25 vitamin D and develop bone disease.

Calcitonin

Calcitonin is a peptide produced by the parafollicular cells of the thyroid. It reduces Ca^{2+} release from bone causing a decrease in ECF Ca^{2+} concentration.

Hypocalcemia

Causes
- Hypoparathyroidism.
- Rickets and osteomalacia (low vitamin D).
- Hypomagnesemia.
- Pancreatitis.
- Alkalemia, which reduces the amount of H^+ available to bind to serum albumin, increasing its negative charge so that more Ca^{2+} can bind to

Renal Function

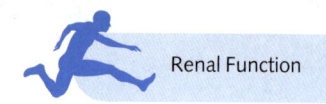

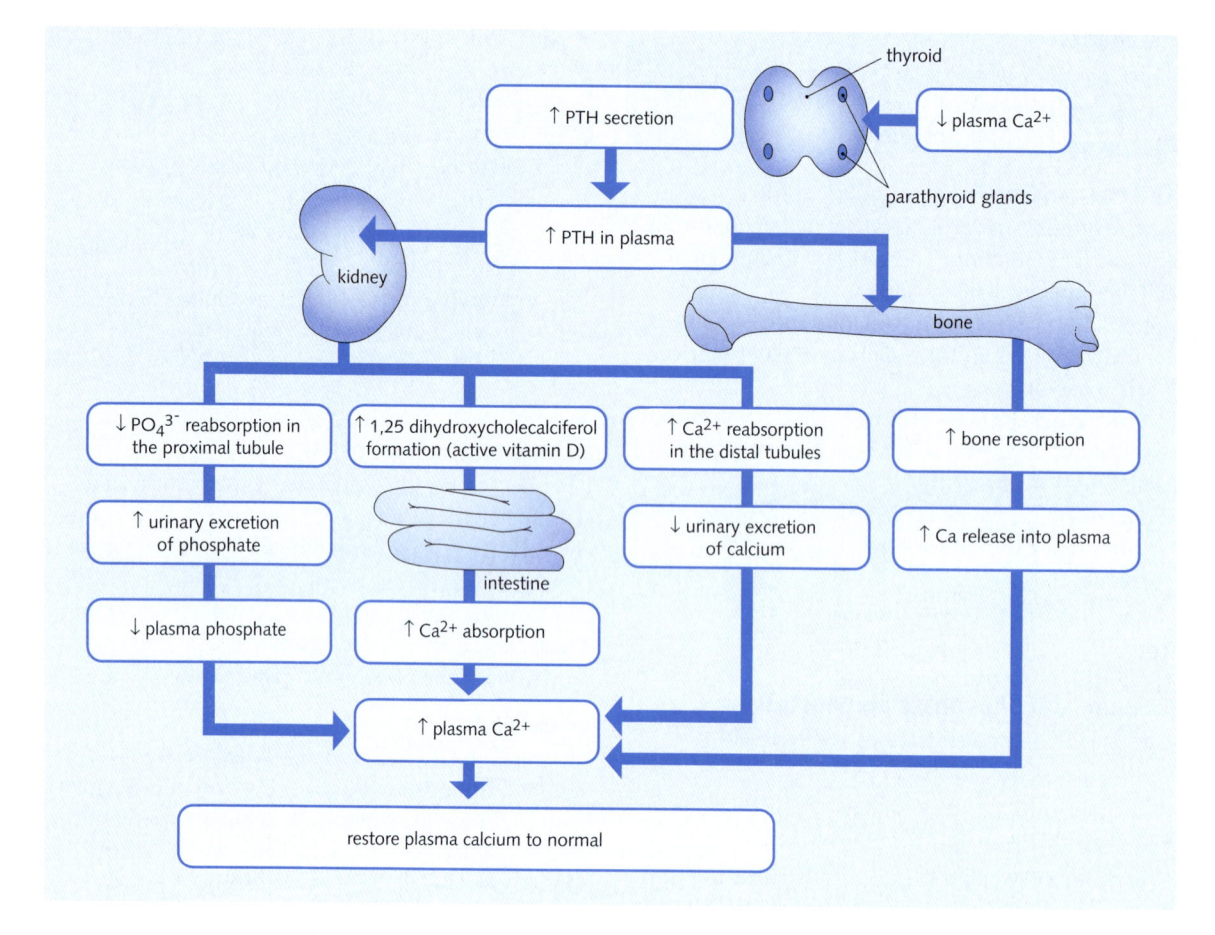

Fig. 3.38 Mechanisms of Ca^{2+} and phosphate homoeostasis. PTH, parathyroid hormone.

protein. This results in decreased ionized Ca^{2+}, although total Ca^{2+} remains the same.
- Chronic renal failure, due to hyperphosphatemia (if PO_4^{3-} rises, Ca^{2+} must fall proportionally) and low levels of activated vitamin D.

Consequences
- Tetany with convulsions.
- Hand and foot muscle cramps (leading to paralysis).
- Cardiac arrhythmias.

Treatment
Treatment may include oral or IV calcium, plus repletion of causes (replace magnesium, administer vitamin D, etc.).

Hypercalcemia
Causes
- Primary hyperparathyroidism.
- Malignancy or myeloma: bone destruction resulting in increased Ca^{2+} release from bone or tumor production of humoral hypercalcemic agents.
- Granulomatous disease (sarcoidosis).
- Increased intestinal absorption due to excess vitamin D or ingestion of calcium (milk–alkali syndrome).
- Thiazide diuretics: reduce intracellular Na^+ in the DCT, increasing Ca^{2+} reabsorption.
- Secondary or tertiary hyperparathyroidism in chronic renal failure.
- Hypermagnesemia.

Consequences
- Renal calculi.
- Altered mental status.
- Constipation due to decreased intestinal mobility.
- Acute renal failure (from vasoconstriction).
- Calcification outside the skeletal system.
- Polyuria and polydipsia (nephrogenic diabetes insipidus).

Treatment
Treatment may include forced diuresis with loop diuretics and saline, calcitonin, binding agents such as pamidronate, and treatment of underlying causes (chemotherapy for malignancy, remove parathyroid glands, suppress secondary hyperparathyroidism with vitamin D therapy, etc.).

Phosphate
Plasma phosphate concentration is 3–4.5 mg/dL. Phosphate is present in the plasma and interstitial fluid as:
- "Acid" phosphate $H_2PO_4^-$.
- "Alkaline" phosphate HPO_4^{3-}.

The proportion of the two forms depends on plasma pH. In cells, both inorganic forms (acid phosphate and alkaline phosphate) and organic forms (ATP, ADP and cAMP) are found.

Renal handling of phosphate
The kidney handles PO_4^{3-} as follows:
- Alkaline phosphate and acid phosphate are filtered by the glomerulus in a ratio of 4:1. Alkaline phosphate is converted to acid phosphate in the tubule as a result of H^+ secretion (see Fig. 3.29).
- 95% of the filtered PO_4^{3-} is reabsorbed in the early proximal tubule.
- Renal PO_4^{3-} excretion is increased by PTH, which is the only hormone to regulate phosphate transport.

Hypophosphatemia
Causes
- Malnutrition.
- Refeeding after starvation.
- Alcoholism.
- Diabetic ketoacidosis (osmotic diuresis).
- Burns.

Consequences
Decreased PO_4^{3-} results in muscle weakness and may impair oxygen delivery in sick patients, since it results in low 2,3-DPG levels on erythrocytes, leading to an inability to release oxygen to tissues in times of stress. It may also cause a cardiomyopathy and respiratory muscle weakness.

Treatment
Phosphate may be repleted orally or intravenously.

Hyperphosphatemia
Causes of hyperphosphatemia are:
- Chronic kidney disease (decreased filtration).
- Rhabdomyolysis, hyperthermia, or cell lysis (release from damaged cells).

Chronic effects are hypocalcemia and increased parathyroid hormone, leading to renal osteodystrophy.

Magnesium (Mg^{2+})
The plasma concentration of magnesium is 1.5–2.4 mg/dl; about 20% is protein-bound.

The total body magnesium has:
- 55% in bone.
- 40% in intracellular fluid.
- Up to 10% in plasma at any one time.
- 0.6% is in ECF.

Magnesium is an intracellular cation that:
- Controls mitochondrial oxidative metabolism and so regulates energy production.
- Is vital for protein synthesis.
- Regulates K^+ and Ca^{2+} channels in cell membranes.

Renal handling of Mg^{2+}
- In the glomerulus ionized Mg^{2+} (75% of total Mg^{2+}) is filtered.
- 15% is reabsorbed in the proximal tubule.
- 60% is reabsorbed in the thick ascending loop of Henle—the $Na^+/K^+/Cl^-$ cotransporter system enables Mg^{2+} absorption through the paracellular route.

There is intrinsic regulation by the cells of the thick ascending loop of Henle—if Mg^{2+} decreases, cell transport of Mg^{2+} increases. PTH increases reabsorption of Mg^{2+} in the thick ascending loop of Henle.

Hypomagnesemia
Causes
- Malnutrition, alcoholism.
- Diarrhea.
- Absorption disorder including fat absorption defects.
- Renal losses (diuretics, amphotericin).

Consequences
The main clinical consequences are neuromuscular disease (tremors, tetany) and hypocalcemia; the mechanism for this is unknown. There often are no symptoms.

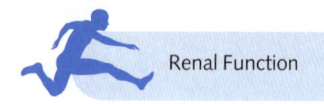

Uric acid: regulation and clinical disorders

Production and excretion
Uric acid is not ingested; it is produced in the liver from the degradation of dietary and endogenously purines, then is eliminated by the gut and the kidney. GI tract bacteria break down uric acid; this is responsible for approximately one-third of total urate metabolism.

The kidney accounts for the remaining two-thirds of excretion. Nearly all urate is filtered at the glomerulus. There is then tubular reabsorption of about 90 percent of the filtered urate in the proximal tubule, accomplished by a complex mixed process of reabsorption and secretion that is poorly understood. Reabsorption is indirectly linked to sodium reabsorption.

Hyperuricemia
Hyperuricemia is an excess of uric acid (end-product of purine degradation) in the blood. The normal serum urate is <7.0mg/dl, depending on the lab.

Causes
Causes of hyperuricemia are:
1. Overproduction:
   - Idiopathic gout.
   - Lymphoma, leukemia.
   - Tumor lysis syndrome.
   - Congenital metabolic syndromes (e.g., Lesch-Nyhan syndrome).
2. Underexcretion:
   - Idiopathic gout.
   - Renal failure.
   - Syndrome X (metabolic syndrome).
   - Drugs (aspirin, thiazides, cyclosporine: these inhibit tubular secretion of urate, thereby decreasing urate excretion and causing hyperuricemia).

Consequences
Hyperuricemia may precipitate gout in susceptible patients. It may also cause uric acid stones and an acute or chronic interstitial nephritis with progressive renal failure.

Diagnostic and therapeutic approach
Investigation of hyperuricemia is summarized in Fig. 3.39.

Renal regulation of erythropoiesis

Action and synthesis of erythropoietin
Erythropoietin (EPO) is a glycoprotein hormone involved in erythrocyte production by the bone marrow. Although it is produced in the liver in neonates, the main sources of EPO in adults (over 80%) are the kidney peritubular interstitial cells. The kidneys secrete EPO in response to hypoxia in an attempt to increase the number of circulating red blood cells and therefore reduce tissue hypoxia. This response is thought to be prostaglandin (PG) mediated, the PG stimulating the renal cells to synthesize EPO. In the bone marrow EPO-sensitive stem cells are converted into proerythroblasts and then into red blood cells.

Erythropoetin deficiency in CKD
Patients with chronic renal failure often have reduced EPO production, leading to a normocytic normochromic anemia. This can be treated by administration of exogenous (synthetic) EPO, which is produced using recombinant DNA technology. Subcutaneous or intravenous injections three times a week are required at a dose of 30–50U/kg to reach a hemoglobin level of 10–12g/dL without the need for blood transfusions.

Iron deficiency is the most common cause of failure in EPO treatment, and is corrected with oral or intravenous supplements. Other reasons for failure include bleeding, malignancy and infection.

The complications of treatment are thrombosis, hypertension and seizures. These are associated with rapid increases in hemoglobin concentration.

Fig. 3.39 Investigation of hyperuricemia. *Both a xanthine oxidase inhibitor and a uricosuric agent are needed in tophaceous gout. Xanthine oxidase is an enzyme in the metabolic pathway that produces urate from purines (from Green HL: *Clinical medicine*, 2nd ed. Mosby Year Book, 1996).

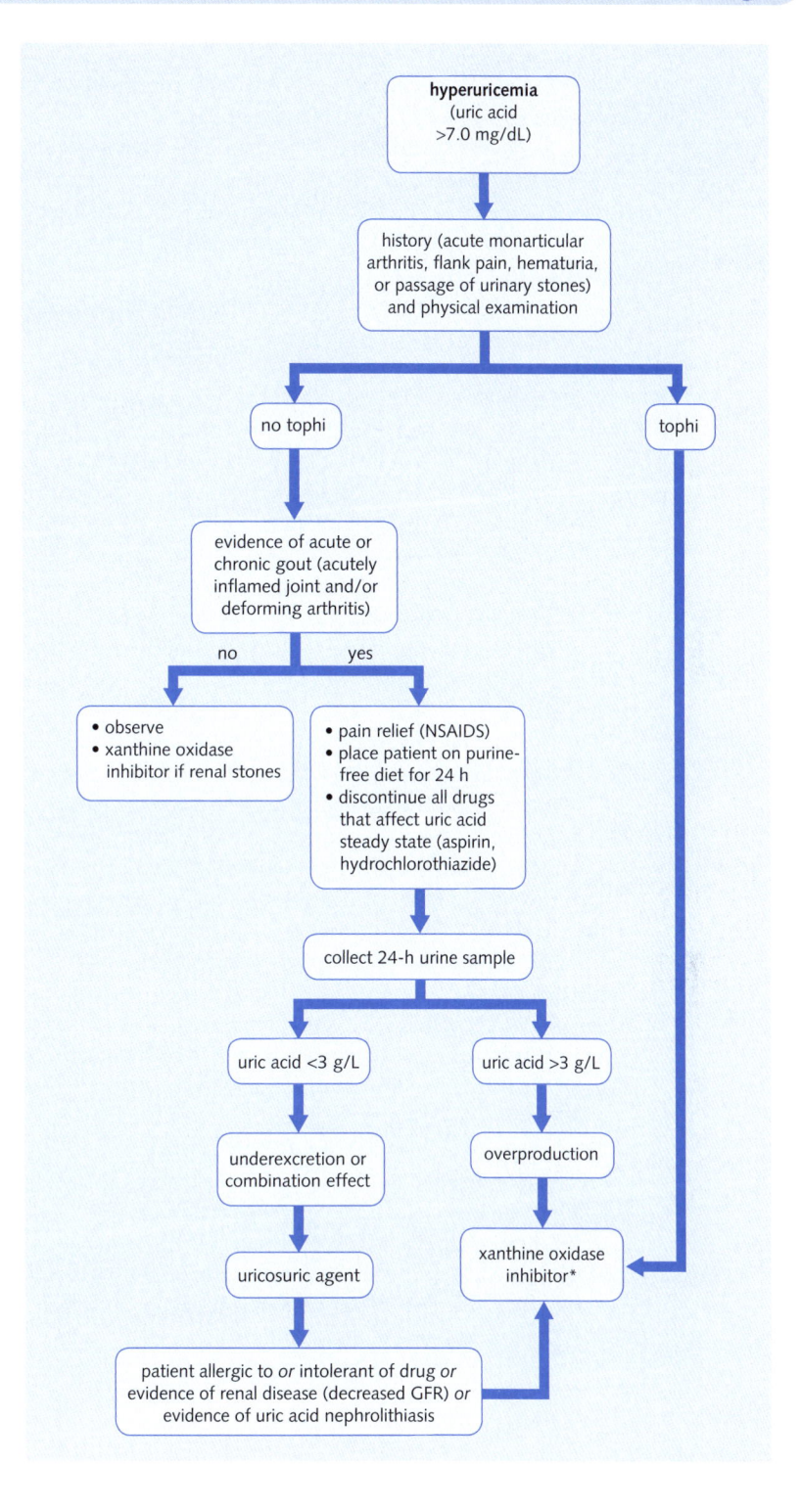

- Define clearance. Explain how it is measured and what its units are.
- Describe how to measure the GFR. Discuss how this varies with age.
- Outline the factors that affect creatinine clearance.
- Define autoregulation of GFR and explain how it is achieved.
- List the three types of acute renal failure and the most common causes of each.
- Describe how to use the urinalysis and urine electrolytes to diagnose ARF.
- Discuss the common sequellae of chronic kidney disease.
- Explain how to prevent the progression of chronic kidney disease.
- Explain how the two common types of dialysis differ, and what is the indication for using them.
- Summarize the importance of the renin–angiotensin–aldosterone system.
- Outline the mechanisms controlling Na^+ reabsorption.
- Describe the effective circulating volume and explain how this is regulated.
- Describe the therapy of extracellular volume depletion and excess.
- Describe the mechanism, utility, and side effects of the common diuretics.
- Explain what osmoreceptors are, where they are located and what their function is.
- Briefly describe the synthesis, storage and function of ADH.
- Summarize the countercurrent mechanism of the loop of Henle.
- Describe how the kidneys' ability to concentrate or dilute urine is altered in disease.
- Discuss the site and mechanism of action, uses and side-effects for each of the different diuretics.
- Describe how hyperglycemia leads to hyponatremia.
- Describe how to evaluate hyponatremia, distinguishing etiologies with appropriate examination and lab findings.
- Distinguish the two types of diabetes insipidus and explain how they differ.
- State the normal pH range. Outline how and why it is tightly controlled.
- Explain what a 'buffer' is. Name the main buffering system in the body and describe how it works.
- Explain how the kidney retains filtered bicarbonate.
- Explain two ways the kidney rids the body of excess acid.
- Explain how metabolic acidosis and metabolic alkalosis are differentiated by arterial blood gas results and outline how you would correct each of them.
- Discuss the significance of the anion gap.
- Describe the distribution of potassium within the body compartments and explain why it is important to keep this distribution constant.
- List the treatments of severe hyperkalemia and their physiologic rationale.
- Explain the relationship between plasma calcium and phosphate. Describe the influence of three factors involved in their regulation.
- Explain the clinical consequences of hypo-and hypercalcemia, and hypophosphatemia.
- Outline the diagnosis and treatment of hyperuricemia.
- Discuss how and where erythropoietin release is stimulated and what its effects are.

4. The Kidneys in Disease

Congenital abnormalities of the kidney

Congenital structural abnormalities can develop within the kidney, as described below.

Agenesis of the kidney
Absence (agenesis) of the kidney can be unilateral or bilateral. Unilateral agenesis occurs in 1 in 1000 of the population. Agenesis occurs if the collecting system (from the ureteric buds) fails to fuse with the nephrons (from the metanephric mesoderm). The only kidney present gradually hypertrophies and is often abnormal with malrotation, ectopia or hydronephrosis. The kidney is at risk of infection and trauma. This disorder is associated with other developmental abnormalities such as absent testes or ovaries, spina bifida, and congenital heart disease. Bilateral agenesis occurs in less than 1 in 3000 pregnancies and is incompatible with life. It is also known as Potter's syndrome, which is associated with pulmonary hypoplasia and oligohydramnios in utero. There is no treatment.

Hypoplasia
The kidneys develop inadequately and are consequently smaller than average. This is a rare disorder, affecting one or both kidneys, which are prone to infection and stone formation.

Ectopic kidney
The incidence of ectopic kidney is 1 in 800. The kidney does not ascend fully into the abdomen, so remains lower than usual (if it remains in the pelvis, it is called a "pelvic kidney"—Fig. 4.1). It is usually unilateral and, the lower the kidney, the more abnormal it is. As a result of the abnormal positioning, the ureters can be obstructed by neighboring structures, leading to obstructive uropathy, infection and stone formation. This disorder can also affect pregnancy and birth.

Horseshoe kidney
The incidence of horseshoe kidney is between 1 in 600 and 1 in 1800, and is more common in boys than girls. The two kidneys fuse across the midline, usually at their lower poles, by renal tissue or a fibrous band (Fig. 4.2). The horseshoe kidney is usually lower than normal because the inferior mesenteric artery limits its ascent. It can also be malrotated and is prone to reflux, obstruction, infection, and stone formation.

Cystic diseases of the kidney

Overview
Cystic diseases of the kidney form a spectrum of diseases comprising hereditary, developmental (but not hereditary) and acquired disorders. They can result if the ureteric bud or kidney tissue fails to develop. Some of these diseases can lead to chronic renal failure. Diagnosis is made by finding multiple cysts on ultrasound. A single simple cyst is not an uncommon finding and should be considered normal.

Simple cysts
These are very common, with incidence increasing with age. They vary in size (usually 2–5cm in diameter) and number, and contain clear fluid. Microscopically, they have a cuboidal epithelial lining and a thin capsule. Renal function is not affected but pain may be felt if there is hemorrhage into the cyst. The cysts can be differentiated from tumors by ultrasound or CT scanning.

Polycystic kidney disease
Adult—autosomal dominant
Incidence and presenting features
This type of polycystic kidney disease accounts for 8–10% of chronic renal failure. Inheritance is autosomal dominant, and three polycystic kidney disease (PKD) genes have been identified:

The Kidneys in Disease

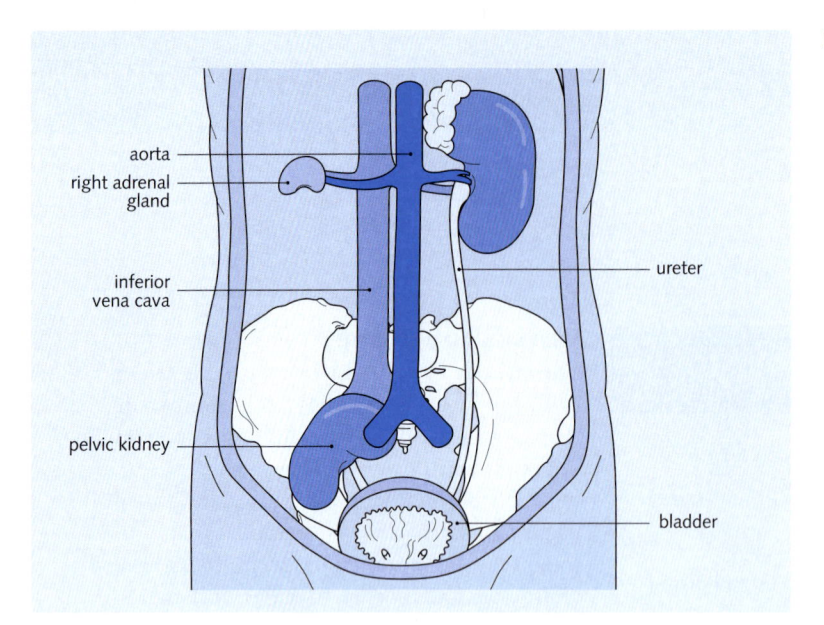

Fig. 4.1 Ectopic (pelvic) kidney.

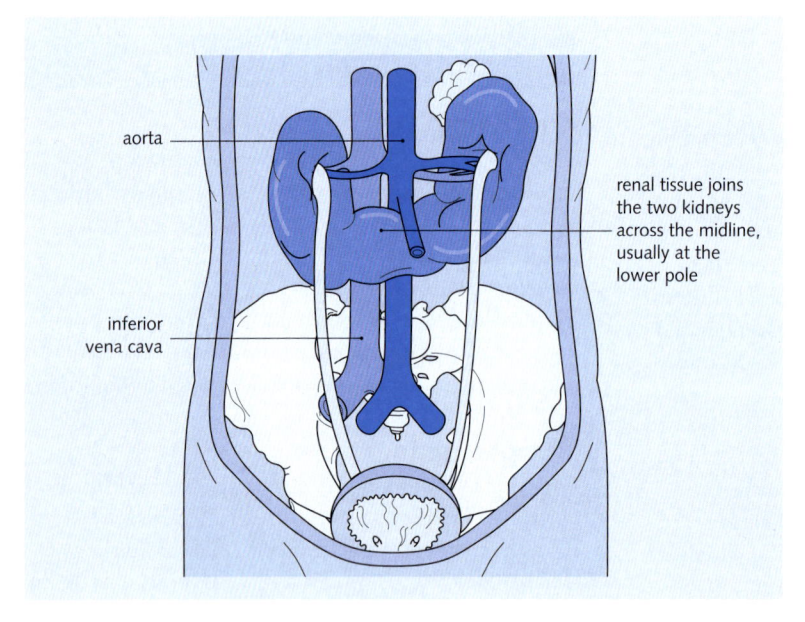

Fig. 4.2 Horseshoe kidney.

- PKD 1: on chromosome 16 (accounts for 85% of cases).
- PKD 2: on chromosome 4 (accounts for 10% of cases).
- PKD 3: accounts for a minority of cases and has yet to be mapped.

These mutations are thought to alter tubular epithelium growth and differentiation. Presentation is at 30–40 years of age with hypertension, urinary symptoms or bilateral large palpable kidneys. End-stage renal failure can develop in up to 50% of patients, usually in the 5th or 6th decade of life. Risk factors for renal failure include male gender, African-American race, and onset by 30–35 of gross hematuria or hypertension.

Pathology

Cysts develop anywhere in the kidney (Fig. 4.3A) and compress the surrounding parenchyma,

Fig. 4.3 Polycystic adult (A) and childhood (B) kidney disease.

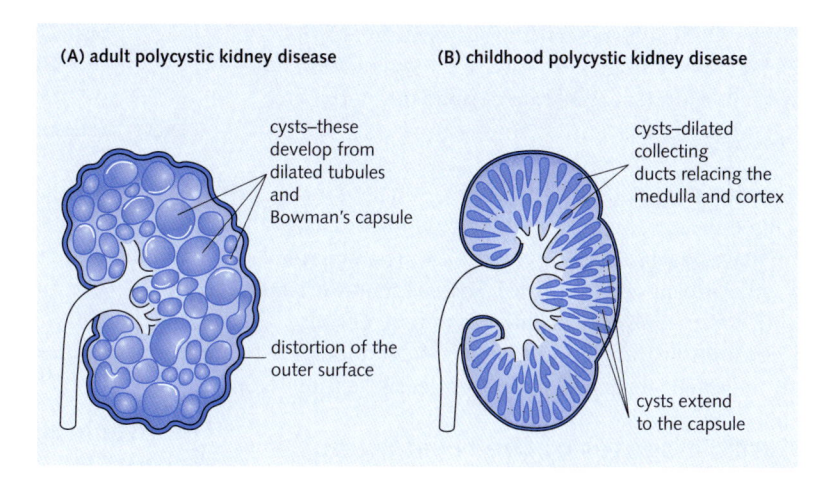

(A) adult polycystic kidney disease

cysts—these develop from dilated tubules and Bowman's capsule

distortion of the outer surface

(B) childhood polycystic kidney disease

cysts—dilated collecting ducts relacing the medulla and cortex

cysts extend to the capsule

impairing renal function. Sites for cyst formation are:
- Both kidneys.
- Liver (lined by biliary epithelium) in 30–40% of cases.
- Pancreas, lungs, ovaries, spleen and other organs.

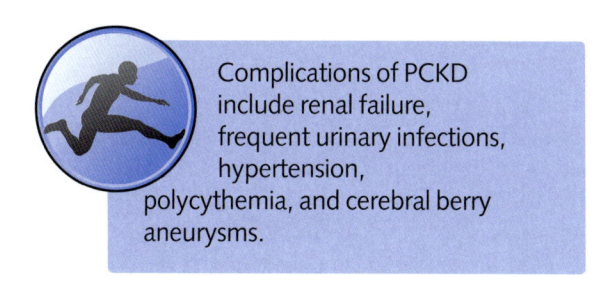

> Complications of PCKD include renal failure, frequent urinary infections, hypertension, polycythemia, and cerebral berry aneurysms.

Berry aneurysms (found in 10–20% of cases) develop as a result of congenital weakness in the arteries and increased blood pressure; they can lead to a subarachnoid or cerebral hemorrhage.

Macroscopically, the kidneys are large with clear yellow, fluid-filled cysts replacing the parenchyma. Hemorrhage into the cysts can occur. Microscopically, the cysts are lined by cuboidal epithelium.

Diagnosis
Diagnosis is made by:
- Ultrasound or computerized tomography (CT): this shows bilateral enlarged kidneys with multiple cysts.
- Genetic testing in families known to carry the PKD gene.

Prognosis
Morbidity and mortality are often the result of hypertension, for example myocardial infarction and cerebrovascular disease. The condition also leads to infections and CRF. Rarely, complications are produced by the extrarenal cysts.

Treatment
Control blood pressure and treat infections. Dialysis and renal transplantation are needed if CRF develops.

Child—autosomal recessive
Incidence and presenting features
This rare condition presents with enlarged kidneys or stillbirth. Both sexes are affected equally, and more than one gene may be involved.

Pathology
Macroscopically, large kidneys with a radial pattern of fusiform-like cysts ("sunburst pattern") are seen. Both kidneys are enlarged by multiple dilated collecting ducts which form the cysts. These replace the medulla and cortex and extend into the capsule (see Fig. 4.3B). The liver is almost always affected, with cysts, bile duct cell proliferation, fibrosis interfering with liver function and eventual portal hypertension.

Diagnosis, prognosis, and treatment
Diagnosis is based on the presence of a palpable mass and ultrasound findings. Treatment involves managing the renal failure, hypertension and respiratory problems.

The prognosis is poor and death usually occurs due to renal or respiratory failure within the first few

81

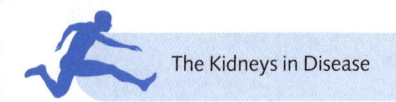

weeks of life, unless renal replacement therapy is given. Some children can survive for several years with independent renal function and develop portal hypertension and hepatic fibrosis.

Cystic renal dysplasia
This is an area of undifferentiated mesenchyme or cartilage within the parenchyma. It can be unilateral (better prognosis) or bilateral, and is often associated with obstructive abnormalities in the ureter and lower urinary tract. Presentation is in childhood as an abdominal mass, treated with surgical excision.

Cystic diseases of the renal medulla
Medullary sponge kidney
Incidence and presenting features
This is uncommon (1 in 20,000). It usually presents at 30–40 years of age with symptoms of urinary tract infection (UTI), stone formation, or hematuria.

Pathology
Dilated collecting ducts in the medulla result in multiple cyst formation, mainly in the papillae. Small calculi can develop within the cysts. One, part of one, or both kidneys can be affected. Macroscopically, some cysts are seen extending into the medulla from the involved calyces. In severe cases, the medulla looks spongy.

Diagnosis, prognosis, and treatment
Diagnosis is by intravenous pyelography (IVP). The prognosis is good, with renal function remaining intact. A partial nephrectomy might be required.

Acquired cystic disease (dialysis-associated)
Acquired cystic disease occurs in patients with CRF who have received dialysis for some time. The damaged kidneys develop many small cysts throughout the cortex and medulla, caused by obstruction of the tubules by interstitial fibrosis. The cysts have an atypical hyperplastic epithelial lining that can undergo malignant change.

Diseases of the glomerulus

Overview
Glomerular disease (usually called glomerulonephritis [GN]) can be classified as:
- Hereditary (e.g., Alport's and Fabry's syndromes).
- Primary: idiopathic disease process originates in the glomerulus.
- Secondary: GN arises from a systemic diseases: e.g., diabetes mellitus (most common GN in U.S.), systemic lupus erythematosus (SLE), bacterial endocarditis.

Four structures within the glomerulus are prone to damage:
- Capillary endothelial cell lining.
- Glomerular basement membrane.
- Mesangium supporting the capillaries.
- Podocytes on the outer surface of the capillary.

The mechanisms of glomerular injury
In situ immune-complex deposition
While there are known mechanisms of glomerular injury, specific etiologies for most glomerular diseases remain unclear. Antigen–antibody immune complexes form within the kidney when antibodies react with intrinsic or planted antigens within the glomerulus (Fig. 4.4A).

Antiglomerular basement membrane (anti-GBM) disease is an example of reaction to intrinsic antigens. Antibodies are formed against an antigen in the GBM to form a complex which stimulates the complement cascade. This damages the glomerulus and leads to rapidly progressing renal failure. The anti-GBM antibodies also attack the basement membrane of the alveoli in the lungs. The triad of anti-GBM antibodies, GN, and pulmonary hemorrhage is known as Goodpasture's syndrome.

Reaction to planted antigens occurs when circulating antigens are deposited within the glomerulus. They can be:
- Exogenous: e.g., bacteria such as group A beta-hemolytic streptococci, which cause post-streptococcal GN. Other antigens include bacterial products, aggregated IgG, viruses, parasites, and drugs.
- Endogenous: e.g., anti-DNA antibodies react with circulating DNA (as seen in SLE).

Circulating immune complex nephritis
This is the most common mechanism of immune-mediated damage. Immune complexes form outside the kidney and become trapped in the glomerulus after traveling to the kidney via the renal circulation (Fig. 4.4B). The antigen can be:
- Exogenous: bacteria (e.g., group A streptococci, *Treponema pallidum*), surface antigen of hepatitis

B, hepatitis C virus antigen, tumor antigens, viruses.
- Endogenous: DNA in SLE.

When trapped in the glomerulus, the immune complexes activate the classic complement pathway, causing acute inflammation of the glomerulus. Immunofluorescence microscopy shows neutrophil deposits along the basement membrane and/or in the mesangium. These increase vascular permeability.

Cell-mediated immunity
Sensitized T cells from cell-mediated immune reactions likely play a key role in the onset and progression of most glomerular diseases (Fig. 4.4C). Glomerular damage is thought to be mediated by macrophages and T lymphocytes.

Cytotoxic antibodies
Antibodies to glomerular cell antigens cause damage without the formation and deposition of immune complexes (Fig. 4.4D). This is uncommon. An example would be antibody fixing to mesangial cells, resulting in complement-mediated mesangiolysis and mesangial cell proliferation.

Activation of alternative complement pathway
Bacterial polysaccharides, endotoxins, and IgA aggregates can stimulate the alternative complement pathway—the products of which deposit in the glomeruli, impairing glomerular function (Fig. 4.4E). This occurs in membranoproliferative GN.

Clinical manifestations of glomerular disease
Glomeruli manifest damage either through increased protein excretion or through appearance of red blood cells in the urine. Therefore, glomerular diseases are generally classified as either nephrotic or nephritic. Patients with nephrotic glomerular diseases will excrete more than 3.5 grams of protein in the urine during a 24-hour period, while those with nephritic glomerular diseases present with hematuria. Some renal diseases present with both nephrotic and nephritic features, such as membranoproliferative glomerulonephritis and SLE.

Fig. 4.4 The five mechanisms of immune complex renal disease. Ab, antibody; Ag, antigen; IC, immune complex.

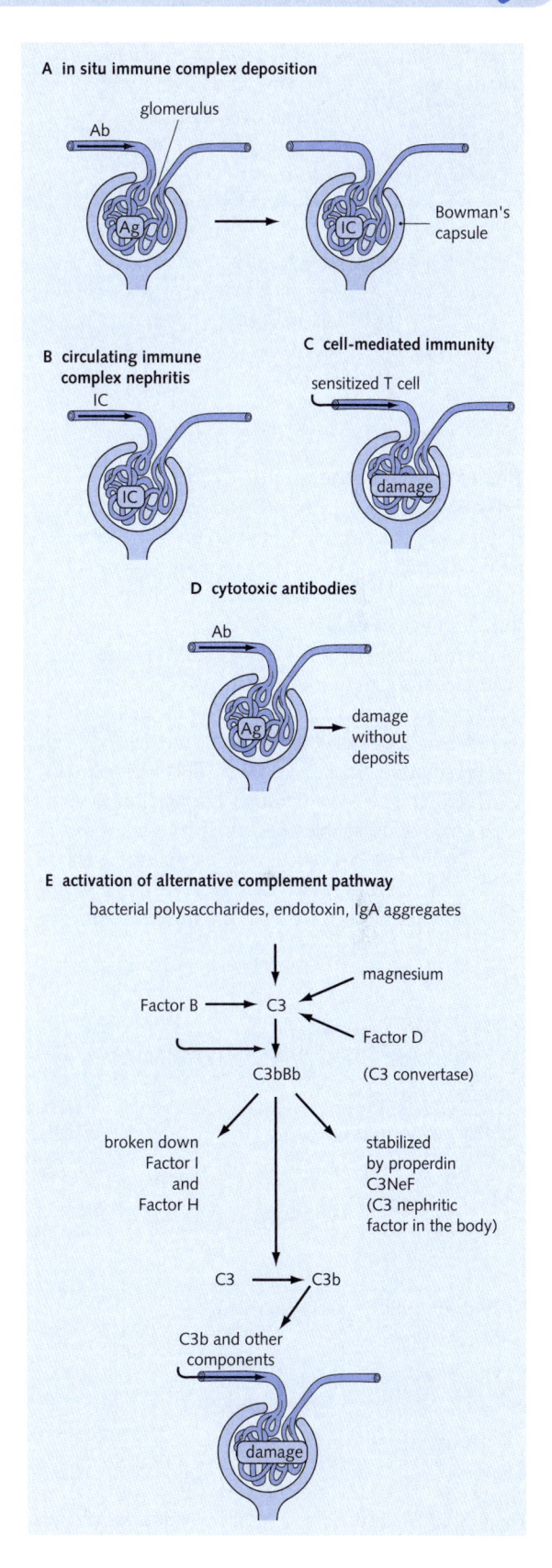

The Kidneys in Disease

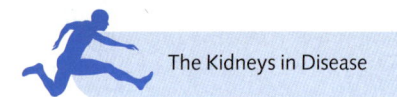

> Pathologically, glomerular disease is classified as:
> - Focal—affects only some glomeruli.
> - Diffuse—affects all the glomeruli.
> - Segmental—affects only part of the glomerulus.
> - Global—affects the entire glomerulus.

Proteinuria and the nephrotic syndrome

Proteinuria of over 150mg/24 hours is abnormal. Proteinuria of less than 1 gram is very nonspecific and can be seen in a variety of renal and nonrenal diseases. The heavier the proteinuria, the more likely it is due to glomerular injury.

- Proteinuria of over 2 grams per 24 hours usually comes from glomerular injury.
- Proteinuria of >3.5g/24hr is classified as nephrotic, especially in association with hypoalbuminemia and edema. The edema is usually due to renal resistance to natriuretic peptides, but can be worsened by very low serum albumin concentrations with resultant low oncotic pressure. Hyperlipidemia is also present, and may be due to the urinary loss of apolipoproteins that modulate lipoprotein structure, leading to decreased lipoprotein catabolism.

Nephrotic Syndrome

The nephrotic syndrome is characterized by:
- Proteinuria (>3.5g/24hr)
- Hypoalbuminemia (serum albumin <2.5g/dL)
- Edema secondary to tubular resistance to ANP and to hypoalbuminemia with consequent decreased serum oncotic pressure
- Hypercholesterolemia with elevated LDL.

The nephrotic syndrome results when the glomerular capillary wall is excessively permeable to plasma protein. This leads to heavy proteinuria (>3.5g/24hr). The capillary wall becomes permeable to proteins of higher molecular weight as the severity of injury increases, due to glomerular basement membrane damage and increase in pore size. A limited amount of filtered protein can be reabsorbed by proximal tubule endocytosis, but if this is exceeded, protein is lost in the urine.

Most pathologic lesions seen in the nephrotic syndrome come in primary and secondary forms. These are summarized in Fig. 4.5.

In an adult a loss of more than 3–5g of albumin per day can cause hypoalbuminemia, but some patients can have nephrotic-range proteinuria without being overtly nephrotic, because the rate of hepatic albumin synthesis compensates for the albumin loss.

Summary of types of glomerular diseases and their clinical presentations		
Clinical presentation	**Primary glomerular diseases**	**Secondary glomerular diseases**
proteinuria and nephrotic syndrome	FSGS membranous GN minimal change disease membranoproliferative GN (rare)	diabetic nephropathy severe hypertension amyloidosis hepatitis C-related MPGN eclampsia Henoch-Schönlein purpura drugs (NSAIDs)
hematuria and nephritic syndrome (these often present with concurrent proteinuria)	IgA nephropathy	postinfectious GN SLE hepatitis C-related MPGN polyarteritis nodosum (PAN) Wegener's granulomatosis Goodpasture's syndrome Henoch-Schönlein purpura

Fig. 4.5 Summary of types of glomerular diseases and their clinical presentations.

Complications of nephrotic syndrome
- Chronic kidney disease with decreased GFR, from glomerular scarring and excessive protein trafficking through the nephron.
- Hyperlipidemia: increases risk of vascular disease and ischemic heart disease.
- Immunosuppression: increases risk of infection.
- Hypercoagulable state: increases risk of deep vein thrombosis (DVT), pulmonary embolus (PE) and renal vein thrombosis.

Renal vein thrombosis should be suspected if proteinuria increases or renal function deteriorates suddenly. Diagnosis is by ultrasound, and treatment involves anticoagulation.

Treatment of nephrotic syndrome
Management includes:
- Treatment of underlying causes, e.g., prednisone in minimal change disease.
- Blood pressure control.
- Reduction of proteinuria, using ACE inhibitors.
- Control of hyperlipidemia with HMGCoA reductase inhibitors.
- Anticoagulation if hypercoagulable (risk of thrombosis increases as albumin decreases).

> The nephrotic syndrome is managed by use of ACE inhibitors, hypertension control, and anti-hyperlipidemic agents.

Hematuria and the nephritic syndrome
Hematuria is a common finding in glomerular disease. However, not all patients with hematuria have glomerulonephritis, since urologic problems may also result in hematuria. Glomerular hematuria can be seen alone or with signs and symptoms of the nephritic syndrome. Common primary and secondary causes of the nephritic syndrome are summarized in Fig. 4.5.

The symptoms and signs of acute nephritic syndrome are:

- Hematuria—microscopic or macroscopic. RBCs appear dysmorphic on microscopy, and RBC casts may be seen.
- Oliguria/anuria.
- Hypertension.
- Edema.
- Renal failure.
- Proteinuria.

Rapidly progressive GN (RPGN)
This is a severe subset of nephritic disease. It occurs when there is severe glomerular injury. It presents with hematuria, oliguria and hypertension, eventually causing renal failure in weeks to a few months. The causes are the same as for the nephritic syndrome, with PAN, Goodpasture's, and Wegener's most frequently presenting with this syndrome.

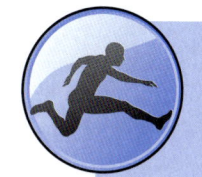

> Suspected RPGN requires urgent consultation with a nephrologist for renal biopsy.

Chronic glomerulonephritis
In chronic GN, advanced CKD or chronic renal failure results from any glomerular disease causing progressive loss of renal function. The kidney shrinks, with cortical thinning. Most of the glomeruli hyalinize and there is almost complete tubular atrophy. This is often asymptomatic in the early stages. Later, symptoms develop as waste products accumulate and erythropoietin or vitamin D production is reduced. Symptoms include:
- Uremia.
- Hypertension.
- Salt and water retention, causing edema.
- Anemia.
- Nausea, vomiting, diarrhea.
- Gastrointestinal bleeding.
- Itching.
- Polyuria and nocturia.
- Lethargy.
- Paresthesias (due to polyneuropathy).
- Mental slowing and clouding of consciousness (terminal stage).

The Kidneys in Disease

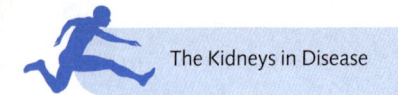

In extreme cases, oliguria results. Progression may be slowed by careful blood pressure control and the use of ACE inhibitors. The only treatment is dialysis until renal transplantation is possible.

Specific glomerular diseases
Hereditary glomerular disease
Alport's syndrome
This is usually X-linked, affecting mainly males (females are usually asymptomatic carriers). Autosomal dominant and autosomal recessive patterns of inheritance have also been described. An abnormality of basement membrane collagen IV is found in all patients, and they lack the Goodpasture's antigen.

Presentation is with hematuria, ocular abnormalities and sensorineural deafness. Ocular lesions include lens dislocation, cataract and conical cornea. It is also associated
with platelet dysfunction and hyperproteinemia.

A few patients develop end-stage renal failure in childhood and adolescence. Females might have microscopic hematuria, but rarely develop end-stage renal failure. Treatment involves dialysis and/or transplantation.

Fabry's syndrome
This is a rare X-linked disorder, with a glycolipid metabolism defect due to the deficiency of galactosidase A. As a result, ceramide trihexoside (a glycosphingolipid) accumulates and is deposited in the kidneys, skin and vascular system. This disorder is associated with cardiac problems such as angina and cardiac failure—consequently, most patients die in the 5th decade of life.

Primary (idiopathic) nephrotic diseases
There are four principal primary diseases that cause the nephrotic syndrome. They are listed in Fig. 4.6, along with systemic diseases that can cause the same glomerular histology.

Focal segmental glomerulosclerosis (FSGS)
This accounts for 10% of childhood and 33% of adult nephrotic syndrome cases in the US. Its incidence is increasing in young African-American men. Secondary causes are:
- Intravenous heroin use.
- AIDS (HIV-associated nephropathy).
- Ureteric reflux.
- Morbid obesity.

Histology reveals focal collapse and sclerosis, with hyaline deposits in glomerular segments. Presentation is with proteinuria or nephrotic syndrome, later developing hematuria and hypertension. Most develop CRF within 10 years. Treatment of the idiopathic form involves steroids, cyclophosphamide, cyclosporine, dialysis and renal transplantation. Recurrence can be seen after a renal transplant.

Membranous glomerulopathy
This accounts for 33% of primary adult nephrotic syndrome in the U.S. and is more common in males. Causes are primary (85%) or secondary. Secondary causes include:
- Infections: syphilis, malaria, hepatitis B.
- tumors: melanoma, carcinoma of the bronchus, lymphoma.
- Drugs: penicillamine, heroin, mercury, gold.
- Systemic illnesses: SLE.

	2° minimal change disease	2° FSGS	2° membranous GN	2° membranoproliferative GN
infection		HIV	hepatitis B	hepatitis C
malignancy	Hodgkin's disease		lymphoma, adenocarcinoma	
drug	NSAIDs	heroin	gold, penicillamine	
connective tissue disease			lupus	
other		ureteral reflux, morbid obesity		

Fig. 4.6 Secondary causes of the four primary patterns of glomerular pathology.

Pathologically the disease is characterized by:
- Subepithelial deposition of immune complexes.
- Basement membrane thickening.

Histology reveals widespread glomerular basement thickening caused by immunoglobulin deposition. Over time, the abnormal excess mesangial matrix causes hyalinization of the glomerulus and death of individual nephrons. Drug treatment involves corticosteroids, cyclophosphamide, cyclosporine and chlorambucil. Prognosis depends on the cause; 30% of idiopathic cases develop CRF and require dialysis or transplantation. In secondary membranous glomerulopathy, treatment of underlying disease causes disease remission.

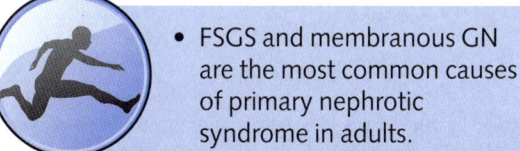

- FSGS and membranous GN are the most common causes of primary nephrotic syndrome in adults.
- Minimal change disease is the most common cause of nephrotic syndrome in children.

Minimal change disease
This is the most common cause of nephrotic syndrome in children under the age of 16. It also accounts for 15% of primary adult nephrotic syndrome in the US. No significant renal changes are seen under the light microscope (hence the name). Under the electron microscope there is podocyte fusion, i.e. foot process effacement. The cause is unknown, but potential mechanisms include a post allergic reaction, circulating immune complexes, or altered T-cell immunity. Secondary causes include nonsteroidal anti-inflammatory drugs and lymphoma.

Treatment involves corticosteroid therapy and cyclosporine or cyclophosphamide (if resistant). The prognosis is good in children (90% respond to steroids) and variable in adults, but usually good. Occasionally, this disorder causes end-stage renal failure.

Membranoproliferative glomerulonephritis
This is common in children and young adults, and more common in females than males. It is characterized histologically by diffuse global basement membrane thickening and mesangial proliferation. Primary membranoproliferative GN is uncommon, has no effective treatment, and has a poor prognosis. The most common form of MPGN is secondary to hepatitis C infection. It is commonly associated with cryoglobulinemia. The treatment is interferon alpha, which treats both the active hepatitis infection and the glomerular disease.

Secondary nephrotic diseases
Diabetic glomerulosclerosis (nephropathy)
The kidneys are the most commonly and severely damaged organs in diabetes. Diabetic nephropathy will likely develop in 25–45% of all diabetics, with similar risks in both types 1 and 2.

Renal manifestations include nodular glomerulosclerosis and arteriosclerosis, including benign nephrosclerosis with hypertension. Diabetic nephropathy presents with microalbuminuria (150–300mg protein per 24 hours), which increases progressively to nephrotic range proteinuria (i.e., >3.5g/24hr). Consequently, GFR gradually declines, leading to CRF. Fig. 4.7 presents a summary of the natural history of diabetes.

Diabetic nephropathy is now the most common reason for initiating dialysis treatment in the USA, and is leading to a growing cost for dialysis and transplantation.

Histological features can include:
- Thickening of the capillary basement membrane.
- Increase in the matrix of the mesangium.
- A diffuse or nodular pattern of glomerulosclerosis (also known as Kimmelstiel–Wilson syndrome).
- Arterial hyalinosis of both the afferent and efferent arterioles—this predisposes to vessel occlusion.

The arteries can also be affected (especially in type 2 diabetes), and severe atheromatous disease in the renal arteries and arterioles leads to renal ischemia and hypertension. Papillary necrosis is a recognized complication, especially in the presence of infection. It is also associated with diabetic complications

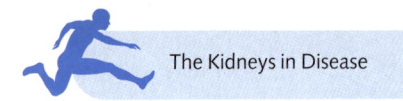

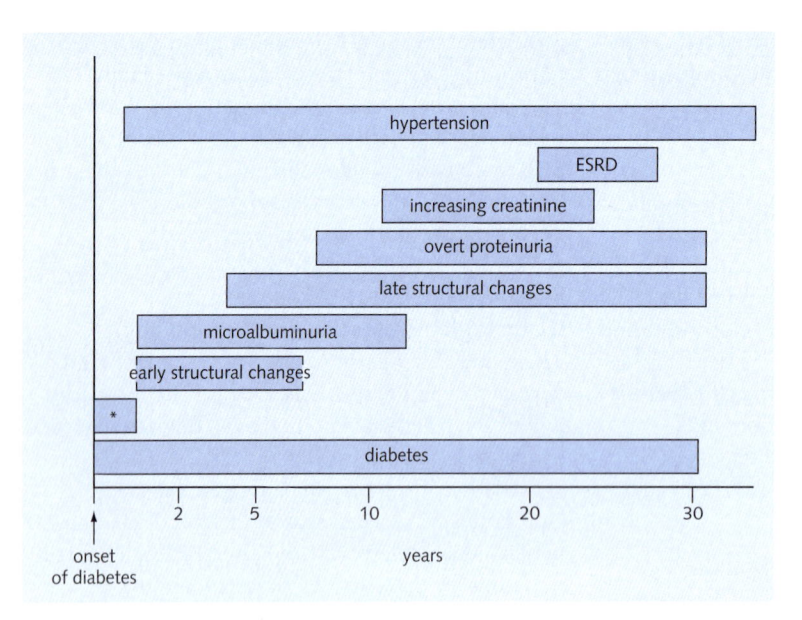

Fig. 4.7 Summary of the natural history of diabetes. *Indicates functional changes in kidney size (increased) and short-term glomerular filtration rate (increased). ESRD, end-stage renal disease.

elsewhere (e.g., retinopathy in the eyes). Chronic renal damage as a result of diabetes is associated and accelerated by hypertension.

Treatment includes ACE inhibitors to reduce proteinuria, strict blood pressure and glycemic control. All these are most effective in the microalbuminuric stage.

Amyloidosis

This disorder is most common in elderly patients. It involves deposition of amyloid (an extracellular fibrillar protein) in the glomeruli, usually within the mesangium and subendothelium, and sometimes in the subepithelial space. Deposits can also be found in the walls of the blood vessels and in the interstitium. Clinically, this results in heavy proteinuria or the nephrotic syndrome, eventually leading to CRF (due to ischemia and glomerulosclerosis). The disease may be primary or secondary to multiple myeloma or chronic infections.

Nephritic glomerular diseases
Postinfectious glomerulonephritis (GN)

Poststreptococcal GN This presents 1–3 weeks following a group A β-hemolytic streptococcal infection of the tonsils, pharynx or skin. Clinical features include proteinuria, hematuria, reduced complement, and a low GFR (this causes fluid retention and hypertension). The anti-strepolysin O titer (ASO) is elevated. All the glomeruli are involved thus resulting in a diffuse proliferative GN—"proliferative" because there is an increase in the cellularity in the glomerulus. Treatment is usually conservative, with antibiotics to treat any remaining infection. The prognosis is excellent in children but only 60% of adults recover completely; the rest develop hypertension or renal impairment.

Nonstreptococcal postinfectious GN
Nonstreptococcal GN follows a similar process to that for poststreptococcal GN except that the causative organism is not streptococcus. It can be triggered by:
- Other bacteria (e.g., staphylococci and pneumococci).
- Parasites (*Toxoplasma gondii*, *Plasmodium* sp.).
- Viruses.

IgA nephropathy (Berger's disease)

This is the most common primary glomerular disease worldwide, causing recurrent hematuria. It is more common in Asia, where it is the leading cause of chronic kidney disease. It is associated with human leukocyte antigen (HLA) DR4. It classically (but not uniformly) affects patients 1–2 days after an upper respiratory tract infection. Presentation is with microscopic hematuria and proteinuria and renal impairment. There is hypertension and plasma IgA levels are raised. Histologically, IgA and C3 deposits are seen in the mesangium of all the glomeruli, with some mesangial proliferation. Eventually, there is sclerosis of the damaged segment.

There is no proven effective treatment, although steroids and fish oil have shown some benefits in small studies. Patients with proteinuria, increased blood pressure and increased creatinine at presentation have a worse prognosis—up to 20% of patients develop end-stage renal failure.

Henoch–Schönlein purpura (HSP)
HSP is a systemic vasculitis that is identical to IgA nephropathy in its renal disease. It is seen predominantly in children, affecting males more than females. It is an immune-mediated systemic vasculitis that affects many parts of the body including:
- Skin: a purpuric rash is seen over on the extensor surface of the legs and arms and buttocks.
- Joints: resulting in pain.
- Intestine: resulting in abdominal pain, vomiting, bleeding.
- Kidney: lesion of IgA nephropathy, resulting in GN (one-third of patients develop IgA nephropathy).

HSP can follow an upper respiratory tract infection. It has an excellent prognosis in children.

Systemic lupus erythematosus (SLE)
SLE is an autoimmune vasculitis characterized by antinuclear antibodies and widespread immune-complex-mediated inflammation. It is more common in females, Asians, and people who are positive for HLA B8, DR2, or DR3. It is a relapsing and remitting condition, usually diagnosed between 30 and 40 years of age. It affects many systems and organs in the body, including the joints, skin, heart, lungs, and kidneys (75% of cases).

The renal lesions are the most important clinically and affect prognosis. Patients present with hematuria, proteinuria (often nephrotic), edema and hypertension. Glomerular changes vary from minimal involvement to diffuse proliferative disease with:
- Immune complex deposition in mesangium.
- Basement membrane thickening.
- Endothelial proliferation.

This results in focal or diffuse proliferative GN, or membranous glomerulopathy. Histologically, SLE is diagnosed by subendothelial and mesangial deposition of immune complexes, which produce a characteristic wire-loop appearance. There may be extrarenal systemic symptoms. Patients may develop CRF, but the prognosis has been improved with immunosuppressive treatment (steroids, cyclophosphamide or mycophenolate).

Rapidly progressive (crescentic) glomerulonephritis (RPGN)
This clinically presents as glomerular disease with renal failure over several weeks. It can be seen as an isolated glomerular disease or as part of systemic illnesses such as SLE, Wegener's granulomatosis and polyarteritis nodosum. As the name suggests, the disease progresses very rapidly and there is a loss of renal function within days to weeks. Histologically, there are usually epithelial crescents seen in the periphery of glomeruli. There is a leakage of fibrin, which stimulates epithelial cells and macrophages within the Bowman's capsule to proliferate and form crescent-shaped masses, reducing glomerular blood supply.

Several serological tests can help clarify the diagnosis:
- Complement levels: reduced in SLE-associated nephritis, membranoproliferative (Hepatitis C associated) and post infectious glomerulonephritis.
- Antinuclear antibodies (ANA): systemic lupus erythematosus (SLE)-associated nephritis.
- ANCA titer: Wegener's granulomatosis (c-ANCA) and polyarteritis nodosum (p-ANCA).
- Cryoglobulin titer: cryoglobulinemia.
- Anti GBM titer: Goodpasture's disease or anti-GBM disease.

Prompt diagnosis and treatment are required to prevent hypertension, kidney scarring, and renal failure. Treatment is high-dose steroids, immunosuppressants, and plasma exchange.

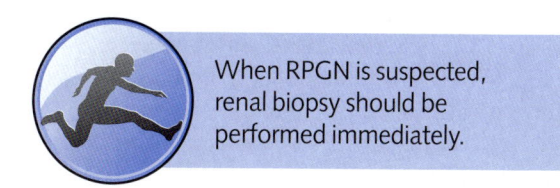

> When RPGN is suspected, renal biopsy should be performed immediately.

Goodpasture's syndrome
In Goodpasture's syndrome, autoantibodies to type IV collagen in the glomerular basement membrane develop, causing inflammation. There may be pulmonary hemorrhage. Renal presentation is with a rapidly progressive "crescentic" GN with acute renal

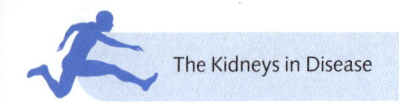

failure and lung hemorrhage. Diagnosis is usually made by lung or renal biopsy. Prognosis is poor without treatment, which involves:
- Plasma exchange (to remove the antibodies).
- Corticosteroids (to reduce inflammation).

Polyarteritis nodosum (PAN; also known as microscopic polyangiitis)
This is a necrotizing vasculitis affecting the small arteries of the body; it is more common in males. There may be abdominal pain, mental status changes, neuropathy, or fevers. Initially, there is a focal, segmental or necrotizing GN followed by RPGN. Histology reveals extensive necrosis, fibrin deposition and epithelial crescents. Microscopic PAN is associated with circulating antineutrophil cytoplasmic antibodies (ANCA), which complex with perinuclear antigen in fixed neutrophils (pANCA). Diagnosis may be made by biopsy of an involved nerve (e.g., sural nerve) or of the kidney.

Wegener's granulomatosis
This is a rare necrotizing vasculitis affecting the nose, upper respiratory tract and kidneys. It typically presents between 40 and 50 years of age. The glomerular disease is similar to that for microscopic PAN, with granuloma formation. Presentation is with asymptomatic hematuria or nephritic syndrome (focal segmental GN) or RPGN. There is often sinusitis. It is associated with ANCA, which characteristically recognizes a cytoplasmic antigen in fixed neutrophils (cANCA).

Diseases of the tubules and interstitium

Overview
The tubules and interstitium are affected by several diseases. Typically, tubules become obstructed (this reduces glomerular filtration) or their transport functions become impaired (reduces water and solute reabsorption). Damage can be acute or chronic.

Acute tubular necrosis (ATN)
ATN is the result of acute tubular cell damage by ischemia or toxins. It is a common cause of acute renal failure (see Chapter 3). It can be oliguric (<400mL/day urine) or nonoliguric. Oliguria results from "backleak," in which tubular fluid leaks out of disrupted tubules and is reabsorbed directly into the blood.

Uremic symptoms develop because there is a significant fall in GFR. This may be due to backleak, hemodynamic changes, or intratubular obstruction. Hyperkalemia can develop as a result of K^+ retention and may trigger cardiac arrhythmias, which can be life-threatening. Recovery is accompanied by a diuretic phase that occurs because of failure of regenerating tubules to concentrate urine.

Mortality is up to 50% but full recovery is possible with prompt treatment—fluid and electrolyte therapy and dialysis if necessary.

Ischemic ATN
This is caused by hypotension and hypovolemic shock following trauma, infections, burns or hemorrhage. There is a rapid fall in blood pressure, which causes hypoperfusion of the peritubular capillaries with consequent tubular necrosis along the entire length of the nephron. The kidneys appear pale and swollen. Histology reveals:
- Infiltration of inflammatory cells and the tubular cells.
- Flattened and vacuolated tubular cells.
- Interstitial edema.
- Cellular debris and protein casts in the distal tubule and the collecting ducts.

NSAIDs can increase the risk of ATN following other renal insults by preventing the synthesis of prostaglandins (PGs). PGs are vasodilators, which protect the kidney from ischemic injury by dilating blood vessels and increasing blood flow.

Toxic ATN
This disorder is caused by agents with specific nephrotoxic activity that damages the epithelial cells. Such substances include:
- Aminoglycoside antibiotics (e.g., gentamicin).
- IV contrast agents.
- Myoglobin (filtered in rhabdomyolysis).
- Organic solvents: carbon tetrachloride in dry-cleaning fluid.
- Heavy metals (gold, mercury, lead, and arsenic).
- Pesticides.

These substances cause the cells to lift away from the basement membrane and consequently collect in and obstruct the tubular lumen. The effect is limited because there is regeneration of the epithelial cells in 10–20 days, which permits clinical recovery and is confirmed by the presence of mitotic figures on biopsy. Damage by nephrotoxic substances is limited to the proximal tubules. The kidneys appear swollen and red.

Tubulointerstitial diseases
Pyelonephritis
This is a bacterial infection of the kidney and results in inflammation and damage to the renal calyces, parenchyma and pelvis. It can be acute or chronic. The urinary tract infections are discussed fully in Chapter 5.

Acute pyelonephritis
This occurs because of infection in the kidney and is spread via two routes:
1. Ascending infection: fecal bacteria enter the kidney from the lower urinary tract if there is an incompetent vesicoureteric valve. This permits vesicoureteric reflux (VUR) and results in ascending transmission of infection.
2. Hematogenous spread: seen in patients with septicemia or infective endocarditis. The pathogens include fungi, bacteria (staphylococci and *Escherichia coli*) and viruses. The kidney is often affected in septicemic diseases because of its large blood supply.

The predisposing factors of acute pyelonephritis are:
- Urinary tract obstruction (congenital and acquired).
- VUR.
- Instrumentation of the urinary tract.
- Sexual intercourse.
- Diabetes mellitus.
- Immunosuppression (HIV, lymphoma and transplants).

Patients present with general malaise, fever, flank pain, tenderness and often rigors with or without symptoms of lower UTI. Infection spreads into the renal pelvis and papillae and causes abscess formation throughout the cortex and medulla.

With retrograde ureteric spread the kidney characteristically contains areas of wedge-shaped suppuration especially at the upper and lower poles. In septicemia there is hematogenous seeding within the kidney and minute abscesses are distributed randomly in the cortex. On histology there is:

- Polymorphic infiltration of the tubules.
- Interstitial edema.
- Focal inflammation.

Uncomplicated cases resolve with 7–14 days of antibiotic treatment and high fluid intake. The important complications of acute pyelonephritis are:
- Renal papillary necrosis.
- Perinephric abscesses.
- Chronic pyelonephritis.
- Fibrosis and scarring.

Chronic pyelonephritis
This condition is characterized by long-standing parenchymal scarring, which develops from tubulointerstitial inflammation. There are two main types:
1. Obstructive: chronic obstruction (stones, tumors or congenital abnormalities) prevents pelvicalyceal drainage and increases the risk of renal infection. Chronic pyelonephritis develops because of recurrent infection.
2. Reflux nephropathy: this is the most common cause of chronic pyelonephritis. It is associated with VUR, which is congenital. The organisms enter the ascending portion of the ureter with refluxed urine as the valvular orifice is held open on contraction of the bladder during micturition. Reflux results from the abnormal angle at which the ureter enters the bladder wall (Fig. 4.8).

The disease process usually begins in childhood and has a silent, insidious onset. Reflux of urine into the renal pelvis occurs during micturition and this increases the pressure in the major calyces. The high intrapelvic pressure forces urine into the collecting ducts, further distorting the internal structure. This is most predominant at the poles of the kidney and results in deep irregular scars on the cortical surface. The tubulointerstitial inflammation heals with the formation of corticomedullary scars that overlie the deformed and dilated calyces, which are characteristic of chronic pyelonephritis.

Renal biopsy is usually not done, but histologically there is interstitial fibrosis and dilated tubules containing eosinophilic casts.

Diagnosis is made by sonography or intravenous pyelography (IVP) (see Chapter 8), which shows distortion of the calyceal system and contraction of the kidney because of cortical scarring. Generally, radiographs are avoided in children and in patients

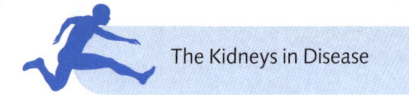

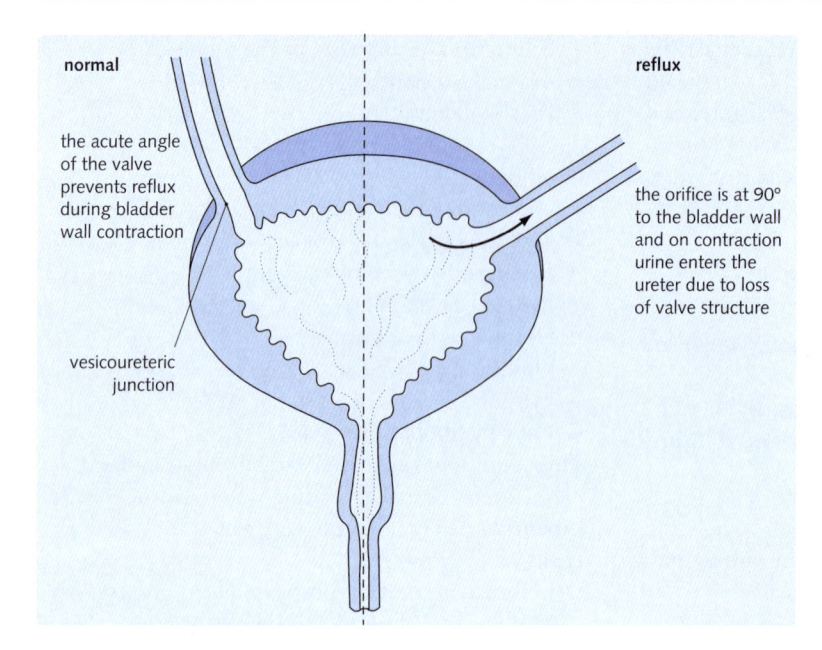

Fig. 4.8 Normal and refluxing vesicoureteric junction.

with renal failure. Ultrasonography is less sensitive than IVP, but is safer.

Drug- and toxin-induced tubulointerstitial nephritis

Drugs (NSAIDs, nafcillin, ampicillin) and heavy metals (mercury, gold, lead) can cause T cell-mediated inflammation in the interstitium. This reaction usually occurs 2–40 days after exposure to the toxin. Clinical features include fever, skin rash, hematuria, proteinuria, and acute renal failure (ARF). Urine eosinophils and WBC casts may be seen. Histology reveals interstitial edema and tubular degeneration with eosinophil infiltration. Withdrawal of the causative agent leads to recovery.

In chronic analgesic abuse with phenacitin, and to a lesser extent aspirin, PG synthesis is inhibited, causing ischemia. This causes papillary necrosis and a secondary tubulonephritis (analgesic nephropathy). It is associated with an increased risk of developing transitional cell carcinomas with chronic analgesic abuse.

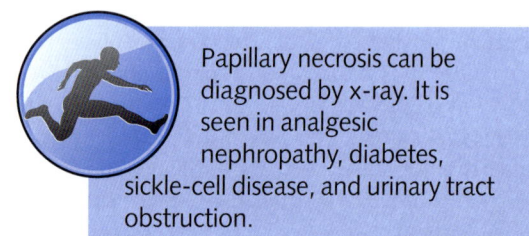

> Papillary necrosis can be diagnosed by x-ray. It is seen in analgesic nephropathy, diabetes, sickle-cell disease, and urinary tract obstruction.

Urate nephropathy

If there is an increased blood uric acid concentration, urate crystals are precipitated in the acidic environment of the collecting ducts, causing inflammatory obstruction and dilatation of the tubules. This eventually leads to fibrosis and atrophy. An increase in urate concentration can be caused by:
- Rapid cell turnover (e.g., in psoriasis or malignancy): in those patients with hematological or lymphatic malignancy who are receiving chemotherapy there is excess cell breakdown and release of nucleic acids, which results in acute urate nephropathy and ARF.
- Reduced uric acid clearance (e.g., in CRF): this is seen in patients with gout, in which there is a long-term deposition of urate in the kidney as a result of the constant high blood urate levels.

Urate nephropathy causes ARF or CKD depending on the time-course of urate deposition:
- Patients with malignancy treated with chemotherapy are prone to ARF.
- Patients with gout are prone to CKD.

Nephrocalcinosis
A persistently high blood Ca^{2+} level causes Ca^{2+} deposition in the kidneys. The hypercalcemia can be due to:
- Primary hyperparathyroidism.
- Multiple myeloma.
- Increased vitamin D activity.
- Bone metastases.

CKD occurs in these patients because of stones (nephrolithiasis) or focal calcification in the renal parenchyma (nephrocalcinosis).

In nephrocalcinosis the Ca^{2+} accumulates in the tubular cells and the basement membrane, resulting in interstitial fibrosis and inflammation. Hypercalcemia also causes a renal concentrating defect, which leads to polyuria, nocturia and dehydration.

Multiple myeloma
Approximately 50% of these patients develop renal damage, sometimes ARF or CKD. They present with proteinuria and urine protein electrophoresis shows a monoclonal Ig spike. Histological changes include:
- Bence-Jones proteins (light chains) enter the urine and these are toxic to the tubular epithelial cells. They precipitate as casts in the tubules, causing inflammation and obstruction to the tubular cells.
- Amyloid lambda (λ) or kappa (κ) light-chain fragments (paraproteins) are deposited in the renal blood vessels, glomeruli and tubules.
- Urate deposition (discussed above).
- Hypercalcemia (discussed above).

Diseases of the renal blood vessels

Hypertensive nephrosclerosis
This is the term given to the changes in renal vasculature in response to long-standing essential hypertension. Renal function usually remains intact, although proteinuria is sometimes detected (usually non-nephrotic) and some patients with poor hypertension control (esp. malignant hypertension) develop chronic renal failure.

The histologic changes consist of hyaline arteriolosclerosis, which is characterized by thickening (due to hyperplasia of smooth muscle) and hyalinization (protein deposition) of the arteriolar wall. This causes narrowing of the lumen of the interlobular arteries, which functionally impairs the smaller branches. The changes are more severe in patients with systemic diseases that affect the renal vessels (e.g., diabetes). The vascular wall lesions gradually reduce the blood supply to the kidney, which leads to ischemic atrophy of the nephrons. This accounts for the small, contracted and granular appearance of the kidneys seen in advanced cases of untreated essential hypertension.

Malignant hypertension
This emergent problem occurs in 1–5% of patients with hypertension. There is a sudden accelerated rise in blood pressure with an increase in diastolic pressure to over 130mmHg. In acute cases the kidney surface appears smooth and is covered in tiny petechial hemorrhages. There are fibrin deposits in the vessel wall, causing necrosis (fibrinoid necrosis), especially in the distal part of the interlobular arteries and the afferent arterioles.

Renal function is impaired because of the ischemia that results from severe arterial damage. Patients have proteinuria and hematuria, which can occasionally be massive. Patients develop renal failure if untreated (in contrast to benign hypertension). Papilledema and cardiac failure are often present. The 5-year survival rate with treatment is 50%.

The trigger for the abrupt and rapid rise in blood pressure is unknown but might be associated with endothelial dysfunction. These patients also have increased plasma levels of renin, angiotensin, and aldosterone. Treatment is aggressive use of IV antihypertensive medication.

Renal artery stenosis
Between 2 and 5% of hypertensive patients have hypertension secondary to renal artery stenosis (RAS) in one or both renal arteries. This is narrowing of the renal arteries caused by atheromatous plaques (70%) or fibromuscular dysplasia within the renal artery wall (Fig. 4.9). Poor renal perfusion stimulates renin secretion. Ischemia of the affected kidney leads to renal failure and a small kidney. Diagnosis is by renal artery Doppler studies, magnetic resonance angiography, nuclear scans, or renal arteriography

The Kidneys in Disease

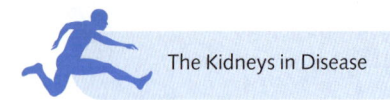

Contrasting clinical findings of fibromuscular dysplasia and atheromatous RAS		
	Fibromuscular dysplasia	Atheromatous RAS
age [years]	<40	>55
sex prevalence	F > M	M > F
bruit heard	80%	40%
vascular disease elsewhere	rare	common
renal failure	rare	well recognized
patient prognosis	good	poor

Fig. 4.9 Comparison between fibromuscular dysplasia and atheromatous renal artery stenosis (RAS).

(the gold standard). Unfortunately, the presence of renal artery stenosis on one of these studies does not predict improved blood pressure control after correction.

Treatment options include:
- **Angioplasty:** to dilate the stenotic region. This can be supplemented with stenting to decrease the risk of restenosis.
- **Bypass surgery** of the narrowed vessels (now uncommon).

Thrombotic microangiopathies

This is a group of diseases that are all characterized by necrosis and thickening of the renal vessel walls and thrombosis in the interlobular arterioles, afferent arterioles and glomeruli. All clinically present with a triad of:
- Hemolysis.
- Thrombocytopenia.
- Acute renal failure.

The main two microangiopathies are:
1. Hemolytic uremic syndrome (HUS).
2. Thrombotic thrombocytopenic purpura (TTP).

Hemolytic uremic syndrome (HUS)

This is characterized by the triad of:
- Microangiopathic hemolytic anemia.
- Thrombocytopenia (decreased platelets).
- Renal failure.

It is classified as:
- **Idiopathic:** this is more common in adults and has a worse prognosis.
- **Secondary:** this more common in children and may be associated with gastroenteritis (e.g., *Escherichia coli* 0157 toxin), drugs (estrogen, cyclosporine A, cytotoxic therapy), or malignancy. HUS can also be caused by accelerated hypertension or, more rarely, there may be a genetic cause.

Clinical features include sudden onset of oliguria with hematuria—occasionally with melena or hematemesis (usually if gastroenteritis is the cause)—and jaundice. Hypertension is seen in 50% of patients.

Treatment involves early supportive therapy with dialysis for renal failure. Fresh frozen plasma can be useful. Approximately 50% of patients later develop hypertension, and a few go on to develop chronic renal failure. Mortality ranges from 5% to 30%.

Thrombotic thrombocytopenic purpura (TTP)

This is a rare and idiopathic condition that is more common in females (usually <40 years) than in males. TTP has a similar disease process to HUS, but affects different sites. The features are thrombocytopenia, microangiopathic hemolytic anemia, fever, neurological signs (CNS involvement), and renal failure. The majority of cases have a CNS component, with thrombosis leading to ischemia in the brain.

Renal involvement occurs in 50% of cases, and presents with:
- Proteinuria.
- Hematuria.
- Renal failure.

Histology shows thrombi consisting of fibrin and platelets in the terminal interlobular arteries, the afferent arterioles and glomerular capillaries. Treatment involves corticosteroid therapy and plasma exchange.

Cholesterol emboli syndrome

Cholesterol emboli syndrome potentially affects all organs in the body because the disrupted cholesterol plaques embolize to all microcirculation. It leads to slowly progressive renal failure. Cholesterol emboli may occur:

Renal and systemic effects of cholesterol embolization	
Kidney effects	**Systemic effects**
hypertension	purple toes
renal failure	livedo reticularis
hematuria	pancreatitis
pyuria	ischemic bowel

Fig. 4.10 Renal and systemic effects of cholesterol embolization.

- Spontaneously.
- During systemic anticoagulation.
- After instrumentation of the arterial system.
- After trauma.

In the latter two cases, mechanical disruption of the cholesterol plaques with resultant showering of the smaller particles is thought to be responsible.

Figure 4.10 lists renal and nonrenal clues to the diagnosis. Renal biopsy is normally not performed. Lab analysis may show eosinophilia, hypocomplementemia, and an increased erythrocyte sedimentation rate.

Although occlusion of blood vessels with emboli is the inciting event, there is evidence that cholesterol emboli cause an immunologic reaction which further damages ischemic as well as normal adjacent tissue.

Treatment is predominantly supportive. Most of these patients develop CKD.

Renal infarction
Embolic infarction
The embolus can come from:
- Thrombotic material from the left side of the heart.
- Atheromatous material from plaques.
- Bacterial vegetations from infective endocarditis.

The emboli lodge in the small renal vessels and cause narrowing of the arterioles and focal areas of ischemic injury. It can be asymptomatic, or present with hematuria and flank tenderness. The areas of infarction appear pale and are characteristically wedge shaped.

Diffuse cortical necrosis
Diffuse cortical necrosis causes ARF and presents with anuria. This is a rare condition that results from profound hypertension caused by:

- Severe hypovolemic shock.
- Sepsis.
- Eclampsia (pregnancy).

In response to hypotension, there is compensatory vasoconstriction that can cause infarction. This can be avoided by prompt resuscitation of the shocked patient. Once the disease is established, no agent has been shown to improve outcome. Prognosis is much better for focal infarction than for generalized cortical infarction. The surface of the kidney appears patchy with irregular yellow areas of necrosis, congestion and hemorrhage (limited to the outer part of the cortex). Infarcts can calcify over time.

Sickle-cell disease nephropathy
Thrombotic occlusion by deformed sickle-shaped red cells causes papillary necrosis. It is precipitated by cold, dehydration, infection and exercise. Presentation is with pain, hematuria and polyuria. Management involves analgesia, warmth and rehydration, blood transfusions and antibiotics (if infection is suspected).

Neoplastic disease of the kidney

Benign tumors of the kidney
These rarely cause symptoms and are usually found on autopsy. They include:
- Renal fibroma or hamartoma (most common).
- Cortical adenoma.
- Angiomyolipoma ("hamartomatous malformation").
- Oncocytoma.

Malignant tumors of the kidney
Renal cell carcinoma (RCC)
Incidence and risk factors
Approximately 90% of renal malignant tumors in adults are RCCs, which arise from the tubular epithelium. RCC is very rare in children and has a peak incidence in 60–70 year olds. The male-to-female ratio is 3:1. It has great geographical variance with the highest incidence in Scandinavia and the lowest in South America and Africa. Risk factors are:
- Smoking.
- Acquired cystic disease in patients who require renal replacement therapy: RCC tends to occur at a much earlier age in these patients.

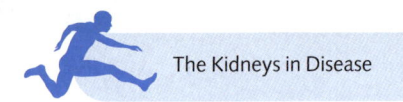

- Von Hippel–Lindau disease: this is a rare autosomal dominant condition caused by a mutation on chromosome 25; 50–70% of these patients develop RCC.

Presentation
Approximately 90% of cases present as hematuria. Nonspecific symptoms include fatigue, weight loss, and fever. There might be a mass in the flank. These are all late manifestations, presenting at an advanced stage of tumor progression, which is why prognosis is poor. RCC often metastasizes before local symptoms develop.

Some RCCs can secrete hormone-like substances such as:
- Parathyroid hormone (PTH), resulting in hypercalcemia.
- ACTH, resulting in a Cushing's-like syndrome.
- Erythropoietin, resulting in polycythemia.
- Renin, resulting in hypertension.

As a result of these hormone-producing tumors, RCC commonly presents with paraneoplastic syndromes.

Diagnosis
Diagnosis is by:
- Ultrasonography: distinguishes between solid and cystic lesions.
- Computed tomography (CT): provides preoperative staging (see Chapter 8).

Pathology
RCC consists of a yellow–brown, well-demarcated mass in the renal cortex, with a diameter of 3–15 cm. Within this area there are patches of hemorrhage, necrosis and cyst formation. The tumors are most common at the upper pole of the kidney. The renal capsule is often intact, although it can be breached and the tumor will extend into the perinephric fat. Spread into the renal vein is often visible and rarely this extends into the inferior vena cava. Histology reveals cells with clear cytoplasm that range from well differentiated to anaplastic.

Spread occurs by direct invasion of local tissues, via the lymph to lumbar nodes (one-third of cases), and via the blood (venous). Metastases are found in the lung, liver, bone, contralateral kidney and adrenals; these may be seen without local spread.

> Renal cell carcinoma commonly presents with painless hematuria; distant metastases and the paraneoplastic syndrome are common.

Prognosis
Prognosis depends on tumor size and the degree of the spread; RCC staging involves assessing local, nodal and metastatic spread (TNM classification).
- T_1: confined to the kidney.
- T_2: enlarging tumor with distortion of the kidney with renal capsule intact.
- T_3: spread through the renal capsule into the perinephric fat with invasion into the renal vein.
- T_4: invasion into adjacent organs or the abdominal wall.
- N^+: lymph node involvement.
- M^+: metastatic spread.

Treatment
If there are no distant metastases, treatment involves a radical nephrectomy with removal of the associated adrenal gland, perinephric fat, upper ureter, and para-aortic lymph nodes. Postoperative radiotherapy is required to decrease risk of recurrence. There is little effective treatment available for metastatic disease. The average 5-year survival rate is 45%, increasing up to 70% if there is no metastatic disease at diagnosis.

Wilms' tumor (nephroblastoma)
Incidence and presentation
This is the most common malignant tumor in children. The peak incidence is in 1- to 4-year-olds, with both sexes affected equally. It is an embryonic tumor derived from the primitive metanephros. It presents with an abdominal mass and occasionally hematuria, abdominal pain and hypertension.

Pathology
The tumors are large solid masses of firm white tissue with areas of necrosis and hemorrhage. They often breach the renal capsule and grow into the perinephric fat. Histology reveals spindle cells or primitive blastema cells with epithelial and mesenchymal tissues, cartilage, bone and muscle.

They are aggressive tumors, often presenting with metastatic disease of the lung.

Treatment and prognosis
Treatment involves nephrectomy, radiotherapy and chemotherapy. The long-term survival rate is over 80%. Prognosis depends upon tumor size and distant spread at the time of diagnosis.

Urothelial carcinoma of the renal pelvis
This is a transitional cell tumor accounting for 5–10% of renal tumors. It can be caused by:
- Analgesic abuse.
- Exposure to aniline dyes used in the industrial manufacture of dyes, rubber and plastics.

Presentation with hematuria or obstruction occurs early, because the renal pelvis projects directly into the pelvicalyceal cavity.

Histology ranges from well-differentiated tumors to diffuse, invasive and anaplastic carcinomas. Poorly differentiated tumors have a poor prognosis and often invade the wall of the renal pelvis and the renal vein. Multiple tumors are also often found in the ureters and bladder. Fragments of papillary tumor and atypical tumor cells can be detected in the urine and this makes cytological diagnosis possible.

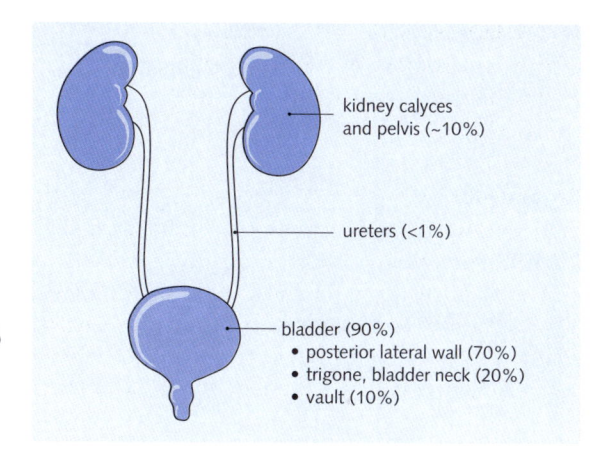

> Metastases from lymphomas, lung or breast cancer, or melanomas can deposit in the kidneys.

Fig. 4.11 Common tumor sites throughout the urinary tract.

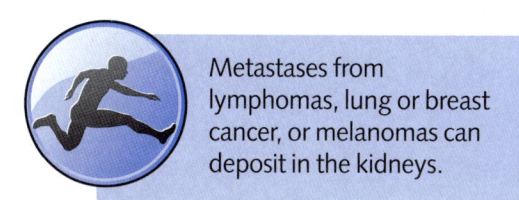

- kidney calyces and pelvis (~10%)
- ureters (<1%)
- bladder (90%)
  - posterior lateral wall (70%)
  - trigone, bladder neck (20%)
  - vault (10%)

Figure 4.11 summarizes the common tumor sites throughout the urinary tract. Bladder and urethral tumors will be discussed in Chapter 5.

Renal responses to systemic disorders

Congestive heart failure (CHF)
CHF occurs when the pump mechanism of the heart cannot cope with its work load (i.e., providing the body with its metabolic requirements) so the cardiac output fails to perfuse the tissues adequately. This results in hypoperfusion of tissues and sodium and water retention. CHF is the common end result of all types of severe heart disease.

> CHF can be caused by:
> - Pump failure (low output heart failure).
> - Increased demand (high output heart failure).
>
> A normal heart can fail under high loads, but an abnormal heart will fail under normal loads.

A fall in cardiac output leads to renal hypoperfusion. The kidney senses this as a sign of hypovolemia and compensates by retaining NaCl and water to increase the circulating volume (Fig. 4.12). As the kidney attempts to increase the circulating fluid volume, peripheral edema develops (left heart failure). This increases pulmonary venous pressure, stimulating fluid transudation from the capillaries in the lungs, which results in pulmonary edema. Hyponatremia may result from excess ADH stimulation. If the cardiac output falls markedly, autoregulation may fail and prerenal acute renal failure may occur.

The Kidneys in Disease

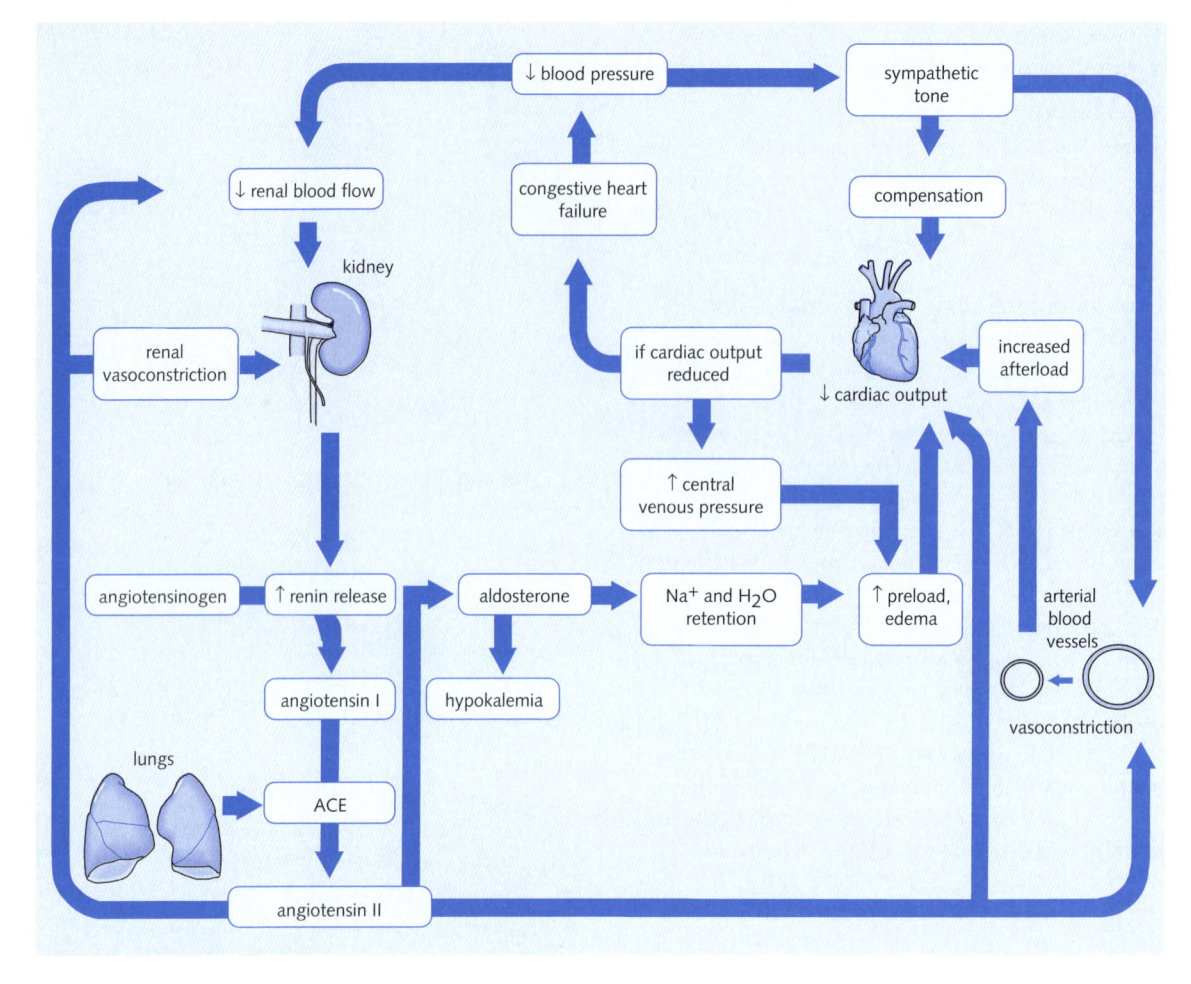

Fig. 4.12 Compensatory mechanisms in congestive heart failure (CHF). ACE, angiotensin-converting enzyme.

Treatment and management

Management involves reducing the fluid load within the body and thereby decreasing the workload of the heart.
- Diuretics: produce symptomatic relief from pulmonary edema.
- Nitrates: produce venodilation, which decreases preload.
- Vasodilators (e.g. hydralazine): these reduce afterload.
- ACE inhibitors: act as afterload-reducing vasodilators (by reducing the synthesis of angiotensin II) and as diuretics (by decreasing aldosterone synthesis).
- Beta blockers
- Spironolactone

Prognosis depends on the overall clinical picture, and the extent of cardiovascular disease. For further information refer to *Crash course: Cardiovascular system*.

Hypovolemia and shock

Shock is a medical emergency in which the vital organs are hypoperfused as a result of either an inadequate circulating blood volume or heart failure. As the amount of oxygen and nutrients delivered to the cells is inadequate, the resulting hypoxic state within the cells leads to anaerobic metabolism and there is inefficient clearance of the metabolites, which build up in the cell. A severe decrease in the circulating volume stimulates sympathetic activity to maintain the blood pressure (BP) by:

- Tachycardia.
- Peripheral vasoconstriction.
- Increase in myocardial contractility.

Vasodilation occurs in the vital organs (heart, lungs, brain) to maintain blood supply, but this is at the expense of perfusion to other organs. If there is inadequate compensation, tissue hypoxia and necrosis can occur in vulnerable organs (e.g. acute tubular necrosis in the kidneys).

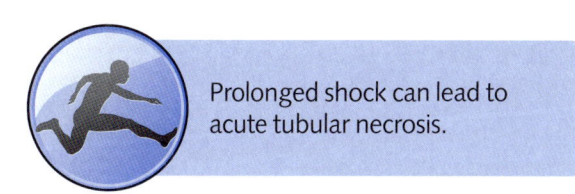

Prolonged shock can lead to acute tubular necrosis.

Types of shock
Cardiogenic shock
This occurs when the heart fails to maintain CO acutely (e.g., ischemic heart disease, arrhythmias). As a result, tissue perfusion decreases dramatically. Venous pressure increases, causing pulmonary or peripheral edema (as described above). Prognosis is poor (90% mortality).

Hypovolemic shock
This occurs when there is an acute reduction in effective circulating blood volume:
- Exogenous losses of plasma (e.g., burns), of blood (e.g., hemorrhage), or of water and electrolytes (e.g., diarrhea and vomiting).
- Endogenous losses of fluid (e.g., sepsis and anaphylaxis).

Figure 4.13 shows the response to a fall in circulating fluid volume. To avoid excessive sympathetic activity in the kidneys (which results in vasoconstriction), more vasodilating prostaglandins (PGE_2 and PGI_2) are secreted within the kidneys. This maintains an adequate blood flow through the kidney to allow sufficient glomerular filtration, unless the shock is severe.

A shift to anaerobic metabolism as a result of hypoxia in the tissues eventually causes a lactic acidosis with an anion gap metabolic acidosis. This is worsened as hypovolemia becomes more severe, as less urine is excreted and H^+ is no longer excreted.

Treatment
Treatment of cardiogenic shock involves inotropes, whereas treatment of hypovolemic shock requires fluid replacement to restore the extracellular volume. Septic shock often requires vasoconstricting pressor agents like dopamine or vasopressin. If blood flow to the kidneys is not restored, renal failure results from tissue anoxia and necrosis and hemodialysis may be needed to support the patient.

Hepatorenal syndrome (HRS)
HRS is an oliguric acute renal failure seen in patients with severe chronic liver disease. It usually portends death without urgent liver transplantation.

Patients with liver disease can have a reduced urine flow (oliguria). This is especially so in patients with portal hypertension and ascites. Portal hypertension results from an increase in intrahepatic resistance to blood flow from the gut and spleen, resulting in venous congestion. There is concurrent splanchnic arterial vasodilation. This stimulates renin release. As there appears to be a fall in arterial blood volume, Na^+ and water are retained. As a result of increased resistance in the liver caused by hepatic cirrhosis, hydrostatic pressure in the portal vein increases. This causes fluid to accumulate in the peritoneal cavity (ascites) as fluid is forced out of the interstitial capillaries. This further reduces the circulating blood volume, which again stimulates release of renin, angiotensin, and other vasoconstricting agents. Thus, a positive feedback loop promoting renal vasoconstriction is set up. An irreversible renal vasoconstriction results in the most severe cases.

Liver disease can also impair albumin synthesis. This decreases the oncotic (colloid osmotic) pressure in the capillaries, favoring fluid movement out and worsening the ascites. Circulating blood volume is further reduced.

Patients present with oliguria, acute renal failure, and urine Na < 10mEq/L. Urinalysis is bland. This can also be seen in reversible prerenal failure, but unlike hepatorenal syndrome, prerenal failure is reversible by volume repletion with albumin. ATN can usually be distinguished from HRS by its active urinary sediment (granular casts, renal tubular epithelial cells.)

The Kidneys in Disease

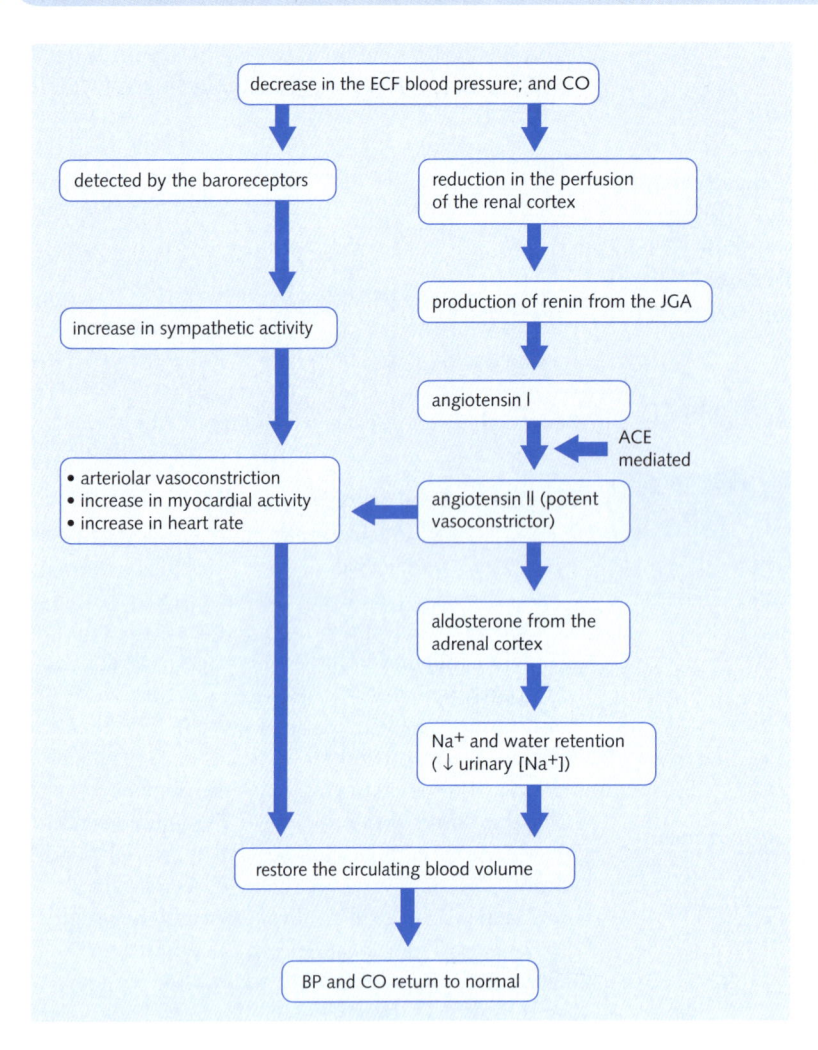

Fig. 4.13 Response to a fall in circulating fluid volume. ACE, angiotensin-converting enzyme; BP, blood pressure; CO, cardiac output; ECF, extracellular fluid; JGA, juxtaglomerular apparatus.

> Because of its poor prognosis, hepatorenal syndrome should be distinguished from reversible prerenal renal failure and from acute tubular necrosis, often seen in sick patients with liver failure.

In HRS, the renal failure may become irreversible and require dialysis. This usually predicts imminent death from liver failure unless liver transplantation can be performed.

Renal responses to systemic disorders

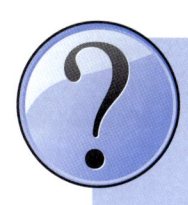

- Compare and contrast unilateral and bilateral renal agenesis. Explain what causes renal agenesis.
- What are common complications of autosomal dominant polycystic kidney disease?
- Outline the system used to classify glomerular disease.
- Define the nephritic and nephrotic syndromes, and list two primary diseases and two secondary diseases for each.
- What are the complications of the nephrotic syndrome, and how are they managed?
- Describe the systemic manifestations of Henoch Schönlein Purpura (HSP).
- Outline the causes of acute interstitial nephritis and how you would make the diagnosis.
- For acute and chronic pyelonephritis, discuss the etiology, predisposing factors, appearance of the kidney and histology.
- Outline the changes seen in the renal vasculature in hypertension. Describe the two main types of hypertension.
- Describe the diagnosis and management of renal artery stenosis.
- What are the thrombotic microangiopathies? Describe the major differences between the two main types.
- Discuss renal cell carcinoma, noting its incidence, the age group affected, predisposing factors, presentation and morphology.
- Describe a Wilms' tumor and clarify which age group it affects.
- Explain the compensatory mechanisms that come into effect in CHF.
- Outline the different types of shock and their effects on renal physiology.
- Explain how to differentiate hepatorenal syndrome from ATN and prerenal azotemia.
- Describe which immune disorders affect the kidney.
- Outline the use of ACE inhibitors in the treatment of glomerular disease.

Fig. 5.1 Anatomy of the male urinary tract.

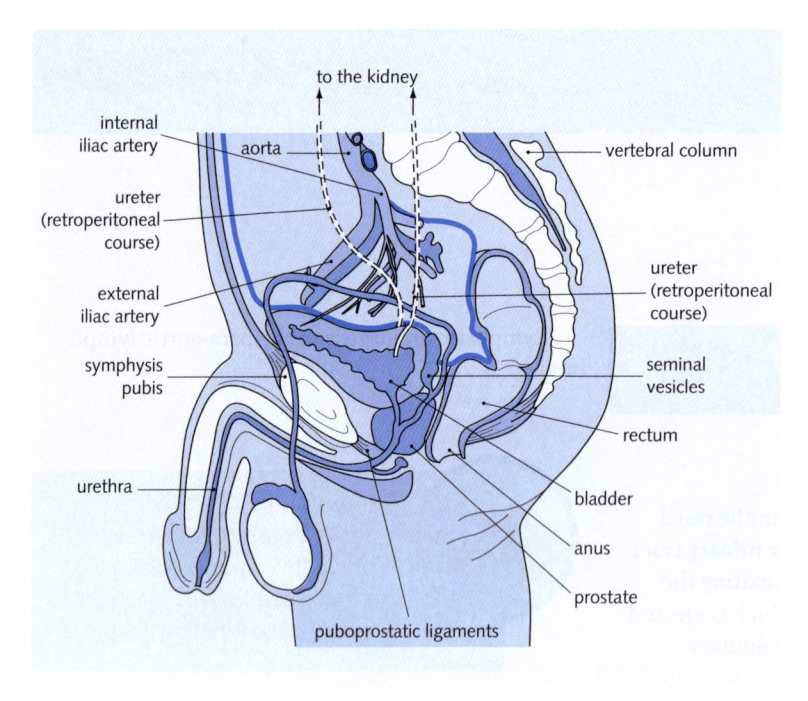

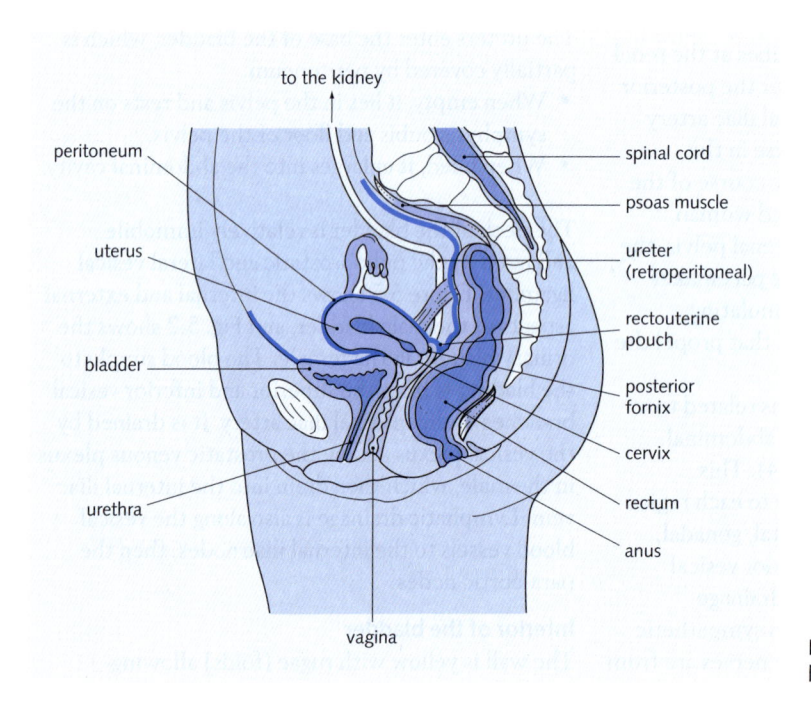

Fig. 5.2 Anatomy of the female lower urinary tract.

Organization of the lower urinary tract

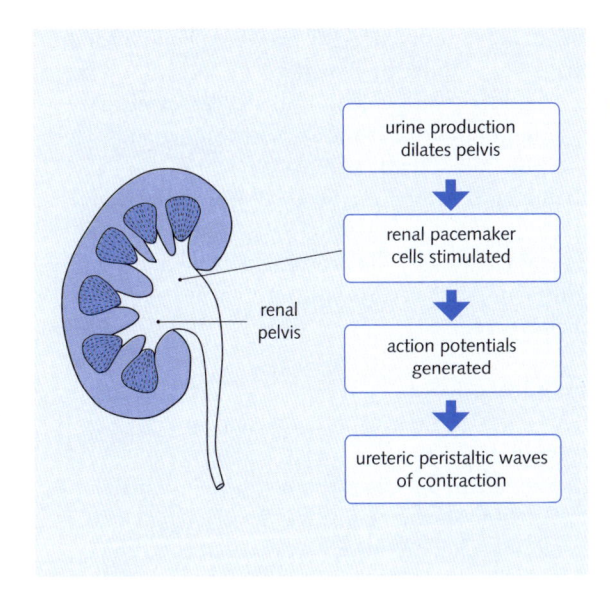

Fig. 5.3 Mechanism of ureteric peristalsis.

- The internal urethral sphincter is not under voluntary control and thus contracts reflexly.
- The external urethral sphincter is under voluntary control.

Bladder innervation (Fig. 5.6) is both:
- **Sensory:** gives sensation (awareness) of a full bladder and also pain from disease. The impulses are suppressed if the bladder is empty.
- **Motor:** parasympathetic activity stimulates the detrusor muscle, so the bladder contracts. It also inhibits the external urethral sphincter, which relaxes to allow micturition. Sympathetic activity inhibits the detrusor muscle, so the bladder relaxes, and stimulates the urethral sphincter (this contracts). Both these actions prevent micturition. Clinically, anticholinergic drugs may cause urinary retention, while α blockers (e.g., terazosin) treat urinary retention.

Male urethra

The male urethra (Fig. 5.7) is longer than the female urethra (male = 20 cm, female = 4 cm). It runs through the neck of bladder, the prostate gland, the floor of pelvis, and the perineal membrane to the

The bladder is lined by smooth muscle, known as the detrusor muscle, which, like the ureter, is arranged in spiral, long and circular bundles. Smooth muscle bundles surround the bladder neck to form the internal urethral sphincter, which is under involuntary control. Slightly further along the urethra there is a skeletal muscle sphincter—the external urethral sphincter. This is under voluntary control.

Fig. 5.4 Regions of the ureter and cross-sectional view, highlighting the normal points of reduced diameter at which stones commonly lodge.

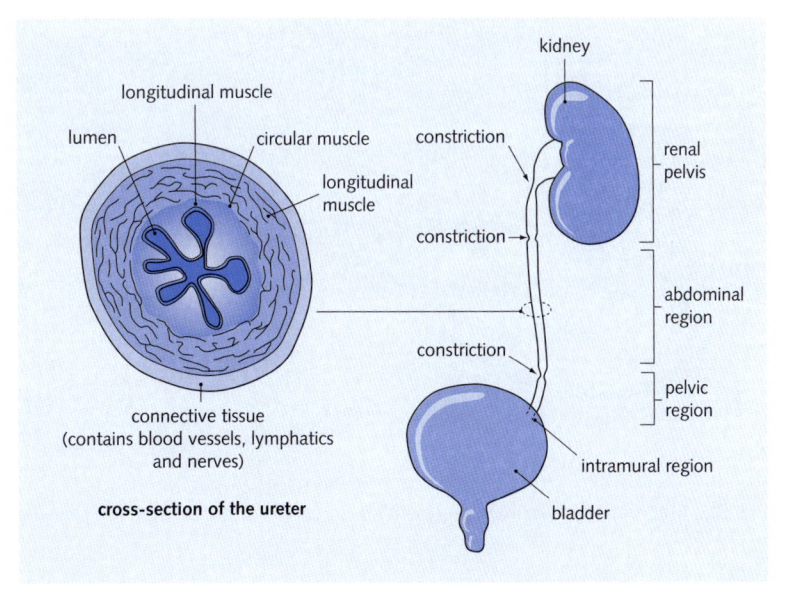

105

The Lower Urinary Tract

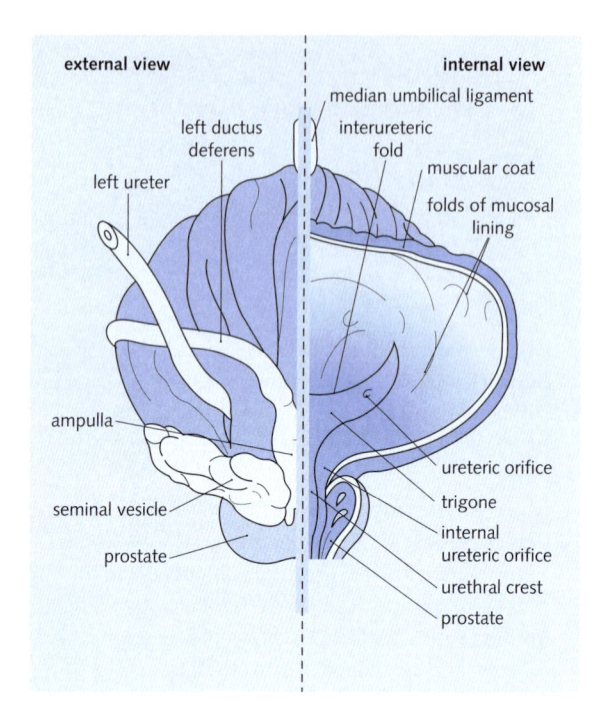

Fig. 5.5 Posterior and interior view of the male bladder.

penis and external urethral orifice at the tip of the glans penis. It has three parts:
1. Prostatic urethra: surrounded by prostate tissue.
2. Membranous urethra: the shortest region, with sphincter activity.
3. Spongy urethra: surrounded by penile tissue.

It is innervated by the prostatic plexus, and lymphatic drainage is to the internal iliac and deep inguinal nodes.

Female urethra
This starts at the neck of the bladder and passes through the floor of the pelvis and perineal membrane to open into the vestibule just anterior to the opening of the vagina. It is 4 cm in length and is firmly attached to the anterior wall of the vagina. Lymphatics drain to the internal and external iliac lymph nodes.

Prostate
This is a gland lying below the bladder in the male and surrounding the proximal part of the urethra (prostatic urethra). It measures $4 \times 3 \times 2$ cm and

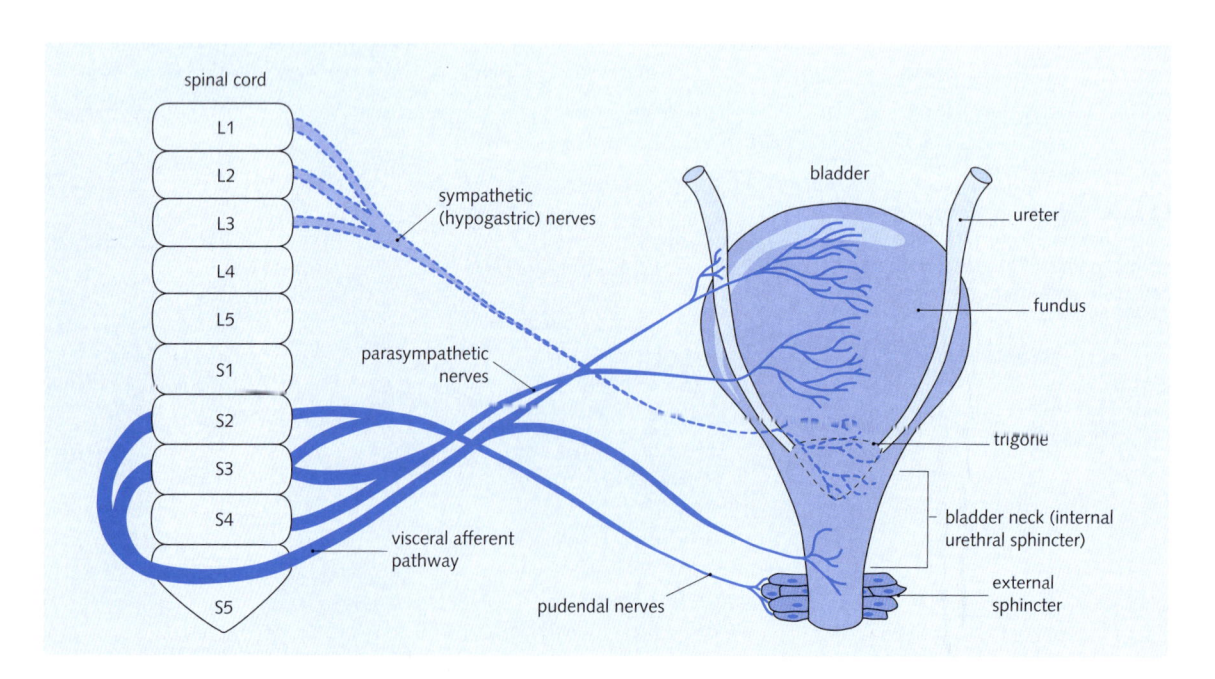

Fig. 5.6 Innervation of the bladder (from Koeppen BM, Stanton B: *Renal physiology*, 2nd ed. Mosby Year Book, 1996).

106

Organization of the lower urinary tract

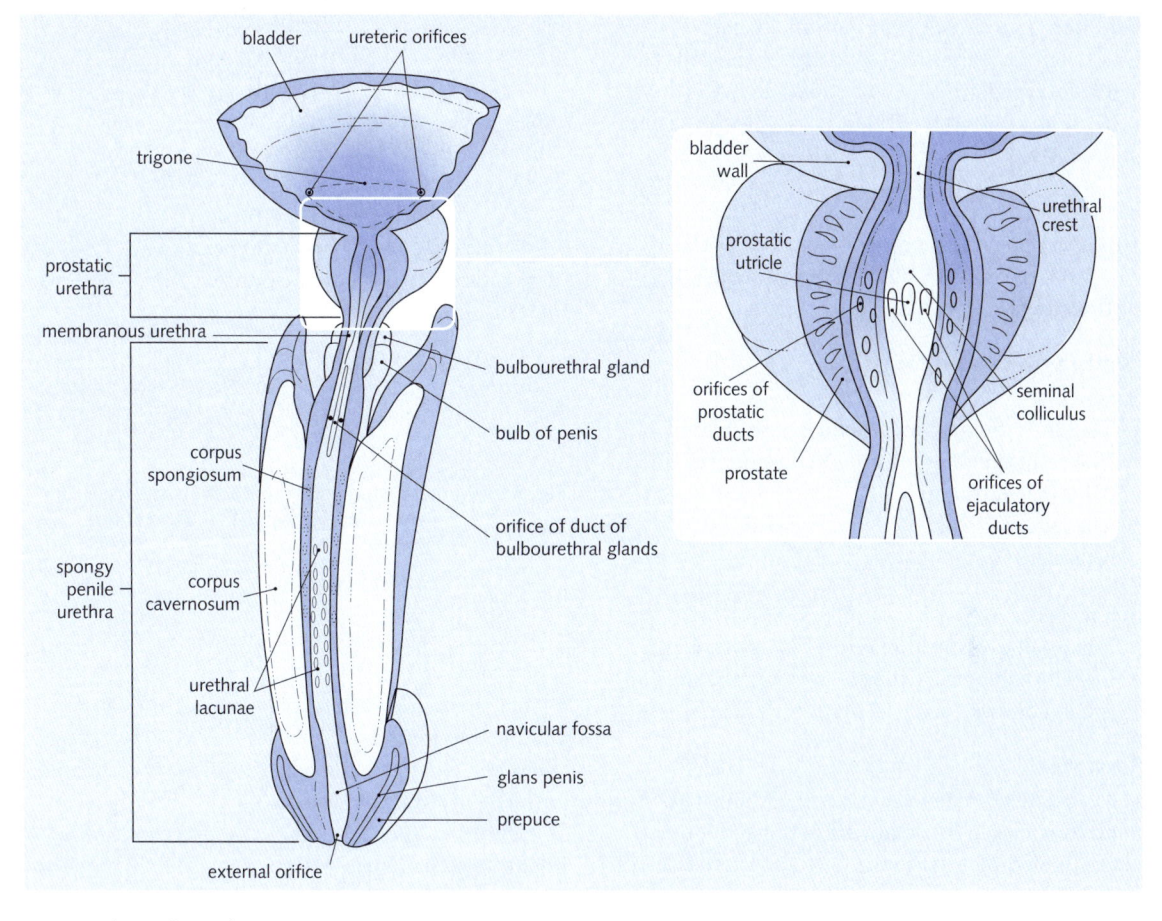

Fig. 5.7 The male urethra.

is conical in shape. It is connected to the bladder by connective tissue stroma and has three lobes.

The prostate has a connective tissue capsule, which is surrounded by a thick sheath from the pelvic fascia. It is influenced by sex hormones resulting in growth during puberty. From the 4th decade onwards, it hypertrophies and nodules of hyperplastic glandular and connective tissue form. As the prostate surrounds the urethra, any enlargement can narrow the urethra and obstruct urine flow.

The prostate is supplied by the inferior vesical artery and blood drains via the prostatic plexus to the vesical plexus and internal iliac vein. Lymphatics drain to the internal iliac and sacral nodes. The prostatic plexus innervates the prostate.

Microstructure of the distal urinary tract
Ureters

The muscular layers are made of smooth muscle arranged in layers (see Fig. 5.4):
- A longitudinal layer just outside the lumen.
- A middle circular layer.
- Another longitudinal layer.

The lumen is lined by urinary epithelium (also known as urothelium or transitional epithelium), which is folded in the relaxed state allowing the ureter to dilate during the passage of urine.

Urothelium (transitional epithelium)
The plasma membranes of urothelium are thicker than other cell membranes, preventing interstitial

fluid from entering the concentrated urine. Urothelium is impermeable to urine. The cells have highly interdigitating cell junctions, allowing the epithelium to stretch without damaging the surfaces of the cells.

Bladder
This is similar to that of the lower third of the ureter, with smooth muscle walls and transitional epithelium.

Urethra (male and female)
In males:
- The prostatic urethra is lined by urothelium.
- The rest is lined by stratified or pseudostratified columnar epithelium.
- The external opening is lined by stratified squamous epithelium.

In females:
- Proximally, the urethra is lined by urothelium.
- Distally and at the external opening, the urethra is lined by stratified squamous epithelium.

Prostate
The prostate contains a central zone of mucosal glands originating prenatally from the endoderm. These drain directly into the urethra. There is also a peripheral zone of mucosal glands, derived from the mesoderm, which drains into the ducts that enter the urethral sinus. Prostatic glandular epithelium can vary from inactive low cuboidal cells to active pseudostratified columnar cells, depending on the degree of androgen stimulation from the testes. The glands secrete 75% of seminal fluid, which is thin, milky and rich in citric acid and hydrolytic enzymes (e.g., fibrinolysin). This prostatic secretion liquefies coagulated semen after deposition in the female genital tract. The prostate is covered by a stroma and capsule made of dense fibroelastic connective tissue with a smooth muscle component.

Micturition

Normal micturition
Micturition is the intermittent voiding of urine stored in the bladder. It is an autonomic reflex that is under voluntary control. The inside of the bladder wall is folded and can expand and accommodate fluid with little increase in pressure. However, it can accommodate only a certain volume of fluid before an increase in intravesical pressure occurs, causing an urge to micturate. Figure 5.8 shows a normal cystometrogram in which pressure rise is compared with rise in volume in the bladder.

Figure 5.6 shows the innervation of the bladder. In infants, micturition is a local spinal reflex where the bladder empties upon reaching a critical pressure. However, in adults this reflex is under voluntary control, so can be inhibited or initiated by higher centers in the brain. Higher-center stimulation of the pudendal nerves keeps the external sphincter closed until it is appropriate to urinate. Bladder distension with urine stimulates bladder stretch receptors, which, in turn, stimulate the afferent limb of voiding reflex and parasympathetic fibers of the bladder, resulting in the desire to urinate. During micturition:
- Perineal muscles and the external urethral sphincter relax.
- The detrusor muscle contracts (parasympathetic activity).
- Urine flows out of the bladder.

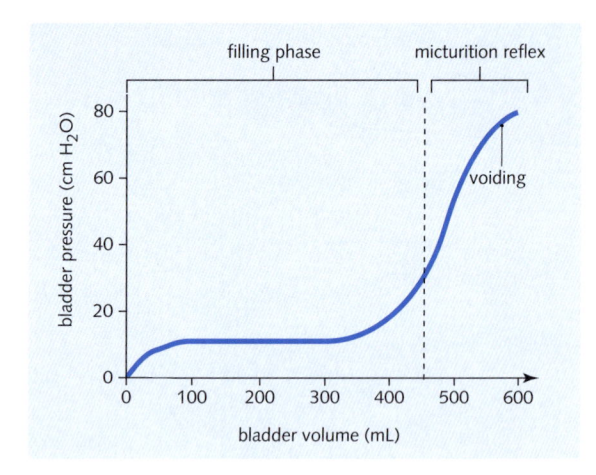

Fig. 5.8 Normal cystometrogram showing the rise in pressure associated with increasing bladder volume.

Figure 5.9 illustrates the voluntary control of micturition.

Abnormal micturition
Neurological lesions
Urinary continence is affected by various neurological lesions along the micturition pathway, as summarized in Fig. 5.10.

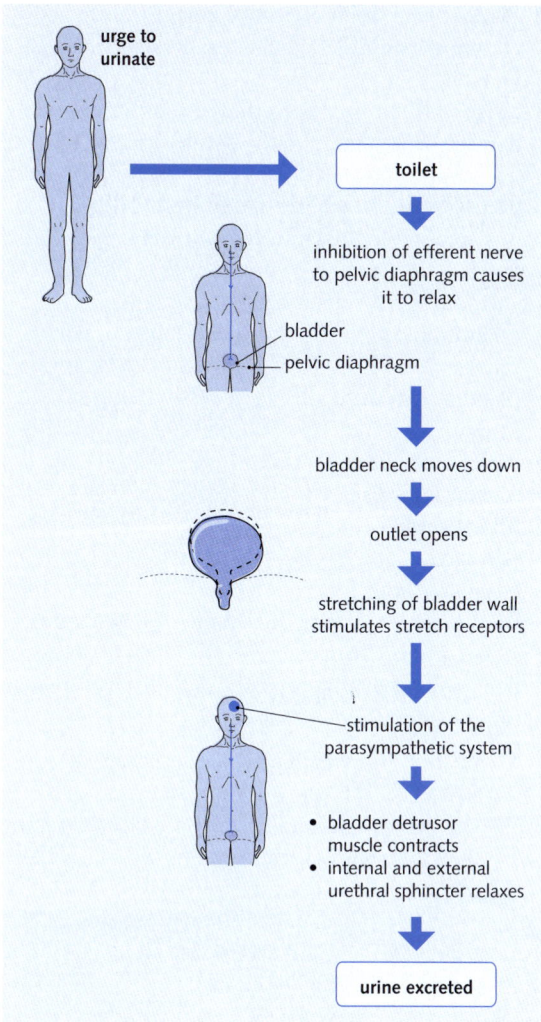

Micturition

Fig. 5.9 Voluntary control of micturition.

Fig. 5.10 Sites of damage along the micturition pathway.

Lesion in the superior frontal gyrus
This can be the result of a stroke, and leads to:
- Reduced desire to urinate.
- Difficulty stopping micturition once started.

Lesion of afferent nerves from the bladder
A lesion of afferent sensory nerves from the bladder (e.g., caused by disease of the dorsal roots such as tabes dorsalis) prevents reflex contractions of the bladder, so the bladder becomes distended, thin-walled, and hypotonic.

Lesion of both afferent and efferent nerves
A lesion of both afferent and efferent nerves (e.g., because of a tumor of the cauda equina or filum terminale) results in:
- Initially: bladder flaccidity and distention.
- Later: bladder hyperactivity with dribbling.

This eventually leads to a shrunken bladder with a hypertrophied bladder wall.

Spinal cord lesion
A lesion to the spinal cord (e.g., spinal shock following trauma) results in:
- Initially (spinal shock): overflow incontinence because of a flaccid and unresponsive bladder. This results in overfill and dribbling.
- After shock has passed: the voiding reflex returns, but with no control from higher centers, so the patient has no voluntary control over voiding.
- Occasionally: hyperactive voiding might be seen.
- Eventually: bladder capacity falls and the wall hypertrophies—spastic neurogenic bladder.

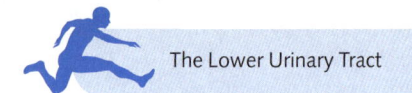

> Spinal cord injuries lead to reflex micturition, as is seen in infants. This occurs because, like infants, patients with spinal cord lesions cannot synchronize detrusor muscle contractions with sphincter relaxation.

Other disorders affecting micturition

Spina bifida
This is a developmental defect in which the posterior neural arches of the spine fail to develop, so part of the spinal cord and its coverings are exposed. It forms a spectrum of defects, resulting in varying degrees of bladder dysfunction.

Diabetes mellitus
Neuropathy is a common complication of diabetes. It can result in a loss of sensation, so there is no desire to micturate and the patient voids infrequently. This eventually leads to bladder distension, with overflow incontinence. The presence of residual urine increases the risk of infection.

Multiple sclerosis
This is demyelination of white matter. The bladder symptoms that develop depend on the level at which demyelination occurs.

Pelvic surgery
The nerve supply to the bladder can be injured during surgery, resulting in postoperative urinary retention. This is usually transient.

Urinary incontinence
Urinary incontinence is the involuntary loss of urine. It affects more women than men and is a socially distressing condition. There are several different types.

Stress incontinence ("sphincter insufficiency")
This is involuntary loss of urine following an increase in intra-abdominal pressure (e.g., cough). It is caused by:
- Pelvic floor laxity (usually seen in multiparous women).
- Bladder neck sphincter impairment (more common in middle-aged, obese, multiparous women).
- Surgery affecting the urethra or prostate causing damage or weakness to the external sphincter.

Urge incontinence ("detrusor instability")
This is involuntary loss of urine, with an urgent "need to go." It is due to sensory or motor dysfunction of the bladder. Causes include:
- Inflammation or infection of the lower urinary tract.
- Bladder hyperreflexia.
- Stroke.
- Parkinson's disease.
- Alzheimer's disease.
- Brain tumor.
- Old age.
- Herniated spinal disc.
- Detrusor overactivity caused by a foreign body, stone, or urethritis.
- Benign prostatic hypertrophy and obstruction (can cause bladder hypersensitivity).
- Loop diuretics.
- Cough or sneeze.

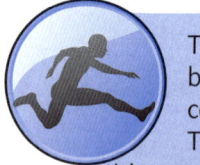

> The detrusor muscle is the bladder muscle and contracts to cause voiding. This is an automatic reflex, triggered by filling of the bladder to a critical pressure.

Overflow incontinence
This is involuntary leakage of urine when the bladder is full. It is usually due to chronic urine retention secondary to obstruction or an atonic bladder. The causes are:
- Outlet obstruction: fecal impaction, benign prostatic hypertrophy (enlarged prostate).
- Underactive detrusor muscle.
- Bladder neck stricture.
- Urethral stricture.
- Alpha-adrenergic agonists.
- Intra- or postoperative overdistention.

- Use of anticholinergics, calcium channel blockers, sedatives.
- Bladder denervation following surgery.

Total incontinence
This is continuous loss of urine with no voluntary control. The causes are:
- Congenital.
- Paraplegia, multiple sclerosis, spina bifida.
- Trauma to the external sphincter, bladder neck and perineal muscles.
- Fistula secondary to radiation, surgery, tumor, invasive neoplasms, obstetric injury.

Functional incontinence
This is incontinence due to severe cognitive impairment or mobility limitations, preventing use of the toilet. For example, there might be difficulty in reaching the toilet or difficulty in undressing, and the patient is "caught short." Bladder function is normal.

Nocturnal enuresis—bedwetting
Nocturnal enuresis is a childhood disorder. It can be primary (since birth) or secondary (acquired). Both can be due to:
- Uninhibited bladder activity.
- Urinary infection.
- Neurological disease.
- Obstruction.

After urinary tract infection has been excluded, no further investigation should be performed if the child is less than 5 years old—unless there are any urinary symptoms. Treatment should focus on behavior therapy, with drug treatment used only as a last resort—sublingual desmopressin is one example.

Diagnostic approach
Figure 5.11 shows an algorithm for the investigation of urinary incontinence.

Congenital abnormalities of the urinary tract

Ureteric abnormalities
These occur in 2–5% of the population. They are frequently bilateral and have usually no clinical relevance. Occasionally, however, they might be associated with an obstruction of urine flow.

Double and bifid ureters
The ureters along with the calyces and collecting ducts are formed from an outgrowth of the mesonephric (Wolffian) duct called the ureteric bud. Early splitting of the ureteric bud or the development of two buds results in the development of double (bifid) ureters (Fig. 5.12). The duplication can be:
- Partial: the two ureters meet before entering the bladder together.
- Complete: the two ureters enter the bladder separately. The upper pole ureter enters the bladder lower and more medially than the lower ureter (see Fig. 5.12).

It is often associated with double renal pelvises with their own renal parenchyma. Renal function is rarely affected. There is a strong predisposition to infection. Urine can reflux from the bladder, especially through the upper pole ureter. Treatment involves excision of the refluxing ureter (usually the upper one).

Ureteropelvic junction obstruction
This often presents in infancy, although milder forms might not present until later in adult life or be found in asymptomatic patients at post-mortem. It is more common in males and in the left ureter. It is bilateral in 20% of cases, and might present as a mass in the flank or pain after drinking. It is thought to result from abnormal smooth muscle organization at the ureteropelvic junction. It can be accompanied by renal agenesis of the opposite kidney; the reason for this is unknown. As a result of the back pressure from the obstruction, the pelvicalyceal system (Fig. 5.13) dilates. If the pressure is transmitted up to the kidneys, the renal tissue atrophies. If bilateral, renal failure can result.

Diverticula
Diverticula are outpouchings of the ureteral wall; they are usually congenital. They are very common and create sites for the stasis of urine. This increases the risk of urine infection because the continuous flow of urine through the urinary tract is a protective mechanism against infection. Acquired diverticula can develop if the pressure in the ureters increases (e.g., because of obstruction).

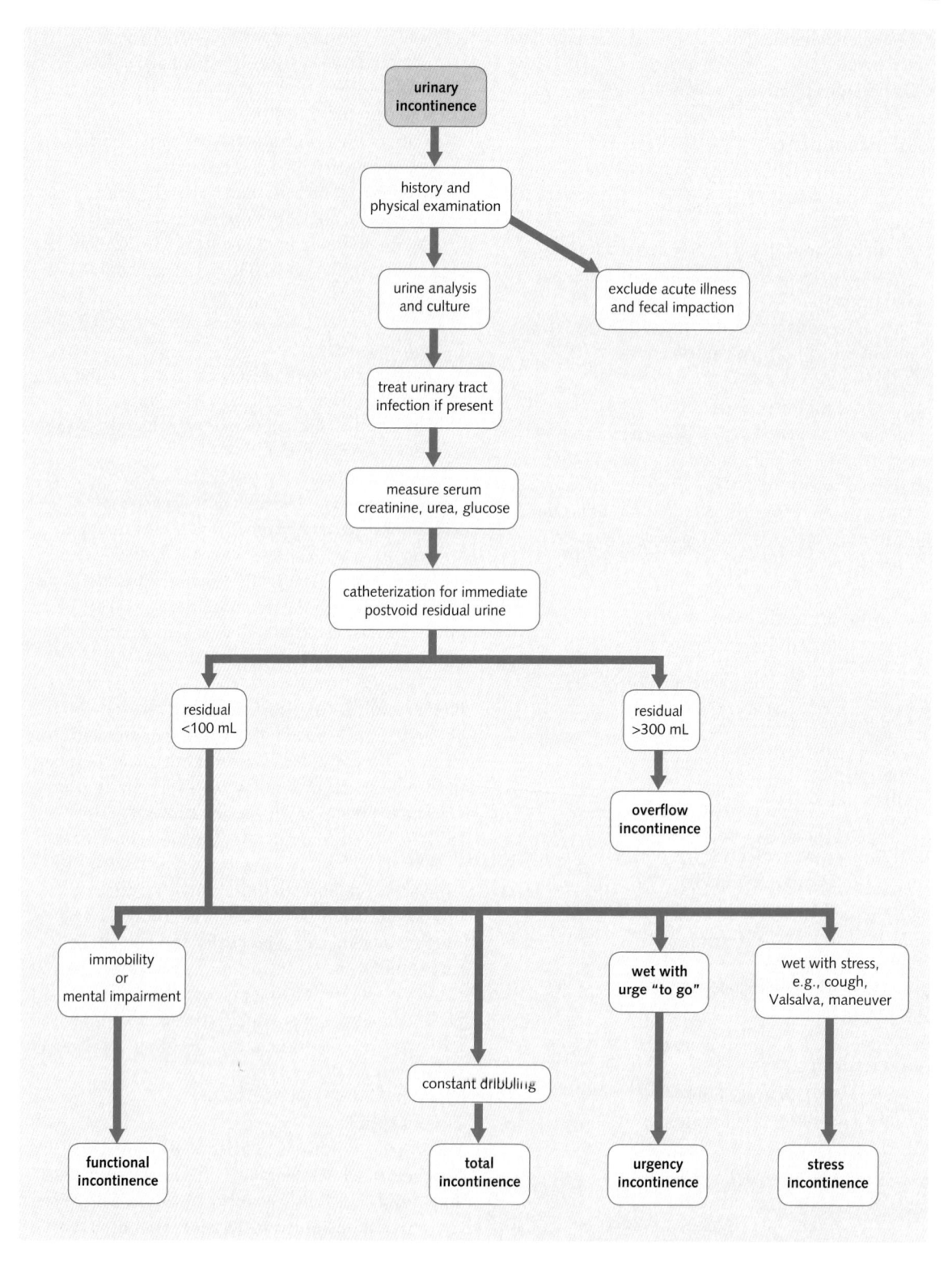

Fig. 5.11 Investigation of urinary incontinence. UTI, urinary tract infection (modified from Green HL: *Clinical medicine*, 2nd ed. Mosby Year Book, 1996).

Congenital abnormalities of the urinary tract

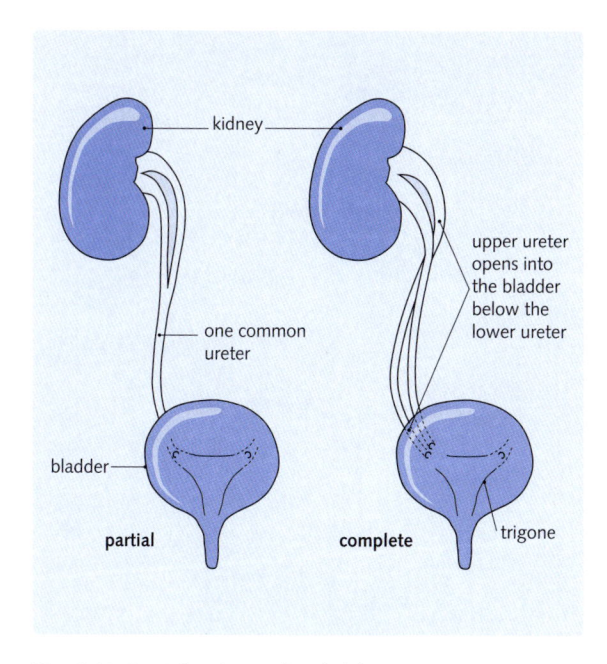

Fig. 5.12 Partial and complete bifid ureter.

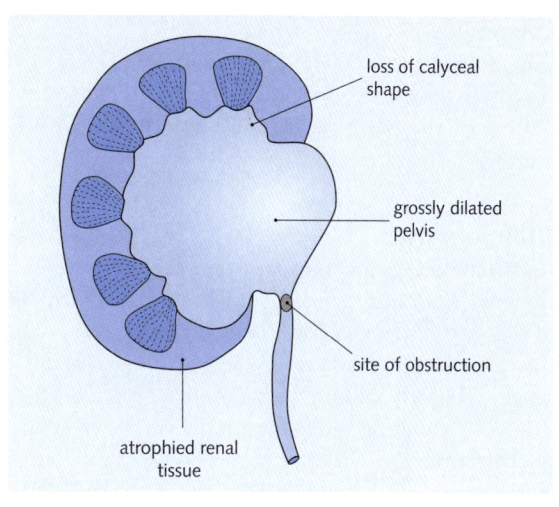

Fig. 5.13 Pelvicalyceal dilatation.

Hydroureter and megaureter
Congenital hydroureters develop if there are neuromuscular defects in the wall of the ureter. They are sometimes associated with other congenital malformations in the genitourinary tract. There is dilatation, elongation and frequently tortuosity of the ureters. Acquired hydroureters develop in adults during pregnancy and lower urinary tract obstruction, where a persistently raised pressure within the bladder impairs ureter emptying. A ureter so dilated that transport of urine by peristalsis is compromised is known as a megaureter.

Bladder abnormalities
Diverticula
These are sac-like outpouchings through a weak point in the bladder wall. They can be either:
- Congenital: these develop in localized areas of defective muscle within the wall or because of urinary tract obstruction in fetal development. They are usually solitary lesions, most commonly occurring close to the ureterovesical junction.
- Acquired: these usually develop much later in life as a result of chronic urethral obstruction (e.g., prostatic hypertrophy). They are clinically significant and, characteristically, occur as multiple lesions.

In both cases, urine stasis increases the risk of bladder infection, leading to vesicoureteric reflux and eventual stone formation.

Exstrophy
Exstrophy of the bladder is a serious condition affecting the anterior wall of the bladder and anterior abdominal wall. It presents in infancy and is more common in males. The anterior wall of the bladder fails to develop, so the posterior wall lies exposed on the lower abdominal wall, causing squamous metaplasia of the mucosa. The mucosa is at high risk of infection. This disorder can vary in severity and can be associated with urethral and symphysis pubis defects. In the male there is epispadias, and in females a split clitoris. Surgical correction allows long-term survival of these infants. Despite treatment, there is an increased risk of adenocarcinomas of the bladder later in life, because of bladder extrusion.

Urethral abnormalities
Hypospadias
This is a spectrum of congenital abnormalities affecting 1 in 400 male infants. The urethra opens on the ventral surface of the penis, usually adjacent to the glans penis, but can open on the penile shaft or perineum. There is a ventral curvature to the penile shaft with a hooded prepuce. Surgical correction is carried out before the age of two to allow micturition with a straight stream.

113

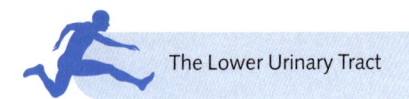

Epispadias

The urethra opens on the dorsal surface of the penis. As with hypospadias, surgical correction is carried out before the age of two to allow micturition with a straight stream.

Urethral valves

Obstruction to urine flow can occur at the level of the posterior urethra in a boy due to the presence of mucosal folds or a membrane extending across the urethra (posterior urethral valve). The patient presents in early infancy with distended bladder, dribbling, vomiting and failure to thrive. As a result of obstruction to urinary flow, male fetuses can have:
- Poor renal growth with reflux and dilated upper urinary tracts.
- Progressive bilateral hydronephrosis.
- Oligohydramnios (reduced volume of amniotic fluid).

Intrauterine intervention has no proven benefit and an early delivery is performed only if there are signs of rapidly progressing renal damage. Postnatal management includes:
- Prophylactic antibiotics from birth to prevent urinary tract infections (UTI).
- Ultrasound scans at birth and a few weeks later to assess the effect of the obstruction.

Surgical treatment is required in all cases. Any male child born with bilateral hydronephrosis must be investigated to exclude a posterior urethral valve.

Urinary tract obstruction

Introduction

Obstruction in the urinary tract can occur at any level. It can be unilateral or bilateral, complete or incomplete, and of gradual or acute onset. It increases the risk of infection, reflux and stone formation. If prolonged or unrelieved, obstruction can cause functional renal impairment and permanent renal atrophy. Imaging techniques involved in the diagnosis of urinary tract obstruction and its location (also see Chapter 8) are:
- Ultrasound: identifies dilatation of the urinary tract (hydronephrosis).
- DTPA (diethylenetriamine penta-acetic acid) renography: confirms any functional obstruction.
- Intravenous pyelography (IVP): highlights anatomical and functional obstruction (cannot be used in patients with renal failure).
- Retrograde pyelography: requires referral for bladder cannulation and cystoscopy.

Careful imaging of the renal tract is essential to determine the site and cause of obstruction (see Chapter 8).

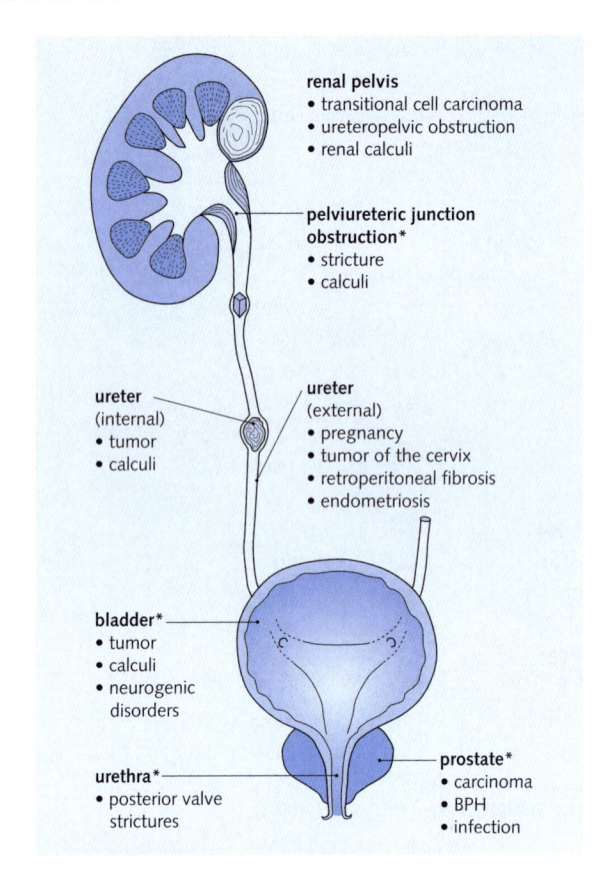

Fig. 5.14 Sites of obstruction in the urinary tract (* indicates the most common sites of obstruction).

Causes of urinary obstruction

Figure 5.14 shows the sites of obstruction in the urinary tract. Obstruction is caused by a congenital defect or, more commonly, by a structural lesion.

Congenital abnormalities

These include the following neuromuscular defects:
- Urethral valves and strictures.
- Meatal strictures.
- Bladder neck obstruction.
- Ureteropelvic obstruction or stenosis.

Mechanical obstruction of the meatus and urethra occurs only in boys. Severe vesicoureteric reflux eventually results in upper renal tract dilatation without obstruction.

Tumors
There are two ways in which tumors can cause obstruction:
1. Internal: tumors within the urinary tract wall or lumen (e.g. bladder carcinoma). These occupy the urinary tract lumen, causing direct obstruction.
2. External: pressure from rectal, prostatic, or gynecological tumors narrows the urinary tract lumen, causing indirect obstruction.

Calculi
Stones in the urinary tract can cause urinary obstruction.

Pregnancy
The high levels of progesterone in pregnancy relax smooth muscle fibers in the renal pelvis and ureters and cause a dysfunctional obstruction. There may also be external compression from the pressure of the enlarging fetus on the ureters.

Hyperplastic lesions
The most common hyperplastic lesion causing urinary obstruction is benign prostatic hypertrophy (BPH).

Inflammation
Any inflammation in the lower urinary tract may cause an obstruction (e.g. urethritis, ureteritis, prostatitis, retroperitoneal fibrosis). Obstruction resolves with the treatment of the inflammation.

Neurogenic disorders
These result from:
- Congenital anomalies affecting the spinal cord (e.g. spina bifida).
- External pressure on the cord or lumbar nerve roots (e.g., meningioma, lumbar disc prolapse).
- Trauma to the spinal cord.

Presentation of urinary obstruction
Hydronephrosis
This is dilatation of the renal pelvis and calyces due to obstruction at any point in the urinary tract causing increased pressure above the blockage. It can be:

- Unilateral: caused by an upper urinary tract obstruction. This is detected late because renal function is maintained by the other kidney. Thus, the affected kidney can be severely impaired by the time obstruction is detected.
- Bilateral: because of obstruction in the lower urinary tract. Renal failure develops earlier and prompt intervention is required to prevent chronic renal failure.

Progressive atrophy of the kidney develops as the back pressure from the obstruction is transmitted into the distal parts of the nephron. The glomerular filtration rate (GFR) declines and, if the obstruction is bilateral, the patient goes into renal failure. Progressive damage to the renal structures results in flattening of the calyces with gradual thinning of the renal parenchyma, eventually leaving a cystic thin-walled fibrous sac with no functional capacity.

- Obstruction at the pyeloureteric junction → hydronephrosis.
- Obstruction of the ureter → hydroureter, eventually developing hydronephrosis.
- Obstruction of the bladder neck/urethra → bladder distension with hypertrophy, eventually leading to hydroureter and thus hydronephrosis.

Clinical consequences of obstruction
This depends upon the site and cause of the obstruction:
- An acute complete obstruction in the ureters (e.g., due to a stone) causes severe renal colic. If bilateral, the patient is at risk of acute renal failure.
- Gradual obstruction (e.g. prostatic hypertrophy) causes bladder distension with hesitancy, terminal dribbling, poor urine flow and a sense of incomplete voiding.
- A unilateral and partial obstruction causing a hydroureter or hydronephrosis might not be apparent for many years because the unaffected kidney maintains adequate renal function.

- A bilateral and partial obstruction presents with nocturia and polyuria caused by tubular cell dysfunction with an inability to concentrate urine. Other chronic manifestations include renal stones, salt wasting, distal renal tubular acidosis and hypertension. If undiagnosed, the patient develops chronic renal failure.
- A bilateral and complete obstruction presents as anuria or oliguria and must be treated for survival. Following removal of the obstruction, there is often a massive postobstructive diuresis that leaves the patient susceptible to dehydration. Any general malaise or fever might be a sign of superimposed infection.

In all cases, management must include relief of the obstruction either with a urinary catheter, urinary stent or a nephrostomy (to allow renal function to improve), followed by surgical intervention.

- Sudden and complete obstruction causes an abrupt, significant fall in GFR.
- Partial or chronic obstruction slowly worsens GFR.

Renal calculi

Overview
Kidney stone disease arises from the formation and movement of stones within the urinary tract. It is more common in males. Different types of stones can form:
- Calcium-containing stones are the most common. They are made of calcium oxalate (spiky), hydroxyapatite, or calcium phosphate (smooth and large).
- Uric acid stones (smooth, brown and soft).
- Struvite or infection stones.
- Cystine stones (yellow and crystalline).

There is no relation between the size of the stones and the severity of the symptoms.

Incidence and risk factors
Urinary calculi affect 1–5% of the population and are more common in men. They are formed by precipitation of urinary components along with a small core of organic material, and form anywhere along the urinary tract, most commonly in the renal pelvis. Calculi vary in size and number. Risk factors for stone formation include:
- Increased solute in the urine as a result of high plasma levels (e.g. calcium and urate) or abnormal tubular function (e.g., calcium and cystine).
- Absence of inhibiting substances (e.g., citrate and phosphate).
- Acidic urinary pH, which reduces solubility of a substance in the urine.
- Urinary stasis or obstruction.

Occasionally, a calculus can grow to take up the shape of the renal pelvis and branch into calyces (staghorn calculus). Stone formation is initiated by a core of mucoproteins or urates (nucleation); as more components deposit on the core, the stone gradually increases in size (aggregation). Figure 5.15 lists the different types of stone and their frequency.

Causes
Causes of kidney stones are:
- Hypercalciuria.
- Hyperuricosuria (of which hyperuricemia is the main cause).
- Hyperoxaluria.
- Cysteinuria.
- Infection.
- Renal tubular acidosis.
- Low urine citrate.
- Renal disease (e.g., polycystic kidneys).

Different types of renal stones and their frequency	
Type	Frequency (%)
calcium-containing stones. • calcium oxalate • calcium phosphate	60–70 10–15
complex triple stones (magnesium, aluminum, phosphate)	15
uric acid stones	5
cysteine stones	1–2

Fig. 5.15 Different types of renal stones and their frequency.

- Dehydration: a concentrated urine is produced, which increases the risk of stone formation.

Symptoms
In acute presentation, pain is usually colicky and localized to one quadrant of the abdomen, radiating from flank to groin. The patient appears sweaty, pale and restless, with nausea and vomiting. There may be gross hematuria.
- Kidney stones cause flank pain.
- Ureteric stones cause renal colic.
- Bladder stones cause "strangulation," i.e., the desire to pass the stone but being unable to do so by voiding.

Diagnostic approach
History
Ask about the following:
- Diet: high dietary calcium intake (e.g., milk, cheese). High dietary oxalate intake (e.g., spinach, rhubarb, tea).
- Fluid intake and urine volume.
- Chronic diarrhea: Crohn's disease or dehydration.
- Personal or family history of gout.
- Family history of renal calculi.
- Number of previous urinary tract infections.
- Medications: check for antacid therapy (contains large amounts of absorbable calcium) and long-term antibiotic therapy.
- Past urological history.

Physical exam
- Look for clinical evidence of gout (tophi, etc.).
- Look for clinical evidence of metabolic bone disease—fractures, short stature.

Lab tests
Figure 5.16 shows an algorithm for urinary investigations of a patient with calcium kidney stones. Examinations and investigations for renal calculi should include:
- Serum Ca^{++}: Exclude hypercalcemia and investigate cause if found (e.g., primary hyperparathyroidism).
- Serum uric acid.
- Urine chemistry: identify and quantify the amount of calcium, oxalate, urate, citrate, and cystine in the urine.
- Stone analysis: urine should be 'sieved' to collect any stones passed for analysis (most pass spontaneously). Ask patient to retain voided stones for biochemical testing or x-ray crystallography.
- Imaging: CT scanning with thin sections is becoming the preferred test. Other possibilities include radiographs showing the kidneys, ureters and bladder (KUB), intravenous pyelography (IVP, the traditional "gold standard") and abdominal ultrasound (less helpful, but might show dilatation of obstructed kidney or acoustic shadow from a stone).

Treatment
Management involves adequate analgesia and a high fluid intake. Stones less than 5 mm in diameter usually pass spontaneously; larger stones may require surgical intervention. If obstruction or infection develops, the stones must be removed urgently. In the long term, the mainstay of treatment is a high fluid intake.

Surgical treatment
- Extracorporeal lithotripsy: shockwaves are used to fragment the calculi into small pieces which will then pass naturally. Used for stones <2 cm.
- Percutaneous endoscopic surgery: removal of larger stones.
- Open resection: used rarely for the largest or most complex stones.

Medical treatment
- Thiazides for hypercalciuria as they decrease urinary calcium excretion.
- Allopurinol for hyperuricemia.
- Penicillamine for cystinuria.

Prevention
- High fluid intake to produce a dilute urine.
- Correction of any underlying metabolic abnormality.
- Low sodium, low protein diet.

Inflammation and infection of the urinary tract

Urinary tract infection (UTI)
Incidence and risk factors
UTIs are very common. They can involve the bladder (cystitis) or the kidneys (pyelonephritis) or both. They are more common in boys in infancy because of congenital abnormalities; this reverses at puberty,

The Lower Urinary Tract

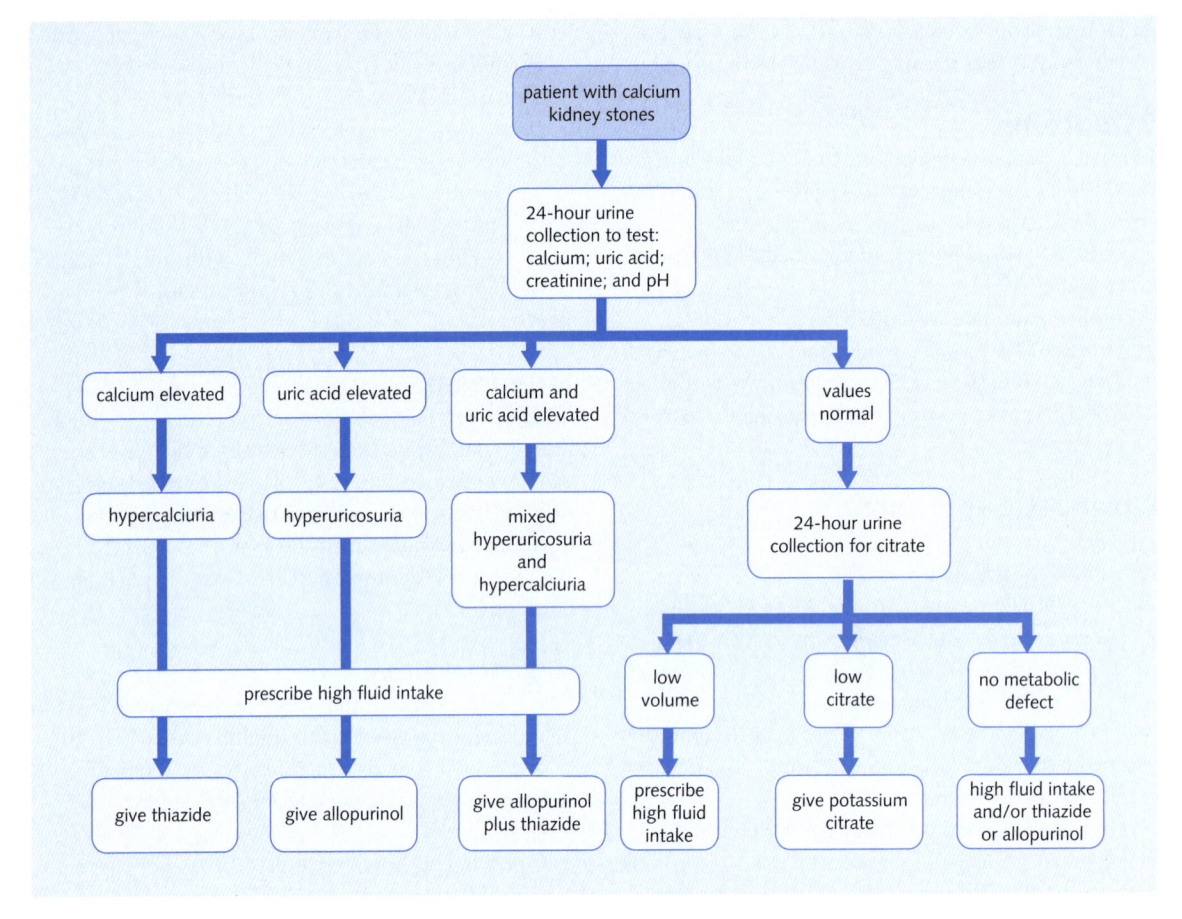

Fig. 5.16 Urinary investigations of a patient with calcium kidney stones (from Green HL: *Clinical medicine*, 2nd ed. Mosby Year Book, 1996).

with more females being affected thereafter because of urethral trauma and pregnancy. Women are particularly at risk of lower UTIs because they have a short urethra, but further investigation is required if infections are recurrent. Any UTI in children and adult males should be investigated to exclude an underlying renal tract abnormality. UTI rarely progresses to renal damage in adults if the renal tract is normal. Treatment involves a high fluid intake, regular bladder emptying and prophylactic antibiotics. After the age of 40, UTI is again more common in men because of prostatic disease, causing bladder outflow obstruction. Risk factors for UTIs include:
- Long-term catheterization.
- Diabetes mellitus.
- Lower urinary tract obstruction (congenital abnormalities or calculi).
- Pregnancy.
- Tumors.
- Immunosuppression.
- Vesicoureteral reflux.

Presentation
UTIs present silently (asymptomatic bacteriuria) or with dysuria (pain on passing urine), frequency and urgency of micturition. Involvement of the kidneys causes flank pain and fever.

Diagnosis
A diagnosis of UTI requires over 10^5 organisms/mL from a midstream urine specimen on culture. In the majority of UTIs the infecting organism comes from the patient's own fecal flora (Fig. 5.17). *E coli* is most common. Hospitalized patients exhibit more varied pathogens, esp. *Pseudomonas*.

Incidence of community- and hospital-acquired UTIs caused by bacteria in the U.S.		
Organism	Community (%)	Hospital (%)
Escherichia coli	70–80	45–55
Proteus	5	10–12
Klebsiella	6	15–20
Enterococcus	5	10–12
Enterobacter	—	2–5
Pseudomonas	—	10–15
Acinetobacter	—	<1
coagulase-negative *Staphylococcus*	1–2	1–2
Staphylococcus aureus	—	<1

Fig. 5.17 Incidence of community- and hospital-acquired urinary tract infections (UTIs) caused by bacteria.

Pyelonephritis

Pyelonephritis is discussed in Chapter 4, "Tubulo interstitial Diseases" (p. 91).

Cystitis

This is inflammation of the urinary bladder and is common in UTI. It can be acute or chronic. The pathogens that cause cystitis are:
- Most common: *Escherichia coli* and *Proteus* species, followed by *Enterobacter*.
- *Candida albicans* in patients on long-term antibiotics.
- *Cryptococcus* species in immunosuppressed patients.
- *Schistosoma* species, particularly in Middle Eastern countries.
- *Mycobacterium tuberculosis*: tuberculous cystitis usually suggests tuberculosis in the upper urinary tract.

Sterile cystitis can be caused by radiation damage, drugs and instrumentation.

The most serious complication of cystitis is pyelonephritis (see Chapter 4).

Acute cystitis

In acute cystitis the mucosa becomes hyperemic, often producing an exudate. There are various forms:

- Hemorrhagic cystitis: occurs if the hyperemia becomes excessive, resulting in bleeding.
- Exudative cystitis: yellow areas of fibrinous exudate develop on the mucosa.
- Suppurative cystitis: large quantities of exudate accumulate.
- Ulcerative cystitis: large areas of ulceration occur in the bladder mucosa.
- Gangrenous cystitis: as a result of ischemia, which results in areas of black necrotic bladder mucosa.

Chronic cystitis

This results from recurrent or persistent infection of the bladder. Chronic infection leads to fibrous thickening, so the bladder wall is less distensible. This affects the ability of the bladder to store urine and contract during micturition.

Interstitial cystitis

This type of cystitis is often associated with SLE, so is thought to be an autoimmune condition. As with all autoimmune conditions, it has a much higher incidence in women than in men. It can also result from recurrent and persistent infection that leads to fibrosis of all the layers of the bladder wall. There is often localized ulceration of the mucosa.

Schistosomiasis (bilharzia)

Schistosomiasis is the most common helminth infection worldwide, although it is rare in the U.S. It is a common cause of cystitis and hematuria in the Middle East, Africa, the Far East, and in parts of South America. The pathogen is a blood fluke (*Schistosoma hematobium*). Humans are infected via freshwater snails, which contain cerecariae—parasites in the cercarial phase of development. The schistosomes penetrate intact skin to enter the venous system, and thus migrate to the liver and bladder. They settle in the bladder to lay eggs causing chronic irritation of the transitional cells of the bladder. The eggs are excreted into local water supplies and transmitted through freshwater snails (Fig. 5.18).

People infected with cercariae can present with an itchy papular rash accompanied by myalgia, abdominal pain and headache. The most common presentation of infection with *S. hematobium* is recurrent hematuria. Eventually, obstruction within the urinary tract, bladder calcification (predisposing to squamous carcinoma) and renal failure occur.

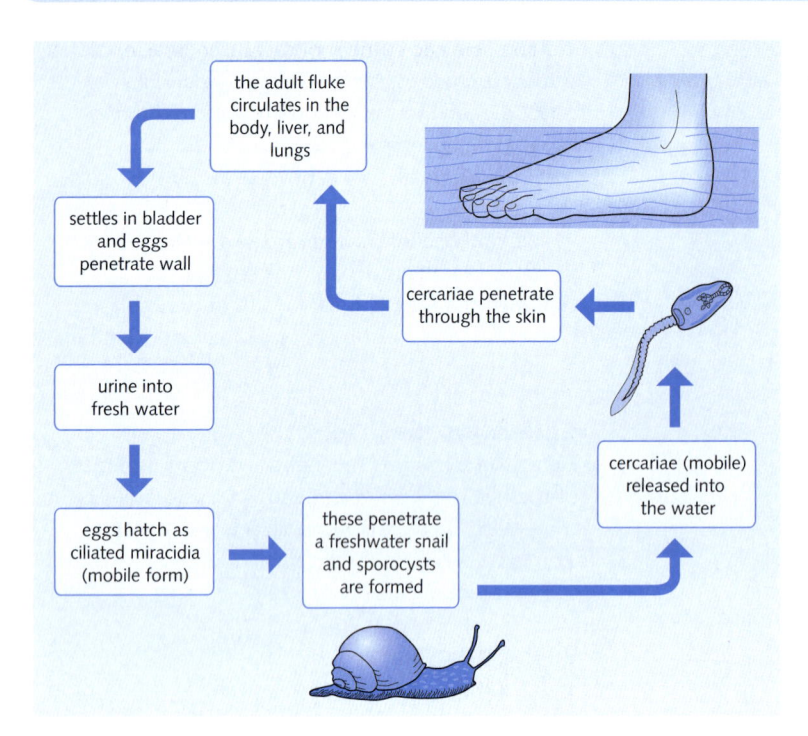

Fig. 5.18 Infestation with *Schistosoma hematobium*.

Diagnosis involves:
- Urine sample to detect the eggs in the urine.
- Enzyme-linked immunosorbent assay (ELISA) to detect a response to infection.

Treatment is with praziquantel given once daily.

Presentation and treatment
The classic symptoms of all types of cystitis are:
- Urgency and frequency of micturition.
- Dysuria.
- Lower abdominal pain and tenderness.

There may be associated systemic signs of fever, general malaise and rigors.

Treatment of cystitis involves a 3- to 7-day course of antibiotics with a high fluid intake. Fluoroquinolones or trimethoprim-sulfa is preferred. Young healthy women may be treated with a short course, while those with diabetes or pregnancy need 7 days. Men require a longer course for eradication of the infection. Recurrent infection should always be investigated.

> Metaplasia associated with bladder extrophy, chronic bladder inflammation, and schistosomiasis are premalignant conditions.

Urethral discharge
A urethral discharge is secretion passed through the urethra at times other than voiding. The female equivalent is vaginal discharge. The secretion may be clear, purulent, bloody, itchy or foul smelling.

Causes
Causes of urethral discharge are:
- Non-infectious: irritation (mechanical or chemical), urethral stricture, non-bacterial prostatitis, phimosis, urethral diverticulum, urethral carbuncle. Occasionally, it can be caused by Reiter's syndrome.
- Infectious (i.e., sexually transmitted infections): gonococcal urethritis (characteristically "canary yellow" discharge) or, more commonly, nongonococcal urethritis (e.g., *Chlamydia*

trachomatis, *Trichomonas vaginalis*, herpes simplex virus).

Diagnostic approach
An algorithm for diagnosing urethral discharge is given in Fig. 5.19.

Neoplastic disease of the ureters and bladder

Tumors of the ureters
These are very rare.

Tumors of the bladder
The most common site for bladder tumors to develop is the posterior and lateral walls (70%), followed by the trigone and bladder neck (20%).

Benign tumors of the bladder
These are rare, accounting for 2–3% of bladder epithelial tumors. Transitional cell papilloma can be the first stage (grade I) of transitional cell carcinoma. These papillomas are often multiple and are found all over the mucosal lining. They are small projections (0.5–2.0 cm in length) with uniform cellular structure. They attach to the mucosa by a small stalk with a fibrovascular core covered in urothelium.

The other benign lesions are inverted papillomas. These consist of solitary nodules in the mucosa and measure 1–3 cm in diameter.

Metaplasia
The transitional cell lining (urothelium) of the bladder can undergo metaplastic changes during any period of infection or inflammation as a result of stones, drugs, and radiation. There are two main types of metaplasia:
1. Squamous metaplasia: occurs in areas of long-term chronic inflammation in bladder extrophy, bladder calculi, and schistosomiasis. It is a risk factor for squamous cell carcinoma.
2. Intestinal or glandular metaplasia: associated with chronic cystitis and leads to the formation of slit-like glands of columnar epithelium.

Transitional cell carcinomas
These are malignant tumors that arise from the transitional cell epithelium that lines the bladder. They account for over 90% of bladder epithelial cell tumors, and the number of cases is increasing. They are uncommon under 50 years of age and more commonly affect males (4 males : 1 female). Risk factors include:
- Smoking.
- Exposure to chemicals in the rubber industry (e.g. naphthylamine and benzidine).
- Analgesic abuse.

> Transitional cell carcinomas are the most common urinary tract malignancies. The most common site is the bladder.

Presentation
The most common presentation of any tumor of the bladder is painless hematuria. This is often accompanied by symptoms of a UTI (i.e. dysuria, frequency and urgency). Symptoms can also be caused by local invasion of the tumor causing ureteric obstruction.

Pathology
There are two main types of transitional cell tumor (Fig. 5.20):
1. Papillary tumor (70%): wart-like lesion covered in a thick layer of urothelium branching off a stalk that attaches it to the mucosa (as described above).
2. Sessile (flat) tumor: plaques of thickened mucosa with a well-defined border.

Both these types of tumor can be in situ or invasive:
- In situ carcinomas: flat lesions that are confined to the mucosa of the upper urinary tract or bladder. They are the precursors of the invasive tumors.
- Invasive tumors: infiltrate the basement membrane of the bladder mucosa and the lamina propria and can penetrate adjacent structures once through the mucosal wall.

Transitional cell carcinomas can be graded according to the degree of cellular abnormalities on histology:
- Grade I: there is an increase in the number of well-differentiated epithelial cell layers (>7) and there is some cell atypia.

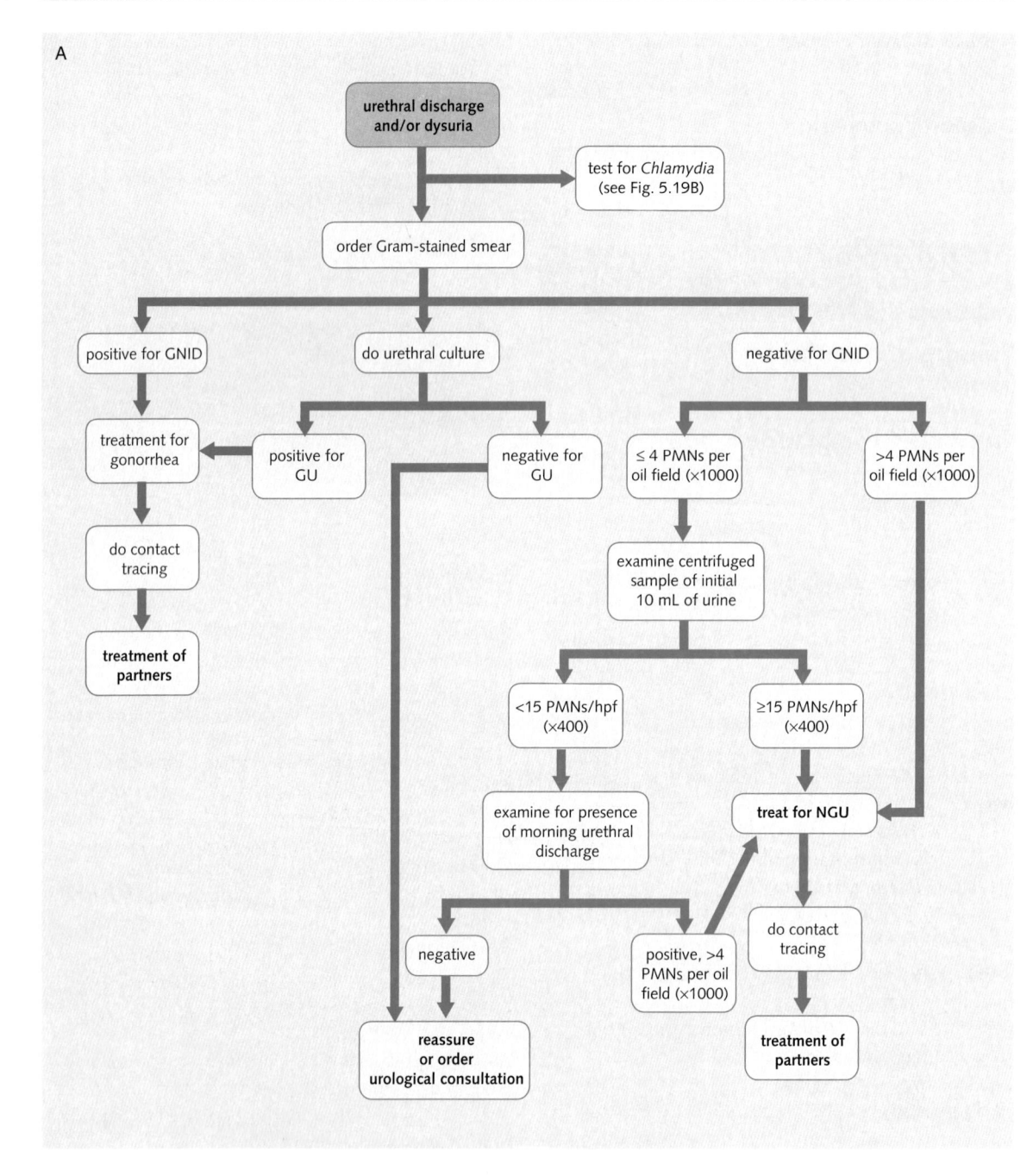

Fig. 5.19 (A) Diagnosing urethral discharge. GNID, Gram-negative intracellular diplococci; GU, gonococcal urethritis; hpf, high-power field; NGU, non-gonococcal urethritis; PMNs, polymorphonuclear leucocytes (from Green HL: *Clinical medicine*, 2nd ed. Mosby Year Book, 1996).

Fig. 5.19 (B) Investigation for *Chlamydia trachomatis*.

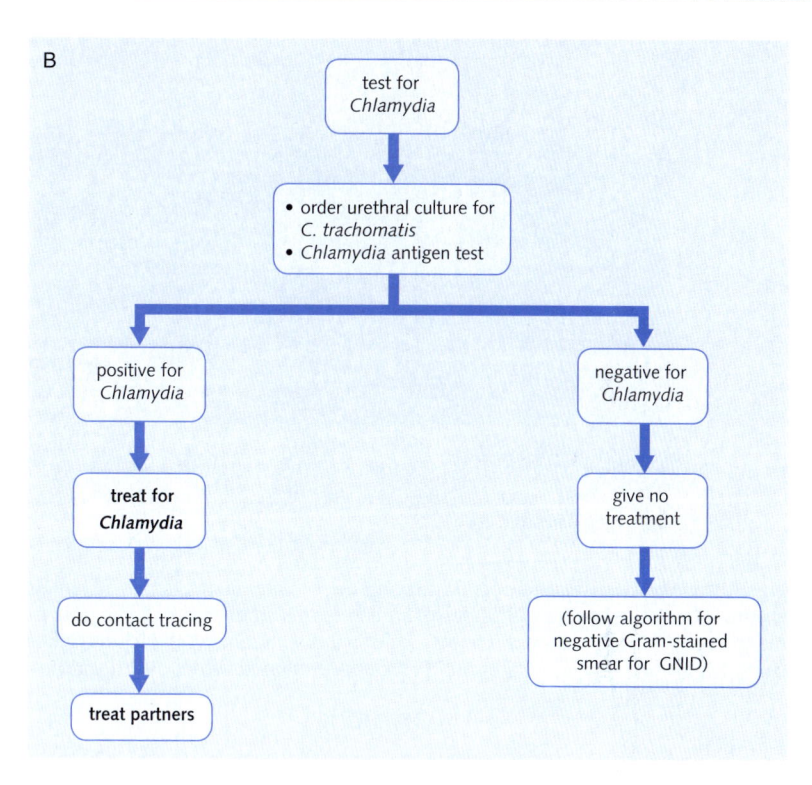

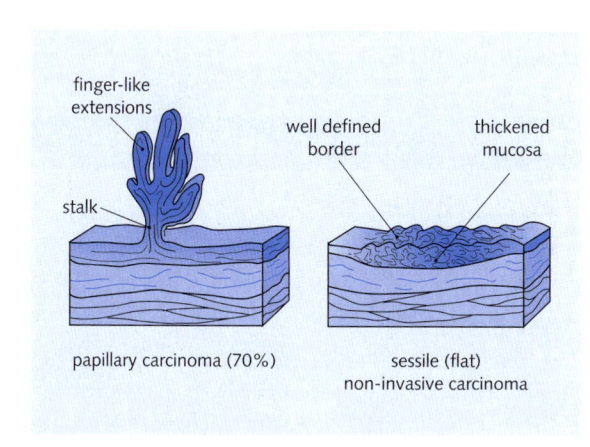

Fig. 5.20 Papillary and sessile transitional cell tumors.

As tumor growth progresses, the relatively benign, well-differentiated papillary growths (grade I) can eventually form solid plaque-like anaplastic tumors (grade III). Grade III tumors are often ulcerated and have penetrated though the bladder muscle wall. They are associated with the worst prognosis.

Carcinomas with over 5% squamous or glandular metaplasia are called mixed tumors.

The TNM system is used for the staging of transitional cell tumors, i.e. to assess the extent of spread (Fig. 5.21). This has been correlated to grade. tumor spread can be:
- Local: invasion into the bladder wall and to adjacent pelvic structures.
- Distant: lymphatic spread to the periaortic lymph nodes or hematological metastases to the liver and lungs.

- Grade II: there is an increase in cell layers (>10) and there is a large variation in cell size and in nucleus shape and size (i.e. moderately well differentiated).
- Grade III: the cells have no resemblance to their cells of origin (poorly differentiated), with breakdown of connections between the cells causing them to fragment.

Investigation via cystoscopy and biopsy allows histological examination, which confirms whether there is muscle involvement. The distinction between the lamina propria invasion and submucosal invasion is correlated with the prognosis.

Most of the tumors are situated on the posterior and lateral walls of the bladder, and are often multiple. This suggests that the entire epithelium is

The Lower Urinary Tract

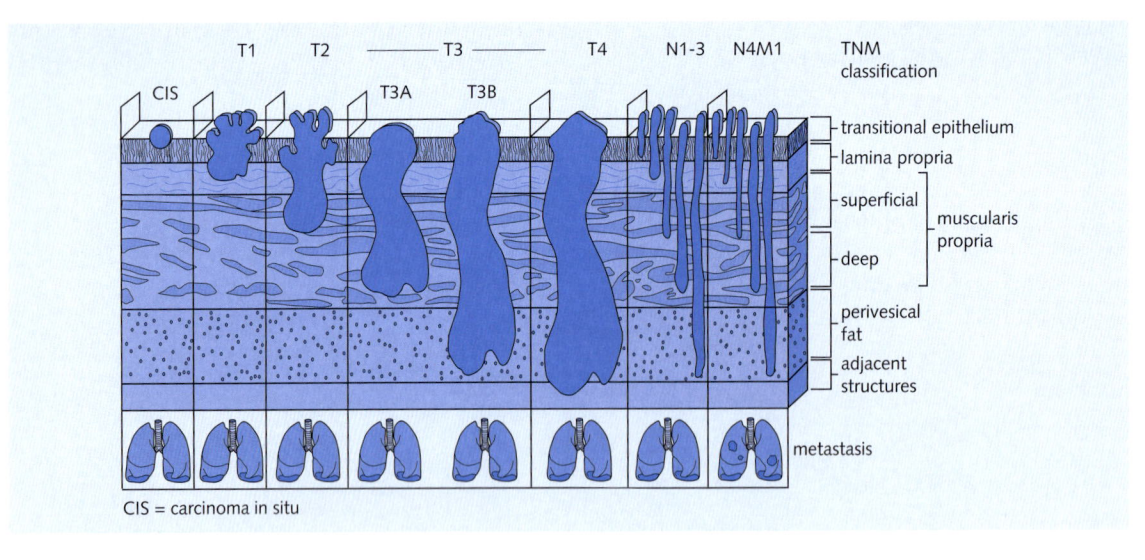

Fig. 5.21 TNM staging system for transitional cell carcinoma of bladder. T staging describes tumor invasion of the tissue layers. N staging describes the degree of spread to the lymph nodes: 1 = local nodes; 2 = distant nodes below the diaphragm; 3 = distant nodes on both sides of the diaphragm. M staging describes the presence or absence of metastases: 0 = none; 1 = present (from Bahnson RR: *Management of urologic disorders*, Mosby Year Book, 1994).

unstable as a result of the constant exposure to the carcinogens being excreted in urine.

Diagnosis, treatment, and prognosis
Diagnosis is made by cytological examination of the urine to check for the presence of malignant cells and by cystoscopy of the lower urinary tract.

Treatment depends upon the stage and histological grade of the tumor:
- T1 tumors: tumor resection using diathermy (via cystoscopy) with close follow-up.
- T2/3 tumors: radiotherapy and cystectomy.
- T4 tumors: palliative radiotherapy.

The average 5-year survival rate is 80% if the bladder wall is not involved and 5% if there is local invasion on presentation. Patients with fixed tumors and metastases have a median survival of 1 year.

Squamous cell carcinoma
These usually arise in areas of squamous metaplasia of the bladder mucosa and account for <10% of bladder carcinomas. Risk factors include bladder extrophy, chronic inflammation, calculi, and schistosomiasis, which cause chronic irritation to the transitional cells of the bladder, leading to squamous metaplasia. This becomes dysplastic, resulting in carcinoma in situ, which can progress to invasive squamous cell carcinoma.

The tumors are solid, ulcerative, invasive, and fungating masses and are often very extensive on discovery. Their prognosis is worse than that of transitional cell carcinoma.

Disorders of the prostate

Prostatitis
There are three subgroups of inflammation of the prostate.

Acute prostatitis
The main pathogens are *E. coli*, *Proteus* and *Staphylococcus* species and sexually transmitted pathogens, including *Chlamydia trachomatis* and gonorrhea. Inflammation can be focal or diffuse. Infection is usually spread from an acute infection in the urethra or bladder because of:
- Intraprostatic reflux of urine.
- Urinary catheterization.
- Surgical manipulation of the urethra (e.g., cystoscopy).

Occasionally, acute prostatitis is caused by a blood-borne infection.

On histology there is an acute inflammatory infiltrate of neutrophils and damaged cells, often resulting in abscess formation.

Patients present with:
- General symptoms: malaise, rigors, and fever.
- Local symptoms: difficulty in passing urine, dysuria, and perineal tenderness.

Rectal examination reveals a soft, tender, and enlarged prostate. Diagnosis is based on the clinical features and a positive urine culture. Treatment is 3–4 weeks of oral trimethoprim sulfa or a fluoroquinolone.

Chronic prostatitis

This results from inadequately treated acute infection. This can occur because some antibiotics cannot penetrate the prostate effectively. There is often a history of recurrent prostatic and urinary tract infections. Causative pathogens are the same as for acute prostatic infection.

Patients present with dysuria and low back and perineal pain, with no preceding acute phase. Some patients are asymptomatic.

Chronic prostatitis is difficult to diagnose and treat. Diagnosis is confirmed by a positive culture from a sample of prostatic secretion.

Chronic nonbacterial prostatitis

This is the most common type of prostatitis and results in enlargement of the prostate, which can obstruct the urethra. The usual pathogen is *Chlamydia trachomatis*; typically, sexually active men are affected. Often there is no history of recurrent UTIs.

Presentation is similar to that of chronic prostatitis, and histology shows fibrosis as a result of chronic inflammation.

Diagnosis is confirmed by the presence of 15 white blood cells per high power field (this indicates inflammation) and repeated negative bacterial cultures.

Tuberculous prostatitis

Tuberculosis is a cause of chronic infection and can affect the kidneys or epididymis. Histology reveals focal areas of caseation and giant-cell infiltrates.

Benign prostatic hypertrophy (BPH)
Incidence

BPH is detectable to some extent in nearly all men over the age of 60. It is a nonneoplastic enlargement of the prostate gland, which can eventually lead to bladder outflow obstruction. The cause is unknown but may be related to levels of male sex hormones (testosterone).

Presentation

Symptoms develop as the enlarging gland compresses the prostatic urethra and the periurethral glands (known as the median lobe) swell, affecting the bladder sphincter mechanism. Examination must include:
- Abdominal examination for an enlarged palpable bladder.
- Digital rectal examination for the prostate, which is firm, smooth and rubbery.

Untreated BPH can present with acute urinary retention, which is accompanied by a distended and tender bladder and a desperate urge to pass urine. Alternatively, the patient might have progressive bladder distension, leading to chronic painless retention and overflow incontinence. If undetected, BPH can lead to bilateral upper tract obstruction and renal impairment, with the patient presenting in chronic renal failure (see Chapter 6).

> Patients with prostatic hypertrophy have:
> - Difficulty or hesitancy in starting to urinate.
> - A poor urine stream.
> - Dribbling postmicturition, frequency and nocturia.

Pathology

There is hyperplasia of both the lateral lobes and the median lobes (these lie behind the urethra), leading to compression of the urethra and therefore bladder outflow obstruction. Within the prostate there are solid nodules of fibromuscular material and cystic regions. Histology shows hyperplasia of the:
- Stroma (smooth muscle and fibrous tissue).
- Glands, often with areas of infarction and necrosis.

Complications

The complications of BPH develop from prolonged obstruction to urine flow. There is compensatory

The Lower Urinary Tract

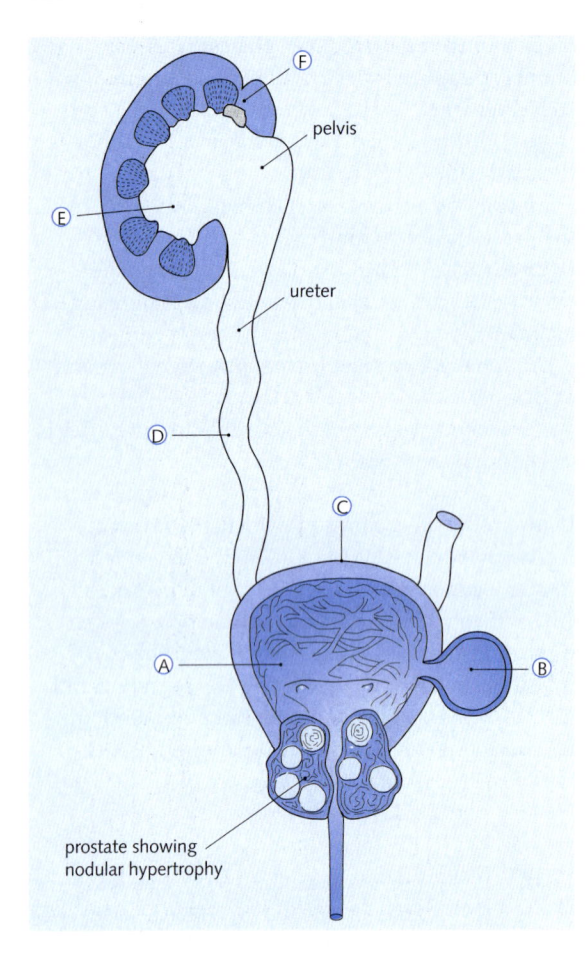

Fig. 5.22 Complications of benign prostatic hypertrophy. (A) Bands of thickened smooth muscle fiber cause trabeculation of the bladder wall. (B) Diverticulae can develop on the external surface of the bladder. (C) Dilatation of the bladder once the muscle becomes hypotonic. (D) Formation of hydroureters resulting in the reflux of urine up to the renal pelvis. (E) Bilateral hydronephrosis. (F) Kidney infection, stones, calculi and renal failure.

hypertrophy of the bladder as a result of the high pressures that develop within the bladder (Fig. 5.22).

Treatment
Medical treatment
- Alpha blockers: relax smooth muscle at the bladder neck, thus improving urinary flow rate.
- Antiandrogens such as finasteride: these prevent the conversion of testosterone to the more potent androgen dihydrotestosterone, which promotes growth and enlargement of the prostate. Inhibition of its production causes gradual reduction in prostate volume, sometimes improving urinary flow rate and obstructive symptoms. However, recent studies show no symptomatic advantages over alpha blockers.

Surgical treatment
- Transurethral resection of the prostate (TURP) is quick and safe with a low mortality rate and a good success rate.
- Open prostatectomy is used for very large prostates only.

Carcinoma of the prostate
Incidence and risk factors
Prostate cancer is the third most common cancer in men (after cancer of the lung and stomach), accounting for 8% of all cancers in men. It is a disease of elderly men, occurring in one in ten men of 70 years of age. It is commonly seen on postmortem exams, indicating that many or most elderly men may have asymptomatic forms. It is rare under 55 years of age and has a strong hereditary component.

The cause is unknown, but there is a link between androgenic hormones and tumor growth. The lesions are most commonly found in the periphery of the posterior part of the prostate compared with the more central and lateral location of BPH—these areas have different embryological origins and often both conditions coexist.

Presentation
It is frequently asymptomatic, and grows very slowly. Patients present with symptoms of UTI, prostatism or metastatic disease in the bone (usually the spine) causing bone pain. Carcinoma can be found coincidentally in autopsies of elderly men who were asymptomatic. About 25% of patients have symptoms of metastatic disease on presentation (anemia, ureteric obstruction or bone pain that is worse at night).

Pathology
The tumors range from well-differentiated single nodules to anaplastic and diffuse involvement of all lobes of the gland. The Gleeson classification is used to grade the tumors on histological appearance. Grade 1 is a well-differentiated tumor composed of uniform tumor cells whereas grade 5 is an anaplastic diffuse tumor with cells showing great variation in their structure and a high mitotic rate.

As for transitional cell carcinoma of the bladder, stage is determined by the universal TNM system:
- T_1: unsuspected impalpable tumor.
- T_2: the tumor is confined to the prostate.
- T_3: there is local extension of the tumor beyond the prostatic capsule.
- T_4: the tumor has fixed to other local structures.

Tumor spread can be by:
- Local invasion of adjacent structures, including the bladder and ureters.
- Lymphatic spread to the iliac and periaortic nodes.
- Hematogenous spread to the bones of the spine and pelvis and occasionally to the lungs and liver.

BPH and prostate cancer are distinct entities that are not risk factors for each other. BPH presents with voiding symptoms, while prostate cancer may be asymptomatic or present with distant metastases.

Diagnosis
- Digital rectal examination: hard and irregular prostate.
- Ultrasound: used to define a prostatic mass.
- Prostatic specific antigen (PSA) level in the blood: this increases in prostate cancer, but a normal result does not exclude the presence of cancer, and elevated values may be seen in BPH. Its use in routine screening is controversial.
- Serum prostatic acid phosphatase: this also increases, especially if there are metastases.
- Radiographs and bone scans: used to stage the tumor. Osteosclerotic lesions on radiographs and increased isotope uptake on bone scans are seen if there is metastatic spread (see Chapter 8).

Treatment and prognosis
Treatment options include surgery, hormone therapy and radiotherapy. Before treatment is started, a histological diagnosis of prostatic carcinoma is required. The specimen is taken by transurethral or transrectal biopsy. Treatment depends upon the stage of the tumor:
- T1/T2 staged tumors: surgical resection of the prostate (prostatectomy). TURP might also be required in advanced metastatic disease to relieve the symptoms of urethral obstruction. Recently some have argued for more conservative management given the slow progression and frequent side effects (impotence, incontinence) after surgery.
- Local radiotherapy can be used if the patient is unfit for surgery, and to treat local or distant spread of the tumor. It can provide useful palliation for bony metastases.
- Advanced tumors: Testosterone promotes tumor growth. Luteinizing-hormone-releasing hormone (LHRH) analogues prevent testosterone release. They are equally effective and are increasingly used for metastatic disease. Antiandrogens are also used to block testosterone action. Removal of both testes (orchiectomy) blocks the source of testosterone, causing the tumor to shrink. This is rarely used.

Prognosis depends on stage. The 5-year survival rate for T1 tumors is 75–90%. However, the 5-year survival falls to 30–45% if there is local or metastatic spread.

- Explain what the trigone is and how it differs from the rest of the bladder.
- Name three differences between the external and internal urethral sphincters.
- Outline the function of the detrusor and sphincter muscles, and their innervation.
- Summarize the common causes and points of neurological damage within the micturition path.
- Describe "spinal shock."
- Outline the difference between a hydroureter and a megaureter.
- Explain how diverticula develop, where they occur and their long-term effects.
- Name three causes of urinary tract obstruction. List the imaging techniques you would use to investigate obstruction.
- Describe how clinical presentation of urinary obstruction is influenced by the site and cause of the obstruction.
- Discuss how bilateral hydronephrosis differs in presentation from unilateral hydronephrosis.
- Summarize the factors influencing stone formation. What is the management for urinary stones?
- Outline the tests required to identify chlamydia in a patient presenting with urethral discharge.
- List the three principles of treating patients with sexually transmitted infections.
- Compare and contrast the three types of inflammation affecting the prostate.
- Define BPH, explaining the histological changes.
- Explain how treatment and prognosis differ according to the stage of prostate cancer.

CLINICAL ASSESSMENT

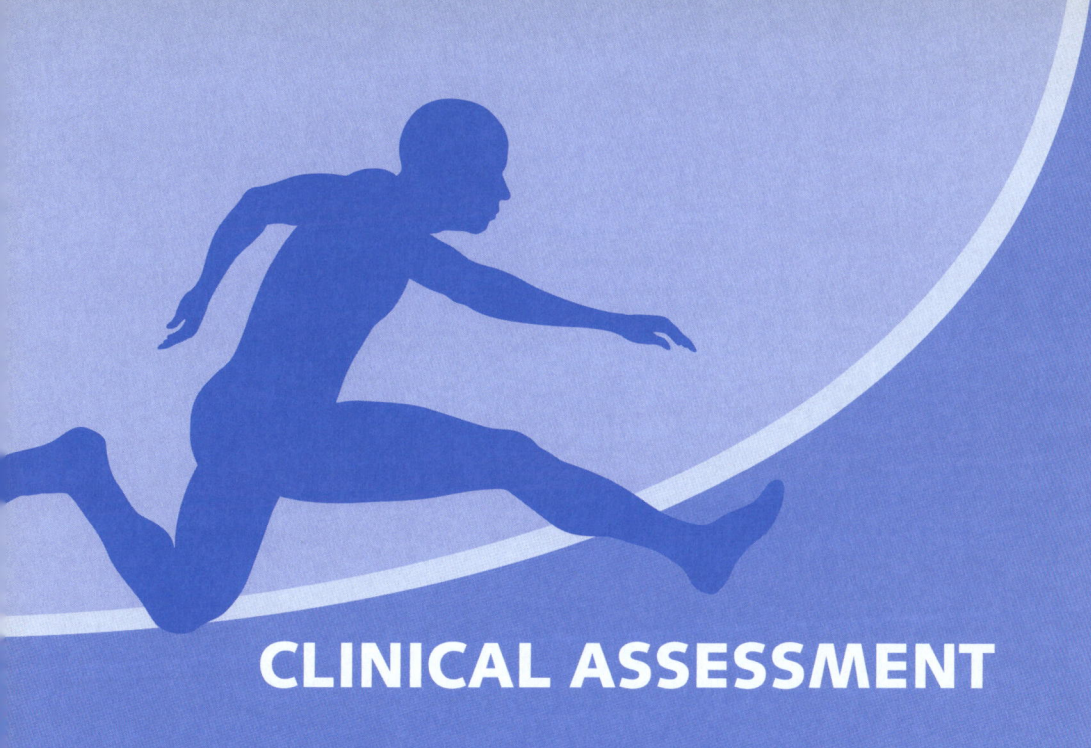

6. Common Presentations of
   Renal Disease   131

7. History and Examination 143

8. Lab Investigation and Imaging 147

6. Common Presentations of Renal Disease

Introduction

There are numerous presenting complaints in renal and genitourinary disease. In this chapter several common ones will be dealt with individually. Many of these, however, are nonspecific for renal disease. In addition, renal disease can be asymptomatic until a very late stage. It is therefore essential to have a routine screening procedure of:
- Blood pressure measurement.
- Urinalysis (midstream urine).

Hematuria

Blood in the urine can be:
- Microscopic: blood is visible only under a microscope or on dipstick analysis.
- Macroscopic ('frank' hematuria): blood is visible with the naked eye (>5 red blood cells per high-power field).

The degree of hematuria does not always reflect the severity of the underlying disorder.

Dipsticks detect hemoglobin (not red blood cells) and will give positive results if there is free hemoglobinuria (from intravascular hemolysis) or myoglobinuria (from rhabdomyolysis). This is because these are filtered freely by glomeruli. This can occur physiologically, after heavy exercise, during pregnancy or with prosthetic heart valves. If hemolysis is severe (i.e. in hemolytic crisis), the urine can become red. Other conditions can cause a red–brown discoloration of the urine that can be confused with hematuria (e.g. porphyria, myoglobinuria, ingestion of some foods (beets) or drugs (phenolphthalein)).

Causes
Causes of hematuria are:
- Renal causes: glomerular disease such as primary glomerulonephritis (e.g., IgA nephropathy), disorders secondary to systemic illness (e.g., vasculitis, systemic lupus erythematosus [SLE]), carcinoma (renal cell carcinoma), trauma, cystic disease, emboli.
- Extrarenal causes: urinary tract infection, (UTI)*, ureteral calculi*, prostatic hypertrophy*, carcinoma of the bladder*, renal stones*, trauma, urethritis, catheterization.
- Systemic causes: coagulation disorders, sickle-cell trait or disease.
- Drugs: anticoagulants, cyclophosphamide.

(*indicates the most common causes)

Diagnostic approach
Figure 6.1 shows the common sites of lesions causing hematuria, and the investigative approach for hematuria is shown in Fig. 6.2. A flow chart summarizing further investigation of hematuria if the CT or ultrasound result is abnormal is given in Fig. 6.3. The significance of urinalysis is summarized in Fig. 6.4.

Patients with negative work-up
Patients who have a negative work-up after following the scheme in Fig. 6.2 can be observed. About 50% will have a glomerular disease (usually IgA nephropathy), but renal biopsy is not necessary unless the creatinine elevates or proteinuria develops. Another 10–20% of these patients may have hematuria related to hyperuricosuria or hypercalciuria (determined on a 24-hour collection) and may be borderline stone formers. Treatment of these patients with allopurinol (↑ uric acid) or hydrochlorothiazide (↑ Ca) will eliminate the hematuria.

Proteinuria

Proteinuria is the presence of excess protein in the urine. Urine usually contains <20mg/L of albumin

131

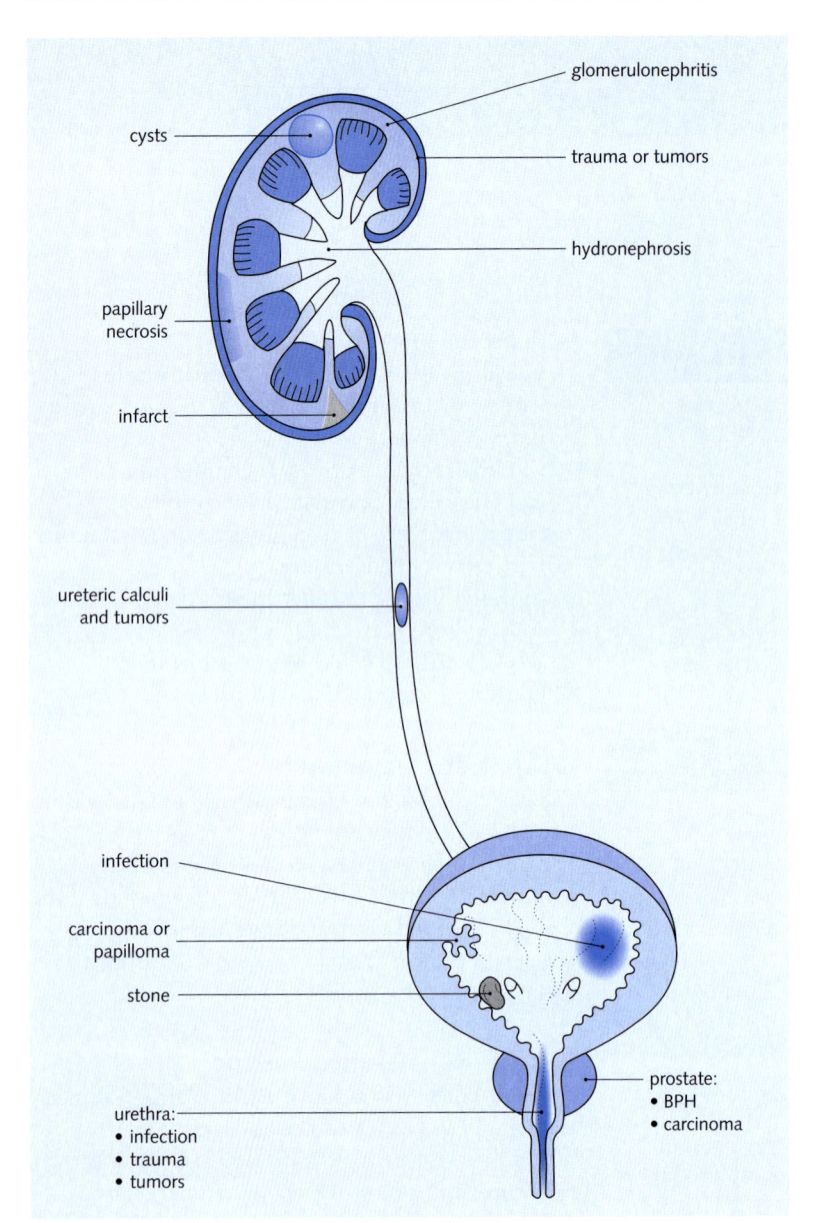

Fig. 6.1 Common sites of lesions causing hematuria. BPH, benign prostatic hypertrophy.

and <150mg/day of protein (exact values vary from laboratory to laboratory according to methods used to measure protein). It is usually assessed with a dipstick, which detects protein levels above 300mg/L. Microalbuminuria is the presence of excess urinary protein (usually albumin) but in amounts insufficient to cause a positive dipstick analysis. It is important to detect in diabetics at risk for renal disease. Dipsticks, therefore, are inadequate to screen these patients.

Proteinuria is measured as follows:
- The amount excreted in 24hr (the amount of protein excreted varies through the day). There may be large errors in this due to collection difficulties.
- A "spot" urine sample. When the urine protein concentration is divided by the spot urine creatinine concentration, this ratio estimates the grams per day of protein that would be found on a 24-hour collection.

Proteinuria

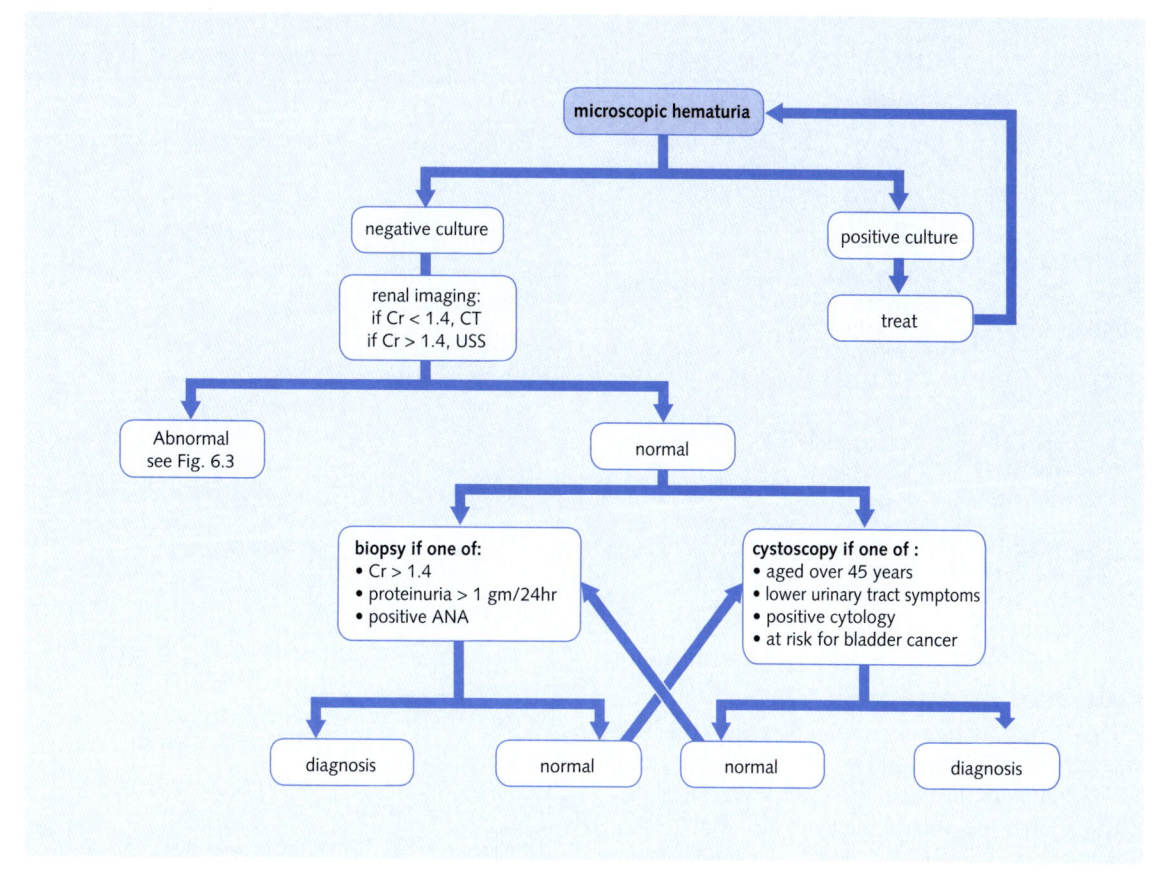

Fig. 6.2 Investigation of hematuria. Cr, creatinine; IVP, intravenous pyelography; USS, ultrasonography.

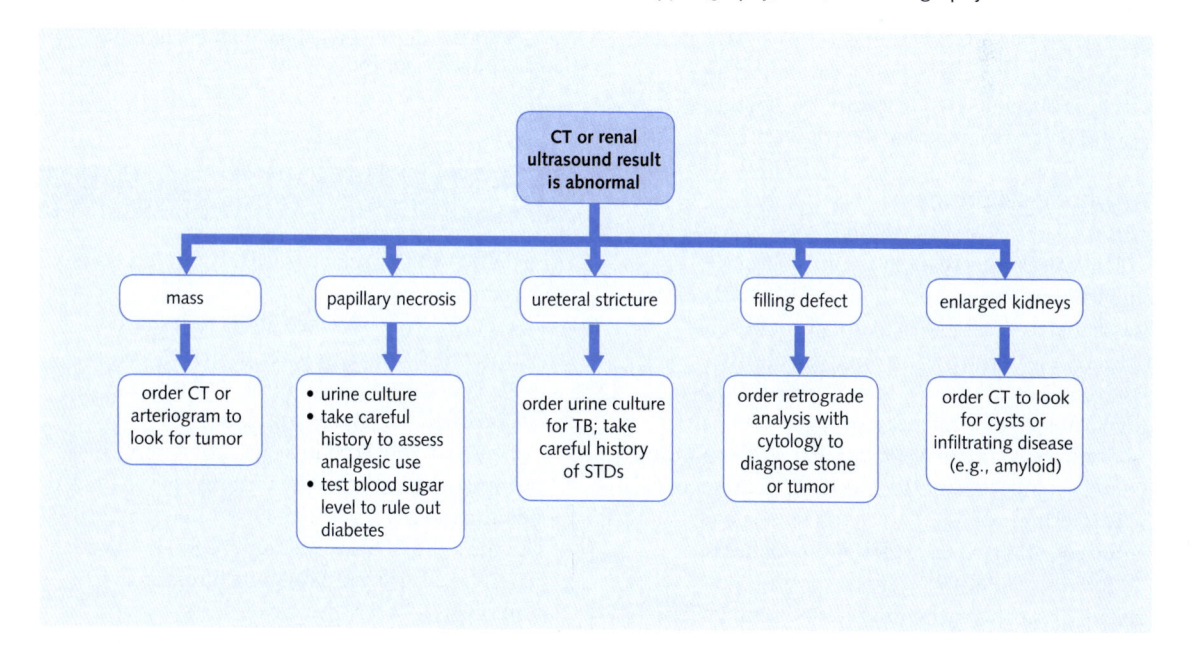

Fig. 6.3 Further investigation of hematuria when the CT or ultrasound result is abnormal. CT, computed tomography; IVP, intravenous pyelography; STDs, sexually transmitted diseases; TB, tuberculosis (from Green HL: *Clinical medicine*, 2nd ed. Mosby Year Book, 1996).

Common Presentations of Renal Disease

Urine analysis—possible findings and interpretation	
Findings	**Possible diagnoses**
clots in urine	carcinoma of the bladder or kidney; clot colic is also a feature of IgA nephropathy
albuminuria and hematuria	glomerular disease
dysmorphic red blood cells or red blood casts	glomerulonephritis—red cell casts are pathognomonic of active glomerular bleeding (e.g., IgA, nephropathy, vasculitis)
hematuria, pyuria, and white blood cell casts	renal tubulointerstitial disease (i.e., pyelonephritis)

Fig. 6.4 Urine analysis—findings and their interpretations.

Causes
Causes of proteinuria are summarized, together with relevant investigations, in Fig. 6.5. Most of these will have <1 gram of protein per 24 hours. Of the listed causes, only glomerular diseases and multiple myeloma normally yield >2 grams of proteinuria per 24 hours. After initial assessment using urine dipstick and spot/24-hour urine collection, investigations are performed to exclude systemic diseases, drugs, and toxins as the cause of proteinuria. Referral for renal biopsy is often needed in suspected glomerular disease or if renal function deteriorates.

Nephrotic syndrome
This is characterized by >3.5g/day proteinuria, which causes a decrease in serum albumin (hypoalbuminemia) and edema (Chapter 4). It is associated with an increase in cholesterol (hypercholesterolemia). Primary nephrotic syndrome results from diseases arising in the glomerulus. These include:
- Commonly, minimal change glomerulonephritis, membranous glomerulonephritis, focal segmental glomerulosclerosis.
- Rarely, other types of glomerulonephritis.

Causes of secondary nephrotic syndrome include diabetic nephropathy, drugs (gold, NSAIDs), amyloidosis, sickle-cell disease, malaria, tumors, and SLE.

Causes and investigation of proteinuria	
Cause	**Investigation**
diabetic nephropathy	blood glucose levels; examination for other diabetic complications
glomerulonephritis	biopsy (for histological diagnosis)
congestive heart failure	clinical signs, blood pressure
hypertension	regular blood pressure measurements
myeloma	complete blood count; serum and urine protein electrophoresis; bone marrow biopsy
amyloid	biopsy and Congo red staining; look for associated splenomegaly, myeloma, infection
pregnancy	HCG pregnancy test
pyrexia	core temperature measurement at regular intervals
exercise	urine sample on waking; to be repeated after exercise
postural proteinuria (rare if >30 years old)	urine sample on waking; repeated at mid-day
vaginal mucus contaminant	repeat urine sample, with sterile technique

Fig. 6.5 Causes and investigation of proteinuria. hCG, human chorionic gonadotrophin.

Pyuria

Urine WBCs can be seen in a variety of infectious or noninfectious conditions.
- Detection in the presence of bacteriuria or symptoms of urinary infection should prompt treatment for UTI or urethral discharge (see Chapter 5).
- Concurrent WBC casts suggest pyelonephritis or interstitial nephritis (i.e., intrarenal inflammation).
- The presence of urine eosinophils (stained with Hansel's stain) suggests allergic interstitial nephritis.
- If no other cause can be detected, and routine cultures are negative, consider tuberculosis as a cause of "sterile pyuria."

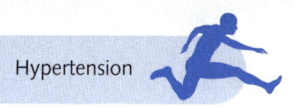

Hypertension

BP is influenced by the interaction of genetic and environmental factors, which regulate CO and total peripheral resistance (TPR):

$BP = CO \times TPR$

The kidneys influence BP by regulating extracellular volume. They also release vasoactive substances:
- Vasoconstrictors: angiotensin II.
- Vasodilators: prostaglandins.

Renal autoregulation maintains renal function despite variations in systolic BP. The kidney compensates for ECF changes by controlling Na^+ and water excretion. If this mechanism is disturbed, there may be uncontrolled Na^+ and water retention, resulting in hypertension. Normal blood pressure is defined by the World Health Organization (WHO) as 120/80mmHg or below, while hypertension is a sustained BP of 140/90mmHg or above. Between these numbers lies "prehypertension," which still may carry increased risk. The cardiovascular risks of hypertension have been found to be continuous, so there may be no "safe" elevated BP.

Essential hypertension

This accounts for about 95% of all cases of hypertension, and the cause is unknown. The typical age of onset is from age 25–45. Initially, there is an increase in cardiac output as a result of sympathetic overactivity. In the later stages the increase in BP is maintained by an increase in the TPR, but cardiac output is normal. When poorly controlled, hypertensive changes seen in the kidney include:
- Arteriosclerosis of the major renal arteries (renal artery stenosis).
- Hyalinization of the small vessels with intimal thickening.

Malignant or "accelerated" hypertension is a rapidly progressing form of severe hypertension. It is characterized by fibrinoid necrosis of the blood vessel walls and ischemic damage to the brain and kidney. This can lead to acute renal failure or heart failure, requiring urgent treatment. Repeated bouts can lead to chronic kidney disease (hypertensive nephrosclerosis) and a reduction in the size of the kidneys.

Secondary hypertension

This is caused by renal (80%) and endocrine diseases and occasionally by drugs (cyclosporine A).
Renal mechanisms causing hypertension include:
- Impaired sodium and water excretion, increasing blood volume.
- Stimulation of renin release.

Renal causes of hypertension are:
- Renal artery stenosis (renovascular hypertension).
- Intrinsic renal disease (renal hypertension).
- Primary hyperaldosteronism (causing renal Na^+ retention and K^+ excretion).
- Excess renin production (e.g., renal tumor).

Intrinsic renal diseases

These account for 75% of renally induced hypertension and include most types of primary and secondary glomerulonephritis (GN), chronic pyelonephritis, and polycystic kidney disease.

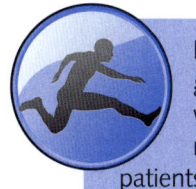

> Patients with primary glomerular disease present with hypertension (which is more severe) earlier than patients with renal interstitial disease.

Renal artery stenosis

This accounts for 25% of renal-induced hypertension cases. There are two types:
- Atherosclerosis: common.
- Fibromuscular dysplasia: uncommon (seen in young women).

Narrowing of the renal vessels reduces the pressure in the afferent arterioles, which stimulates the juxtaglomerular apparatus to secrete renin. This increases plasma angiotensin II, which causes vasoconstriction and aldosterone release. Aldosterone promotes Na^+ and therefore fluid retention (this increases BP), and increases K^+ secretion, causing hypokalemia.
Treatment involves:
- Transluminal angioplasty (to dilate the stenotic region), supplemented with stenting.
- Reconstructive vascular surgery (uncommon).

Endocrine causes

The endocrine causes are:
- Cushing's syndrome.
- Estrogen (i.e., the contraceptive pill and pregnancy).
- Pheochromocytoma (rare).
- Primary hyperaldosteronism (Conn's syndrome, rare).

Primary hyperaldosteronism is a rare condition in which there is chronic excessive secretion of aldosterone because of an adrenal cortical adenoma or adrenal hyperplasia (Fig. 6.6). Patients present with hypertension and hypokalemia. The mechanism of hypertension is unknown, because the increase in extracellular volume is small, and patients have no edema. Diagnosis is made with a triad of:
- Hypokalemia.
- Increased aldosterone.
- Decreased renin.

Treatment is by surgical removal of the adenoma, with a cure rate of 60%.

Management of hypertension

It is difficult to detect and treat hypertension because it is often asymptomatic, and many patients are reluctant to take medication if they feel well. It is very important to exclude an underlying cause of hypertension.

Hypertension is an important risk factor for strokes, cardiac failure, myocardial infarction, and renal failure. Effective treatment will improve the prognosis for each of these conditions.

Lifestyle changes include:
- Weight reduction.
- Reduced alcohol intake.
- Salt restriction.
- Regular exercise.
- Stop smoking.

Drug treatment of hypertension includes:
- Thiazide diuretics (preferred agent overall) and beta blockers as initial therapy.
- Angiotensin-converting enzyme (ACE) inhibitors (preferred in CKD).
- Ca^{2+} channel blockers.
- More potent agents such as minoxidil and hydralazine may be needed for severe cases.

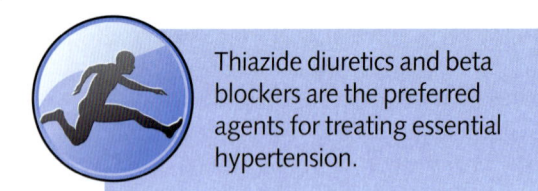

> Thiazide diuretics and beta blockers are the preferred agents for treating essential hypertension.

Angiotensin-converting enzyme (ACE) inhibitors

These agents inhibit ACE and thus block formation of angiotensin II. Angiotensin II is a potent vasoconstrictor and promotes sodium reabsorption in the tubule. ACE inhibitors (e.g., captopril, enalapril) lower BP by:
- Reducing TPR.
- Inhibiting the local (tissue) renin–angiotensin system.

ACE inhibitors also reduce proteinuria and delay the progress of renal disease in glomerular disease. They are also used to treat CHF by reducing afterload.

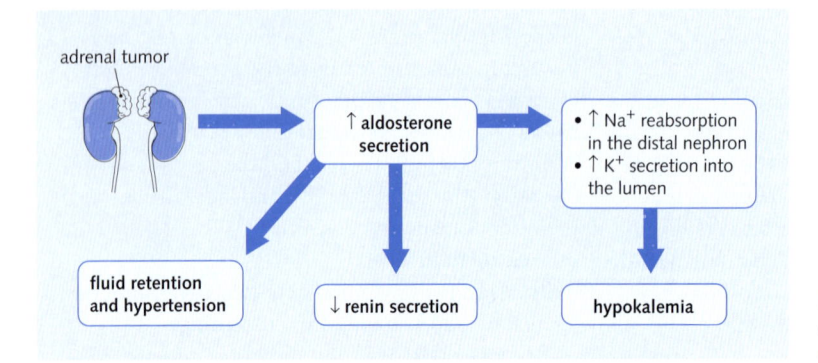

Fig. 6.6 Mechanism by which an adrenal tumor (Conn's syndrome) causes secondary hypertension.

The side-effects of ACE inhibitors include:
- Persistent dry cough.
- Hyperkalemia.
- Allergic reactions or rashes.
- Changes in the sensation of taste.
- Severe hypotension especially in patients who are hypovolemic.
- Acute renal failure in patients with renal artery stenosis (consider this before giving ACE inhibitors).

ACE inhibitors are contraindicated in the final two trimesters of pregnancy because of the risk of:
- Developmental abnormalities in the fetal kidney.
- Oligohydramnios (reduced amniotic fluid).
- Neonatal hypotension and anuria.

The effects of ACE inhibitors are shown in Fig. 6.7.

Dysuria

Dysuria with pyuria suggests either a sexually transmitted disease or a urinary tract infection. Figures 6.8 and 6.9 summarize the evaluation and treatment in women and men.

Dysfunctional voiding

In dysfunctional voiding there are abnormal characteristics of micturition. It is important to find out how the symptoms differ from normal for the patient. They can be:
- Irritative: producing frequency, nocturia, urgency and dysuria.
- Obstructive: producing hesitancy, diminished force, dribbling and increased residual urine.

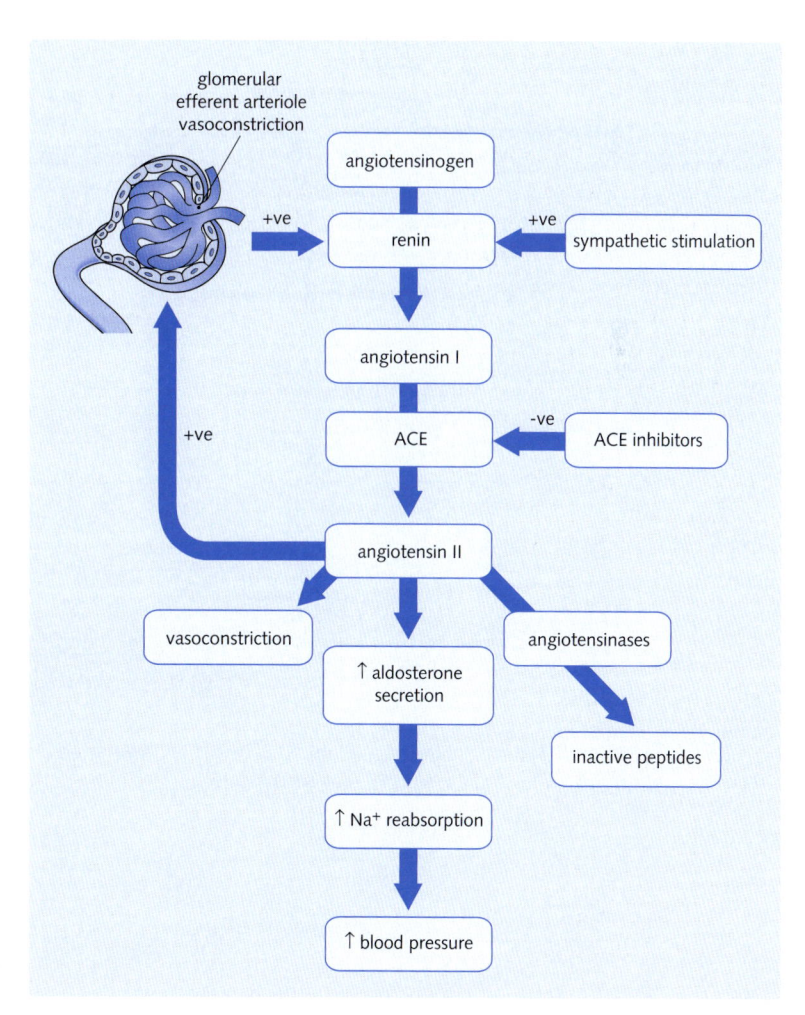

Fig. 6.7 Effects of ACE inhibitors. +ve, positive feedback; –ve, negative feedback.

Common Presentations of Renal Disease

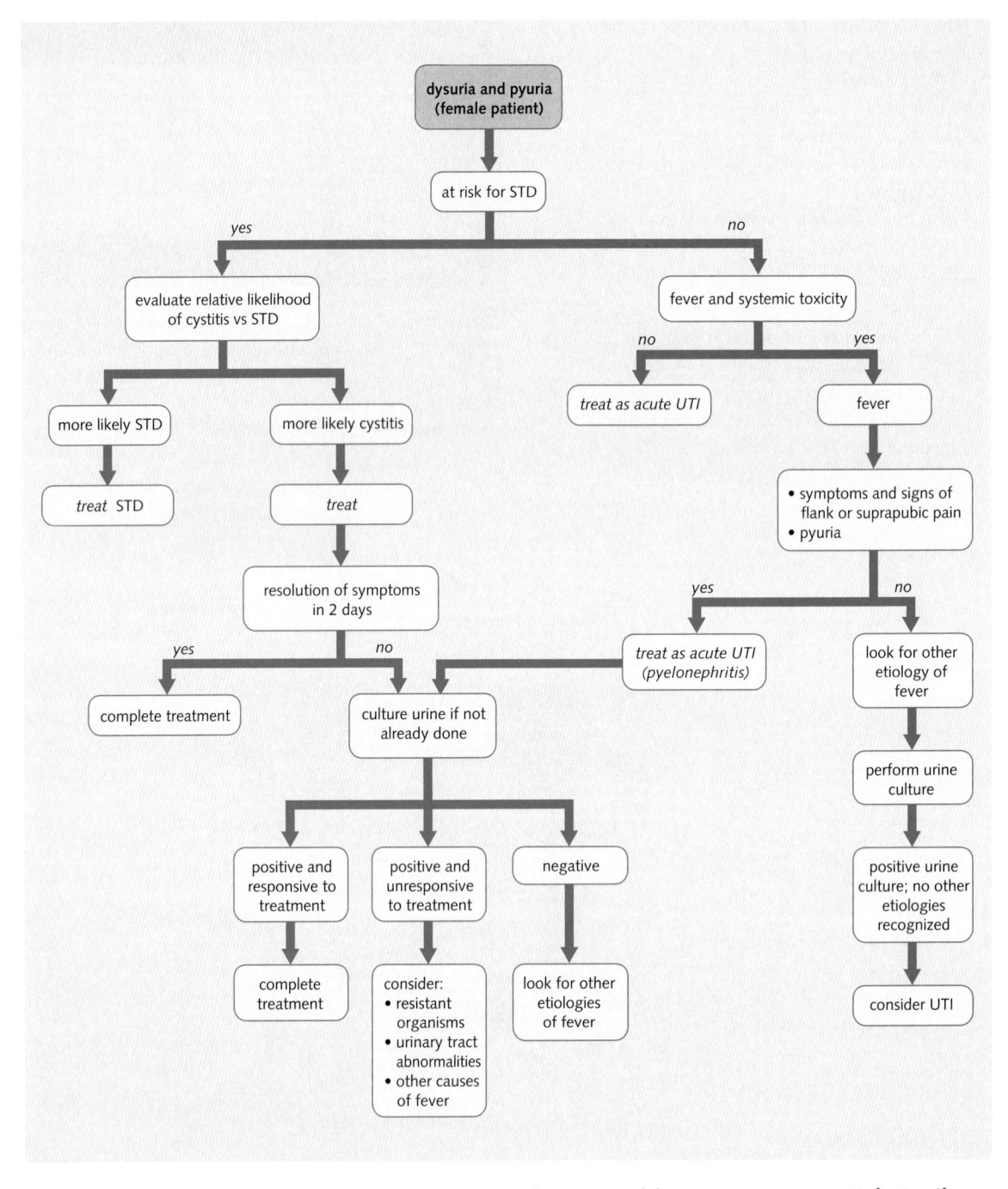

Fig. 6.8 Investigation of dysuria in a female patient. STD, sexually transmitted disease; UTI, urinary tract infection (from Green HL: *Clinical medicine*, 2nd ed. Mosby Year Book, 1996).

Dysfunctional voiding

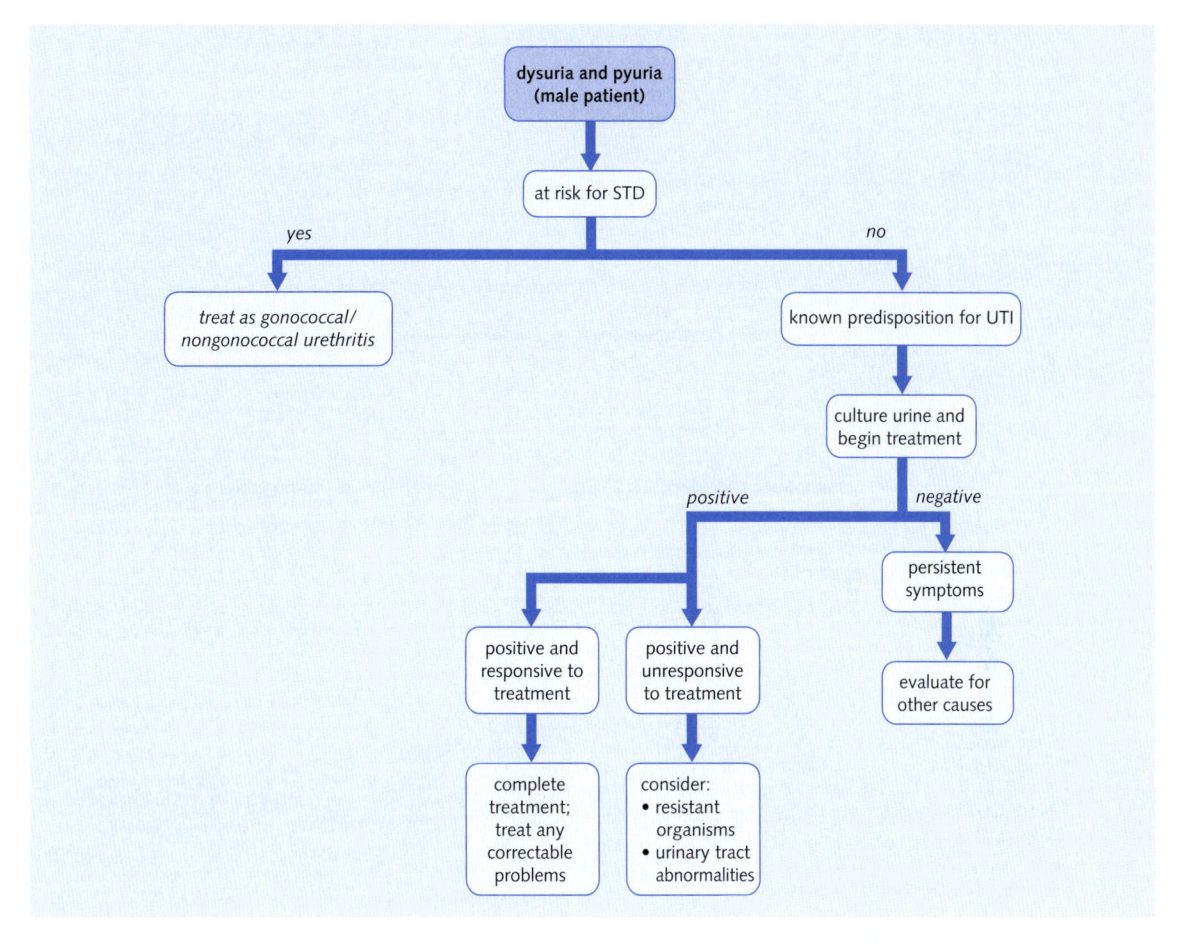

Fig. 6.9 Dysuria and pyuria in a male patient. STD, sexually transmitted disease; UTI, urinary tract infection (from Green HL: *Clinical medicine*, 2nd ed. Mosby Year Book, 1996).

Causes

Irritative bladder symptoms can be caused by:
- Local abnormality with decreased bladder capacity: this can be the result of infection, inflammation or fibrosis. Causes include acute cystitis, chronic infections (e.g., tuberculosis), chlamydia, chronic fungi, foreign body, stones, trauma, radiation, cyclophosphamide, interstitial cystitis, and chronic obstruction.
- Neurological abnormality: this can be the result of stroke, cerebral atrophy or multiple sclerosis, all of which damage the cortex or upper spinal cord.

Obstructive bladder symptoms are more common in men because they have a longer urethra, which is easily compressed or narrowed. Causes are summarized in Fig. 6.10.

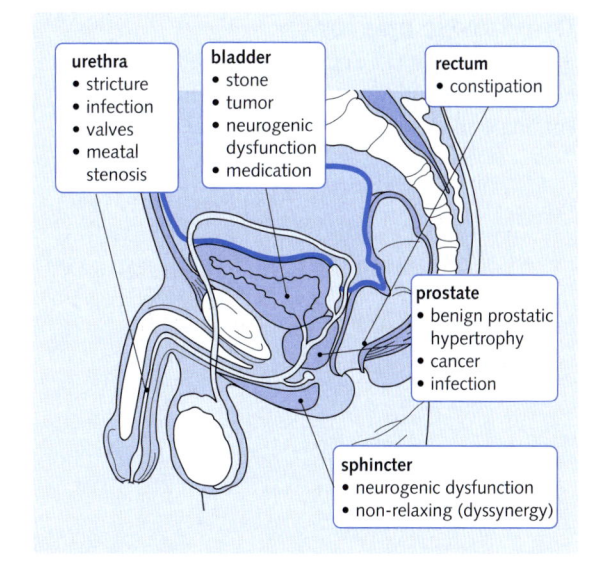

Fig. 6.10 Causes of obstructive bladder symptoms.

Common Presentations of Renal Disease

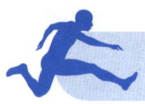

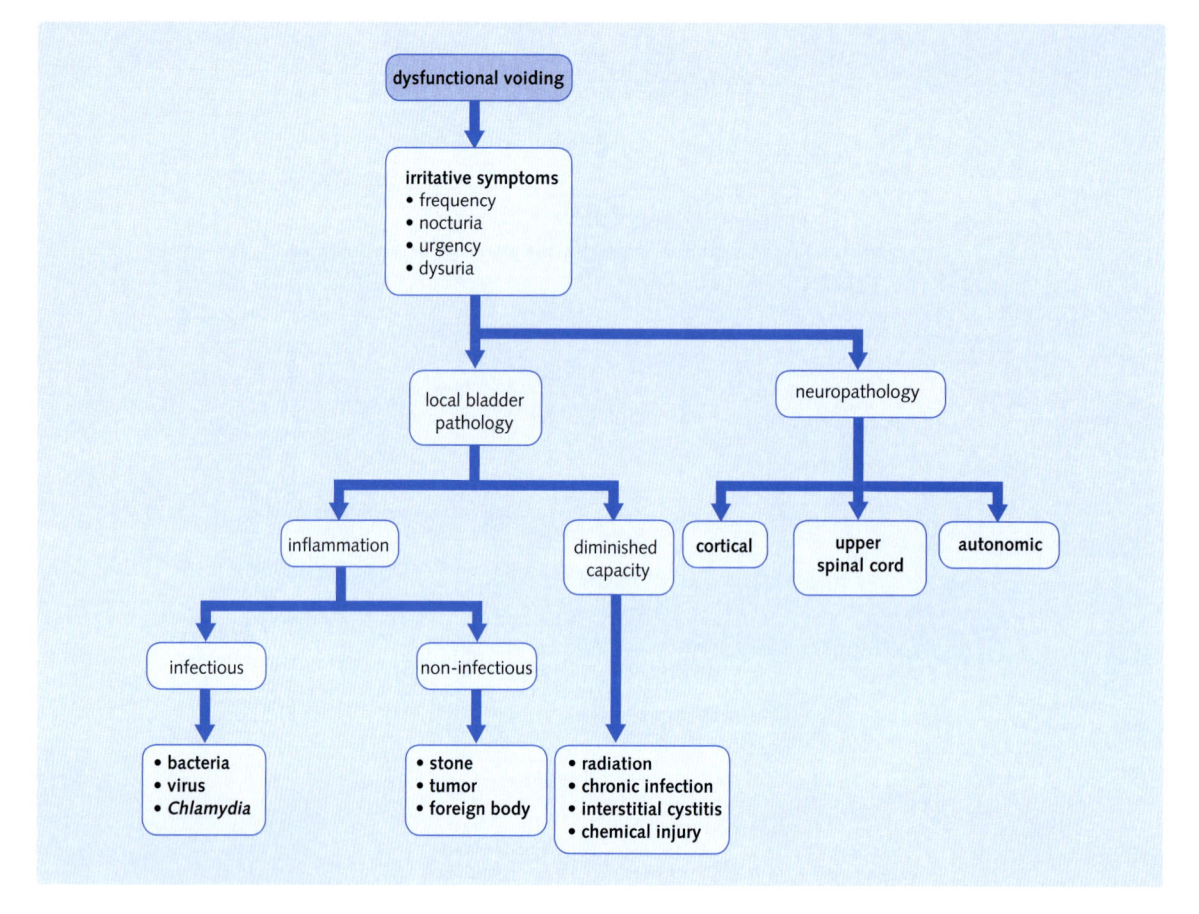

Fig. 6.11 Causes of irritative symptoms in dysfunctional voiding (from Green HL: *Clinical medicine*, 2nd ed. Mosby Year Book, 1996).

Diagnostic approach
A comparison of the etiology of irritative and obstructive bladder symptoms in dysfunctional voiding is shown in Figs. 6.11 and 6.12.

Dysfunctional voiding

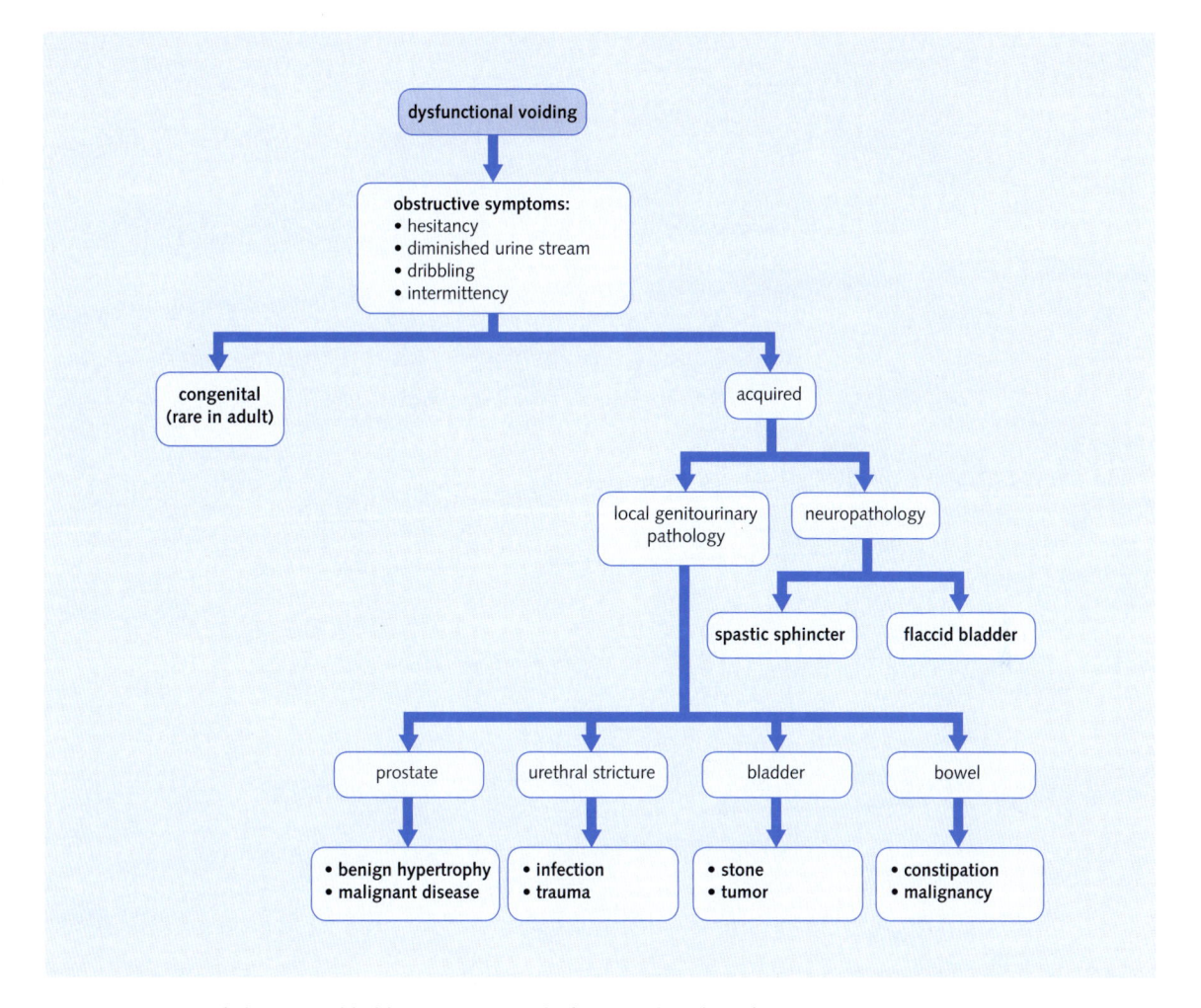

Fig. 6.12 Causes of obstructive bladder symptoms in dysfunctional voiding (from Green HL: *Clinical medicine*, 2nd ed. Mosby Year Book, 1996).

- Outline the workup of hematuria. How are renal vs. nonrenal causes distinguished?
- Summarize the defining features of nephrotic syndrome. Describe how primary nephrotic syndrome differs from secondary nephrotic syndrome.
- What are causes of pyuria with and without bacteriuria?
- What are the diagnostic steps in detecting renal artery stenosis?
- What are the endocrine causes of hypertension, and how are they identified?
- What are the preferred first drugs for hypertension management in the patient with essential hypertension? In the patient with glomerular disease?
- Outline how to distinguish between irritative and obstructive bladder symptoms.

7. History and Examination

Key historical points in renal disease

Symptoms relevant to the urinary system and electrolyte disorders are:
- Hematuria (cancer of the renal tract, urinary tract infection, glomerulonephritis).
- Increased frequency (urinary tract infection).
- Poor stream (bladder outflow obstruction—prostatic hypertrophy).
- Nocturia (chronic renal failure or bladder outflow obstruction).
- Recent infections—in particular, streptococcal throat/skin infections, as this can trigger post infectious glomerulonephritis.
- Vomiting or diarrhea.
- Polyuria (diabetes insipidus, osmotic diuresis).

Past medical history
Medical conditions associated with renal disease include diabetes mellitus, hypertension, chronic urinary infections or inflammatory disease, cancer, urinary tract infections, rheumatic fever, tonsillitis, lupus, and previous renal disease.

Drug history
Important drugs to ask about in renal disease include:
- Diuretics.
- ACE inhibitors or angiotensin receptor blockers.
- NSAIDs.
- Potassium supplements.

Family history
Note any known medical conditions in first-degree relatives—in particular, renal disease, hypertension and diabetes. A history of renal failure most commonly suggests diabetes, Alport's, or polycystic kidney disease.

Key physical exam points in renal disease

General observation
The extracellular volume status of the patient should be examined carefully. Useful physical signs include:
- Orthostatic hypotension or tachycardia.
- Elevated jugular venous pressure (JVP).
- Pleural effusion.
- Pulmonary edema.
- Peripheral pitting edema (most prominent at the ankles and sacrum).

Signs indicating that the patient is on dialysis include the presence of a hemodialysis graft or fistula or continuous ambulatory peritoneal dialysis catheter.

Vital signs
Blood pressure (BP)
Many patients with renal disease will have an elevated BP. When measuring BP (which needs to be done on several occasions) it is important to measure it on the same limb each time to ensure consistent and comparable results. To ensure measurement is accurate:
- Select the correct cuff size.
- Use the cuff on a fully extended arm with the stethoscope applied lightly to the brachial artery.
- Always take the BP with the patient lying, sitting and standing. This is because a 5- to 10-mmHg increase in diastolic pressure is usually seen on standing in a healthy person. Postural hypotension (i.e., a drop in diastolic pressure on standing) can be detected only if both measurements are made.

The World Health Organization (WHO) defines hypertension as a maintained systolic pressure of 140mmHg or above and a diastolic pressure of 90mmHg or above. Renal diseases associated with hypertension include renal artery stenosis, acute, and

143

chronic glomerulonephritis (GN), and polycystic kidneys.

Pulse
Tachycardia (orthostatic or resting) may suggest volume depletion.

Skin
- Scratch marks may indicate pruritus due to chronic kidney disease (CKD).
- Uremic frost is small crystals of urea that may look like dandruff. It is seen in far advanced renal failure.
- Purpuric rashes can be seen in vasculitis, Henoch-Schönlein Purpura.

Lungs
- Pattern and rate of respiration—patients with a metabolic acidosis associated with chronic renal failure often have a deep, sigh-like respiration, with a rapid breathing rate. This is known as Kussmaul's respiration, and is caused by direct stimulation of the respiratory center in an attempt to correct the systemic acidosis. A similar respiratory pattern is seen in severe untreated diabetic ketoacidosis.
- Rales or pleural effusions may indicate extracellular volume expansion.

Cardiovascular system
- Bruits over carotid or other arteries suggest advanced atherosclerotic disease.
- A laterally displaced PMI may suggest longstanding hypertension with ventricular hypertrophy.

Auscultatory findings of significance in renal disease are shown in Fig. 7.1.

Abdomen
Palpation
The kidneys are normally not palpable unless markedly enlarged:
- Bilateral enlargement is seen in polycystic kidney disease and hydronephrosis.
- Unilateral enlargement is seen in tumors, cysts, and unilateral hydronephrosis.

Positive findings on auscultation of the cardiovascular system in renal disease		
Test	Sign	Diagnostic inference
heart sounds: listen for audibility, rate and accentuation of the sound in all four areas	muffled and soft	pericardial effusion
	prominent aortic component of the second heart sound	hypertension
	a low-pitched third heart sound heard after the second heart sound	an early sign of left ventricular failure or fluid overload
	gallop rhythm (two normal heart sounds with a third and tachycardia)	• fluid overload • ventricular failure
murmurs: • low pitch (apex) with the bell • high pitch with the diaphragm feel the carotid pulse—time the murmur with the cardiac cycle	• functional murmurs • murmurs due to coexisting valve disease	• aortic and pulmonary regurgitation due to dilatation of the valve ring secondary to fluid overload • mitral regurgitation due to annular calification of the valve; anemia
pericardial rub: listen carefully over the precordium	a localized or generalized scratchy sound heard in any part of the cardiac cycle heard best if the patient leans forward	this friction rub (two layers of the pericardial layer moving in the presence of an exudate) occurs in: • pericarditis (a terminal feature of CRF) • uremic pericarditis • systemic lupus erythematosus and vasculitis • intermittent illness in a patient with CRF

Fig. 7.1 Auscultatory findings of the cardiovascular system in renal disease. CRF, chronic renal failure.

Key physical exam points in renal disease

The presence of ascites can be seen in nephrotic syndrome, hepatorenal syndrome, and patients on peritoneal dialysis.

Auscultation

Auscultate for bruits by applying the stethoscope firmly on the abdomen or in the flank over the renal artery. Alternatively, they can be heard over the back. However, it can be difficult to distinguish an aortic bruit from one originating in the renal artery. A bruit is heard if there is rapid turbulent movement of blood through a narrowed artery. Causes of bruits include:
- Renal artery stenosis.
- Atherosclerosis.
- Arteriovenous malformation in the kidney.

Digital rectal examination

Always obtain permission and have a chaperone for female patients. The patient should lie on the left side, with the knees drawn up to the chest.

- Inspect the perianal area for hemorrhoids, fissures, inflammation, prolapse and ulcers.
- Put lubricant on the glove and insert finger into the rectum.
- Assess the tone of the anal sphincter, the size and shape of the prostate (normally walnut sized).
- After removing your finger, inspect for any blood or feces.
- Feel for any lateral masses.

Palpable changes in the prostate and their clinical significance are summarized in Fig. 7.2. A vaginal examination should also be performed in female patients.

Extremities/Neuro

Pitting edema may be seen in any intrinsic renal disease.

Patients with CKD may exhibit:
- peripheral neuropathy
- asterixis
- mental status changes

| Prostate findings on digital rectal examination ||
Sign	Diagnostic inference
firm, smooth, rubbery consistency; walnut-shaped and sized	normal prostate
tender, enlarged, and soft	acute infection (prostatitis)
hard, irregular, asymmetric, nodular	prostate carcinoma

Fig. 7.2 Changes of the prostate noted on digital rectal examination.

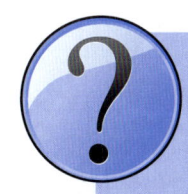

- Describe which symptoms are particularly relevant to the urinary system.
- Describe the skin changes associated with renal disease.
- Explain how you can ensure that blood pressure (BP) measurement is consistent and comparable. Discuss why it is important to measure BP lying, sitting, and standing.
- List the possible findings on auscultation of the heart in renal disease.
- Describe how to examine the kidneys. List the possible causes for unilateral and bilateral kidney enlargement.
- Explain how you can test for ascites, and what the renal-related causes are.
- Outline the possible findings on digital rectal examination.

8. Lab Investigation and Imaging

When considering investigations, always start with the least invasive simple procedures and then progress to second-line investigations if required.

Testing the blood and urine

Renal and urinary tract diseases should be considered if the patient presents with symptoms linked to the urinary tract, abnormal serum urea or creatinine concentration, or abnormal urinalysis. Testing the urine is the simplest investigation and should always be done in suspected renal disease. This is done with a midstream urine sample, and assessment includes appearance, volume, pH, dipstick, microscopy and cytology (Fig. 8.1).

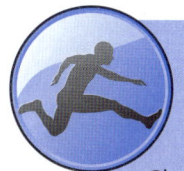

To take a midstream urine specimen:
- The patient must have a full bladder.
- Clean the external urethral meatus with a sterile swab.
- Collect the sample half way through urine flow.

Blood tests that assess the basic renal function include serum urea (BUN) and creatinine. However, a significant amount of renal damage can occur before abnormal values are detected in the blood, so the preferred option is to measure creatinine clearance, which closely reflects the GFR (see Chapter 1). A complete blood count highlights anemia (due to blood loss or impaired renal function) and polycythemia. Other important blood results are shown in Fig. 8.2.

Imaging and other investigations

Radiological imaging of the upper and lower urinary tract can be used to:
- Establish a diagnosis.
- Assess the complications of impaired renal function.
- Monitor the progression of disease.
- Follow the response to treatment.

Imaging of the upper urinary tract includes KUB radiography, ultrasonography, CT, and IVP. The main form of imaging for the lower urinary tract is cystoscopy.

Plain radiography

Plain radiography of the kidney, ureters, and bladder (KUB) is a simple, noninvasive test that can be used before specialized imaging. It is used to detect calcification in the kidney, such as renal and urinary tract stones—uric acid stones cannot be detected, but in general 90% of stones are radio-opaque (Figs 8.3 and 8.4). It also highlights the size and position of the kidneys, and any bony deposits (these can be associated with prostatic cancer).

The main type of radiograph used to visualize the renal system and urinary tract is a KUB—*not* a plain abdominal view, which often does not include the full pelvis.

Ultrasonography

Ultrasonography is another noninvasive technique that involves high frequency sound waves. It is used to assess the size, shape and position of the kidney, and can also distinguish solid masses and renal cysts (Figs 8.5 and 8.6). Dilatation of the pelvicalyceal system and upper ureters can also be detected—indicating the presence of obstruction. This is a major cause of reversible renal failure, and can be treated if detected early enough. Prostate size can also be assessed, and if necessary, a biopsy can be

147

Lab Investigation and Imaging

	Indications	Scientific basis	Normal results	Abnormal results
appearance	any urine sample		clear fluid	**red/pink**: hematuria, beet intake **brown**: cholestatic jaundice **cloudy**: infection
volume	any urine sample		1000–2500 mL/day	**oliguria**: physiological; intrinsic renal disease; obstructive nephropathy **polyuria**: excess H_2O intake; increased solute loss e.g. glucose; diabetes insipidus, diuretics
pH	any urine sample		pH 4.5–8.0	**alkaline urine**: infection with *Proteus*—urea splitting **acid urine**: aminoaciduria; renal calculi
sodium	oliguria altered Na^+ homeostasis	urinary [Na] must be interpreted in context of urine output, sodium intake, and natriuretic drugs	depends on clinical setting; 24-hour urinary Na^+ = 100–250 mEq/L	<20 mEq/L oliguria → prerenal >20 mEq/L renal losses or ATN
creatinine clearance	suspected renal failure	reflects GFR; both the urine and plasma concentration of creatinine is required; requires timed urine collection	125 mL/min per 1.73 m^2 body surface area	decreased levels indicate a decrease in GFR—as see in acute and chronic renal diseases
blood	gross bleeding into urine usually found in patients with renal disease; hypertension; pregnancy; bacterial endocarditis	reagent strips are used—based on a peroxide-like reaction	negative any positive result must be followed by microscopy	**microscopic hematuria**: renal or lower GU disease; gross hematuria: stones, tumors, trauma, UTI, papillary necrosis, IgA nephropathy
protein dipstick and if positive → 24-hour collection	edema	reagent strips impregnated with buffered blue tetrabromophenol—detects [albumin] >150 mg/L; microalbuminuria is used as an earlier indicator of diabetic glomerular disease; the test requires a radioimmunoassay ↑ which is more sensitive than the strips	<150 mg/day	**increased with**: exercise; standing up; renal disease; nephrotic syndrome; fever; diabetic glomerular disease; hypertension; CHF

Fig. 8.1 Urine test results and their significance. MSU, midstream urine; TB, tuberculosis; UTI, urinary tract infection. ESR, erythrocyte sedimentation rate; GFR, glomerular filtration rate; PSA, prostate-specific antigen; UTI, urinary tract infection.

Imaging and other investigations

	Urine test results and their significance—Continued			
	Indications	**Scientific basis**	**Normal results**	**Abnormal results**
glucose	suspected diabetes mellitus; renal disease; pregnancy	reagent strips using glucose oxidase or hexokinase enzyme reactions Clinitest	negative	glucose may be present when: 1. blood glucose above the renal threshold i.e. diabetes mellitus 2. altered renal threshold i.e. pregnancy; Fanconi's
urine microscopy (obtain a clean urine sample) (i) direct (ii) after centrifugation	symptoms of UTIs; suspicion of renal disease	a small amount of unspun urine placed on a slide, covered with a cover slip, and looked at under a microscope Gram stain to look for bacteria counterstained to look at cell cytology	negative	**white cells indicate**: inflammatory reaction; infection in the urinary tract; stones; TB; analgesic nephropathy **red cells indicate**: glomerulonephritis; acute urinary tract infection; calculi; tumor **granular casts indicate**: acute tubular necrosis; **white blood cell casts indicate**: pyelonephritis **red cell casts indicate**: glomerulonephritis **crystals seen indicate**: stones **bacteria seen indicate**: infection **abnormal cells indicate**: cancer of urothelium
urine culture	• must always be performed in suspected complicated UTIs or UTIs in men, elderly. • in cases of TB an early morning sample of urine is required	growing any organisms present; vital to have an MSU specimen	no growth	>10000CFU/mL indicates urinary infection <10000CFU/mL probably indicates contamination of the specimen

Fig. 8.1 *Continued*

taken under transurethral ultrasonography guidance for further investigation (Fig. 8.7). Renal vein thrombosis can be detected with Doppler ultrasonography, and arterial Doppler studies can be used to identify renal artery stenosis. The specificity and sensitivity of ultrasound investigations are very operator dependent.

Renal biopsy

Renal biopsy is used for the histological classification of glomerulonephritis, which can influence the choice of therapy in patients with nephrotic syndrome and acute nephritis. It is also used in the diagnosis and assessment of systemic diseases that affect the kidneys (e.g., SLE). It can aid the investigation of unexplained acute renal failure, proteinuria, and hematuria and is vital in the management of renal transplant patients. A sample of the kidney tissue can be taken by inserting a needle into the back using ultrasound guidance, with the patient lying in the prone position. This is then examined under a microscope, using immunochemical staining to detect complement or immunoglobulins and electron microscopy to define ultrastructure. Relative contraindications to renal biopsy include:
- A bleeding diathesis (absolute contraindication unless corrected).
- Suspected renal carcinoma (hypervascular).
- Obesity (technically difficult).
- Small kidneys (technically difficult).
- Pregnancy.

Lab Investigation and Imaging

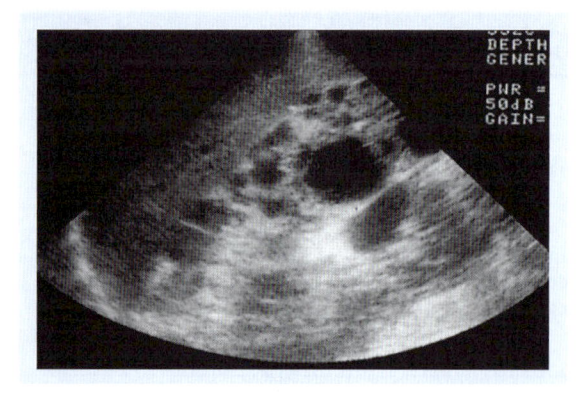

Fig. 8.5 Ultrasound scan showing the typical appearance of polycystic kidneys. There are multiple cysts within the parenchyma (from Lloyd-Davis RW et al: *Color atlas of urology*, 2nd ed. Mosby Year Book, 1994).

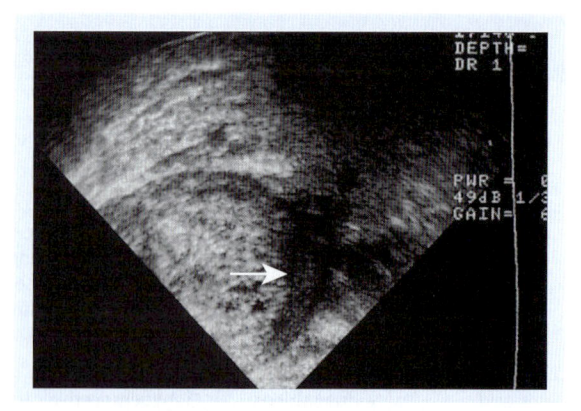

Fig. 8.7 A rectal ultrasound probe is used to define and stage carcinoma of the prostate. The arrow highlights an echo-poor area in the left peripheral zone of the prostate. This extends into the central part of the gland and beyond the capsule (courtesy of Dr. D Rickards).

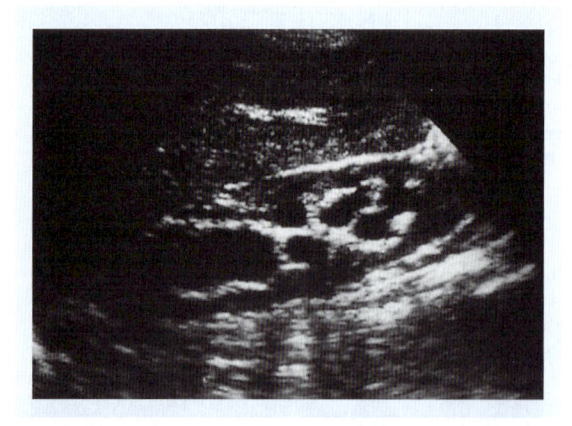

Fig. 8.6 Hydronephrosis of the right kidney demonstrated by ultrasonography. The echo-lucent (black) areas within the kidney are caused by dilated calyces (from Williams G, Mallick NP: *Color atlas of renal diseases*, 2nd ed. Mosby Year Book, 1994).

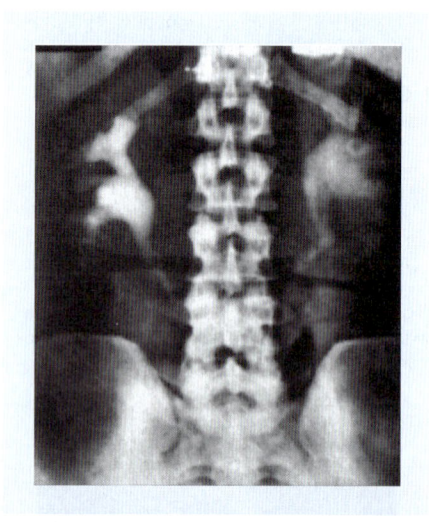

Fig. 8.8 An intravenous pyelogram showing bilateral hydronephrosis in response to bladder neck obstruction caused by dense granulation and fibrous tissue in a patient with schistosomiasis of the bladder (from Williams G, Mallick NP: *Color atlas of renal diseases*, 2nd ed. Mosby Year Book, 1994).

- Chronic renal failure (increased risk of bleeding). The main complications are bleeding (hematuria), infection, pain in the flank, and renal hematoma.

Intravenous pyelography (IVP)

Intravenous pyelography involves serial radiographs taken after intravenous injection of radiopaque contrast medium (Figs 8.8 and 8.9). Normal kidney function is required, and the patient must not be pregnant. These techniques are used to assess kidney size and shape as well as the anatomy and patency of the calyces, pelvis and ureters. It can also be used to localize fistulae and highlight filling defects in the bladder.

Risks of the procedure include allergy to the contrast medium and reaction to the contrast. This ranges from mild (itching, nausea and vomiting) to severe reaction, which could impair renal function—

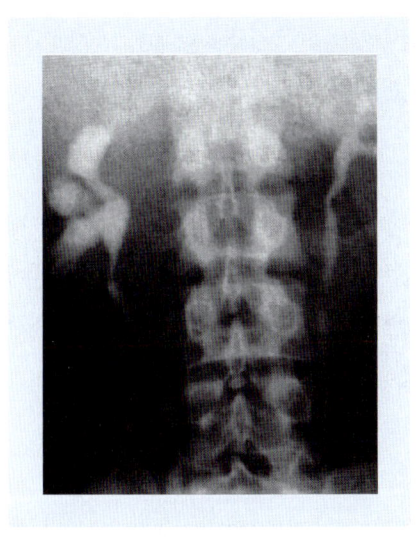

Fig. 8.9 An intravenous pyelogram showing marked calyceal clubbing in the right kidney. There is gross dilatation of the calyces, which is pronounced in all poles of the kidney. These findings are the result of unilateral reflux of urine and chronic infection (from Lloyd-Davis RW et al: *Color atlas of urology*, 2nd edn. Mosby Year Book, 1994).

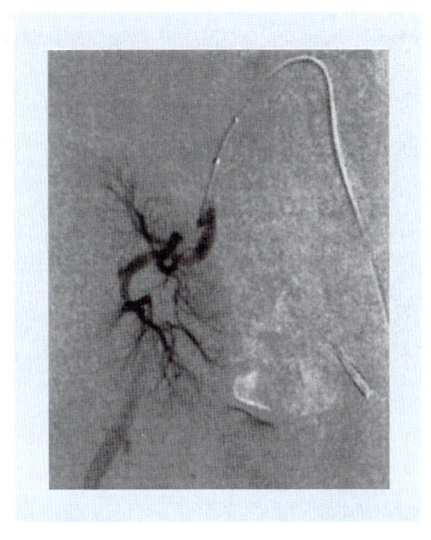

Fig. 8.10 Subtraction arteriogram of a transplanted kidney. The donor renal artery is anastamosed to the internal iliac artery (from Williams G, Mallick NP: *Color atlas of renal diseases*, 2nd ed. Mosby Year Book, 1994).

especially if the patient has pre-existing renal disease. Ensure that the patient is volume replete prior to the procedure. Bicarbonate infusion reduces the risk of ATN.

Renal arteriography

Renal arteriography uses contrast medium to give an anatomical demonstration of the renal arteries. A catheter is introduced into the femoral artery, through which contrast is injected into the renal artery and a series of radiographs are taken. It is used to detect renal artery stenosis or aneurysms (Figs 8.10 and 8.11A) and to investigate renal hypertension. Therapeutic angioplasty may be performed at the same time. It can be used in the diagnosis of tumors, but this is becoming less common with the increasing use of CT.

Renal artery stenosis can be detected without IV contrast using magnetic resonance aided angiography (Fig. 8.11B).

Voiding cystourethrograms

Voiding cystourethrograms are used to demonstrate vesicoureteric reflux from the bladder to the ureters during emptying of the bladder (Fig. 8.12). Reflux can be classified into three grades.

- Grade 1: contrast medium enters the ureter only.
- Grade 2: contrast medium fills the pelvicalyceal system.
- Grade 3: dilatation of the calyces and ureter.

This technique was used to investigate children with recurrent urinary tract infections but has largely been replaced by other techniques because of concerns over ionizing radiation. It is used in the investigation of adults with disturbed bladder function.

Cystoscopy

A rigid or flexible cystoscope is inserted through the urethra to inspect the interior surface of the lower urinary tract (bladder and urethra). This technique is very useful in the diagnosis and treatment of tumors in the bladder. It can also be used to identify and remove stones, take a tissue biopsy and to assess prostatic disease.

Diagnostic cystoscopy can be performed in the outpatient clinic, and involves a flexible cystoscope examination under local anesthesia. Therapeutic cystoscopy uses a rigid cystoscope, with the patient under general anesthesia.

Lab Investigation and Imaging

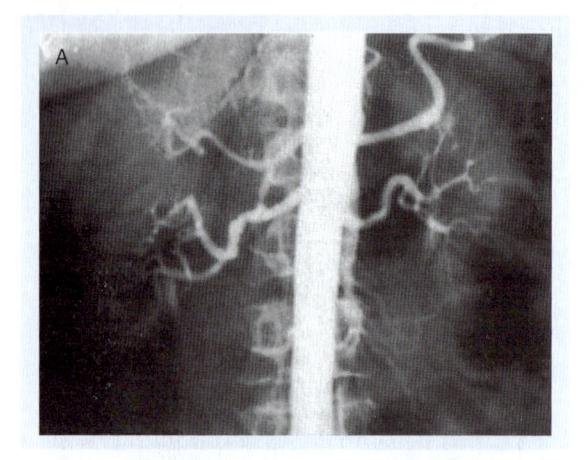

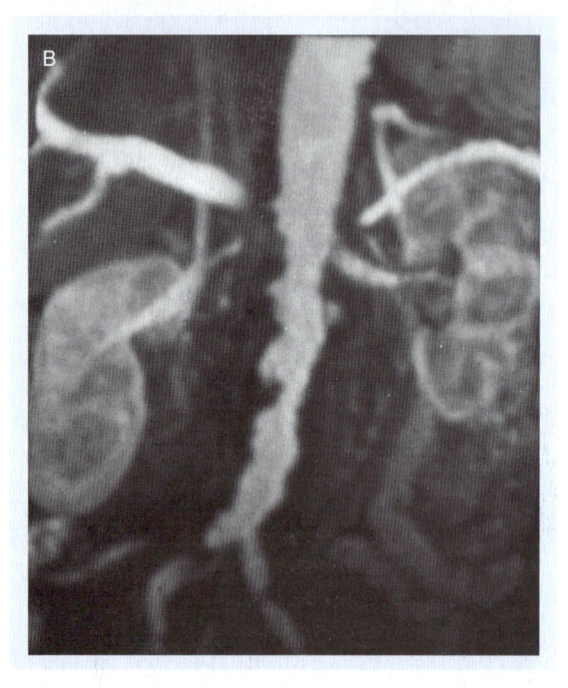

Fig. 8.11 (A) An arteriogram showing a marked renal arterial stenosis on the right, typical of fibromuscular hyperplasia. (B) MR renal angiography demonstrating a tight stenosis at the origin of the right renal artery. The irregularity of the abdominal aorta is due to marked atheroma.

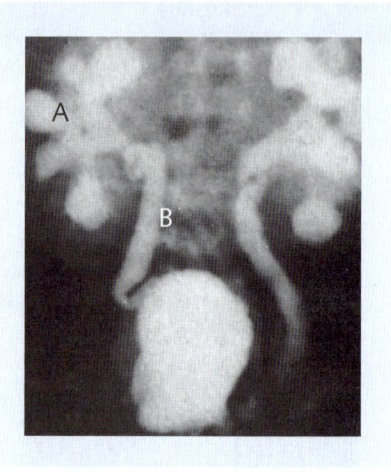

Fig. 8.12 A voiding cystourethrogram showing bilateral ureteric reflux. This patient has early calyceal clubbing (A) and ureteric dilatation (B). This is grade-3 reflux (courtesy Mr. RS Cole).

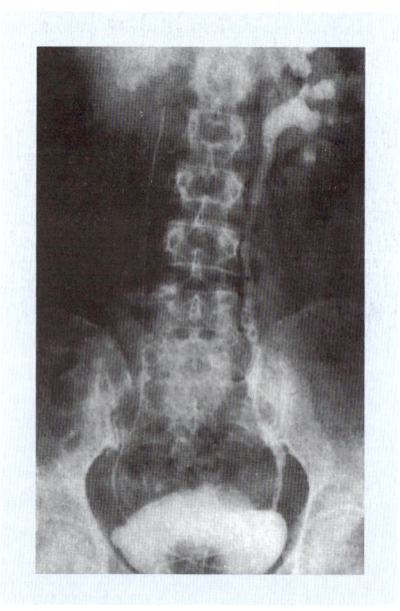

Fig. 8.13 Retrograde pyelogram showing "emphysematous" pyelonephritis caused by gas-forming bacteria (from Catto GRD et al: *Diagnostic picture tests in renal disease*, 1994, TMIP).

Retrograde pyelography

Retrograde pyelography is used to define the site of an obstruction (Figs 8.13 and 8.14) or lesions within the ureter. It does not require functioning kidneys. The patient must be admitted for general anesthesia and a ureteric catheter is then inserted under cystoscopic guidance. Contrast medium is injected into the catheter, to identify any lesions and help dislodge ureteric stones and coax them down the ureter.

Fig. 8.14 Retrograde pyelogram showing a large filling defect in the left ureter (arrow) caused by a tumor (from Lloyd-Davis RW et al: *Color atlas of urology*, 2nd ed. Mosby Year Book, 1994).

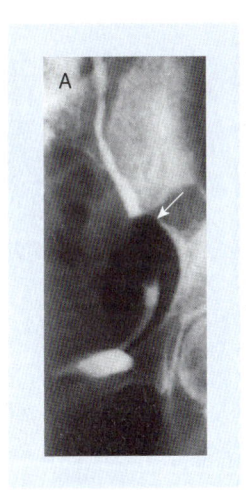

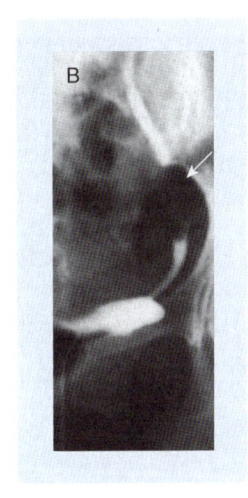

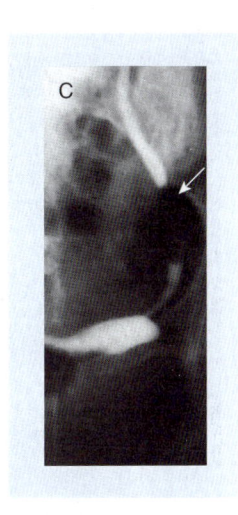

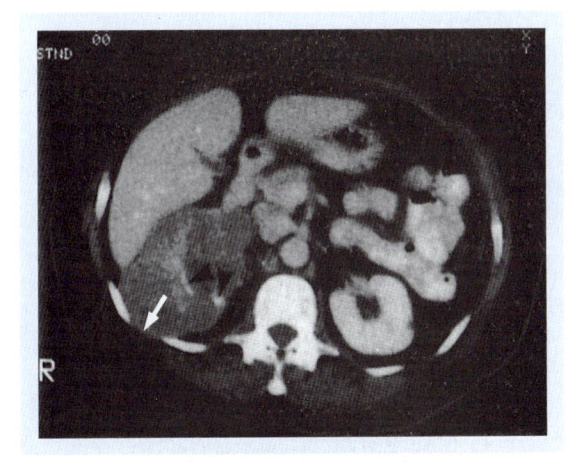

Fig. 8.15 CT scan highlighting a right renal cell carcinoma that extends through the intercostal space between ribs 11 and 12 (arrow) and medially along the renal vein. The high-density (white) areas (arrows) indicate calcification (from Williams G, Mallick NP: *Color atlas of renal diseases*, 2nd ed. Mosby Year Book, 1994).

Antegrade pyelography

This is used to define the site of obstruction in the upper urinary tract, i.e., mainly within the pelvicalyceal system. It involves percutaneous catheterization of a renal calyx and injection of contrast medium as described above for retrograde pyelography. Percutaneous catheterization of the pelvicalyceal system (nephrostomy) is also used therapeutically to relieve obstruction.

Computed tomography (CT)

CT is a quick and non-invasive technique, which can be used with or without contrast. It is used to define renal and retroperitoneal masses and is ideal for locating and staging renal tumors (Fig. 8.15). It is also used to show polycystic kidney disease and has the advantage of also highlighting non-renal pathology. Modern techniques involving spiral CT can be used to visualize the anatomy of the renal arteries, renal vein and inferior vena cava, as well as retroperitoneal studies. Increasingly, thin cut CT is the investigation of choice to diagnose stones and obstruction to the urinary tract, and as the preferred radiologic test for evaluating hematuria (Fig. 8.16).

Magnetic resonance imaging (MRI)

MRI is an imaging technique that does not involve ionizing radiation—unlike CT. Instead, it relies on the measurement of the magnetic fields of atomic nuclei. It is used to differentiate between cystic and solid renal masses and for precise staging of tumors. However, MRI is expensive and cannot be used in patients with pacemakers or other metallic implants. Magnetic resonance has now been developed to provide resolution sufficient to diagnose atheromatous renal artery stenosis (see Fig. 8.11B).

Radionuclide scanning

Radionuclide scans are used in static and dynamic imaging. Technetium-labeled dimercaptosuccinic acid (^{99m}Tc-DMSA) provides static images of the renal parenchyma and shows local renal function. It highlights the localization, shape and function of each

Lab Investigation and Imaging

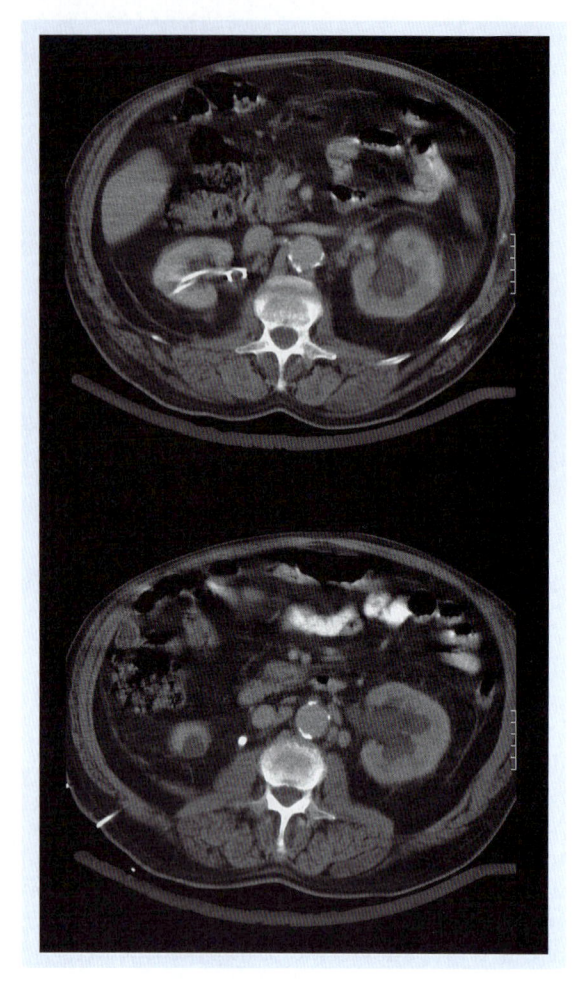

Fig. 8.16 An abdominal CT scan of a patient who presented with acute renal failure and bilateral flank pain. There is bilateral hydronephrosis secondary to bilateral ureteric stones. In the upper image a nephrostomy tube is seen in the right renal pelvis. The lower image demonstrates a dense opacity (calculus) lying in the ureter approximately at the level of L2. Subsequent images demonstrated a similar opacity at L3 on the left.

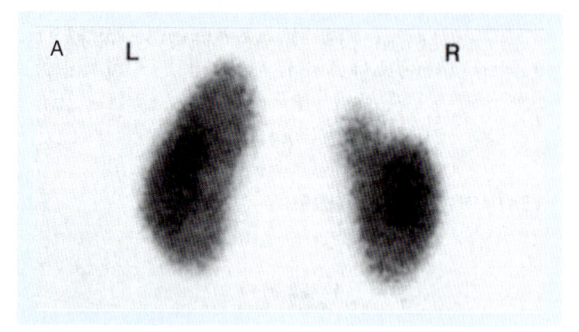

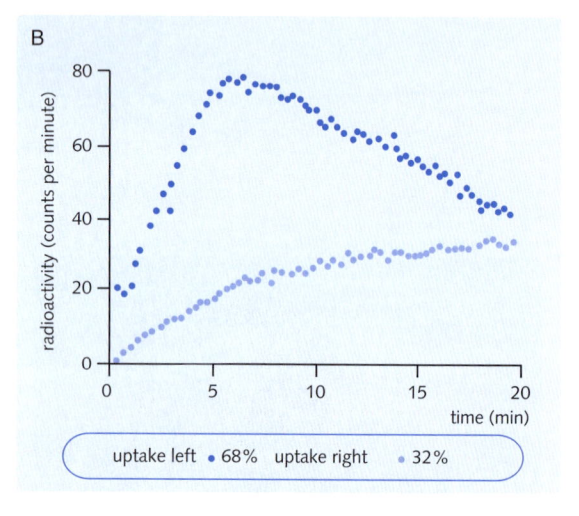

Fig. 8.17 (A) ^{99m}Tc-DMSA scan showing a right upper pole scar (courtesy TO Nunan). (B) The graph shows a diminished uptake of 36% for the right kidney, indicating a degree of loss of function correlating with the scar (from Williams G, Mallick NP: *Color atlas of renal diseases*, 2nd ed. Mosby Year Book, 1994).

individual kidney, and highlights scarring as a result of reflux nephropathy (Fig. 8.17) Technetium-labeled pentetic acid (^{99m}Tc-DTPA) is excreted by renal filtration and the changes in the level of ^{99m}Tc-DTPA in the kidney over time are quantified using a gamma camera. This provides a dynamic index of blood flow to each kidney. It is used to assess transplant function (Fig. 8.18A) and can demonstrate obstruction to the upper urinary tract (by diuresis renogram, Fig. 8.18B). It can also be used to determine the relative function of each kidney. Both ^{99m}Tc-DMSA and ^{99m}Tc-DTPA are injected into the venous circulation. Radionuclide techniques can be used to demonstrate reflux nephropathy.

Urodynamic studies

These are used to distinguish urge incontinence from genuine stress incontinence. They also detect bladder/detrusor muscle instability. The bladder is catheterized and a pressure probe is inserted to measure the bladder pressure. A rectal probe is also inserted to assess intra-abdominal pressure. The detrusor muscle pressure can be calculated by

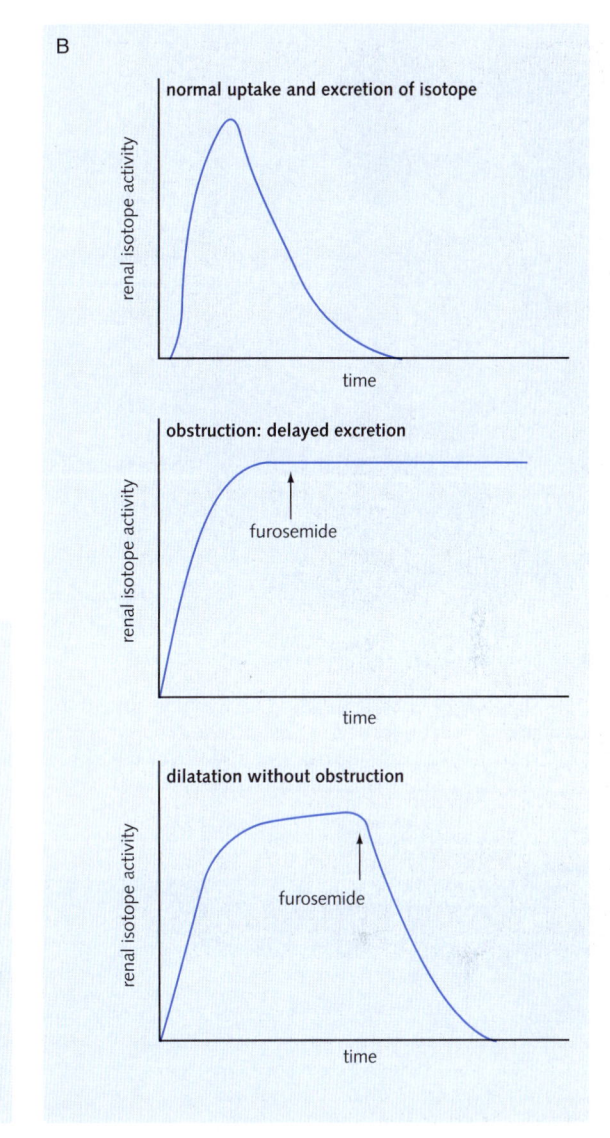

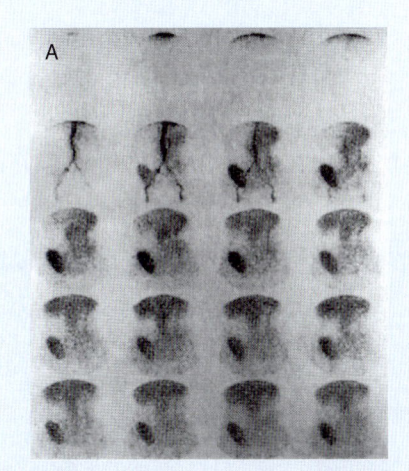

Fig. 8.18 (A) ^{99m}Tc-DTPA diuretic renogram showing a transplanted kidney functioning normally (from Catto GRD et al: Diagnostic picture tests in renal disease. TMIP, 1994). (B) Diuretic isotopic renography showing tracings for normal, obstructed and dilated (without obstruction) upper urinary tract. Obstruction can be distinguished from dilatation by administering furosemide, which promotes excretion of the isotope in dilatation (without obstruction) but has no effect on excretion rates in obstruction (from Johnson RJ, Feehally J: *Comprehensive nephrology*, Mosby Year Book, 2000).

subtracting the bladder pressure from the intra-abdominal pressure. The bladder is then filled with water until the patient feels the urge to void. At this point the relative pressures are recorded. If the patient has stress incontinence, an increase in intra-abdominal pressure (e.g., coughing) leads to involuntary urine leakage, with no bladder/detrusor muscle contraction. If the patient has urge incontinence, the bladder/detrusor muscle contracts either spontaneously or with increased abdominal pressure, and the patient feels an overwhelming urge to urinate immediately (Fig. 8.19).

Lab Investigation and Imaging

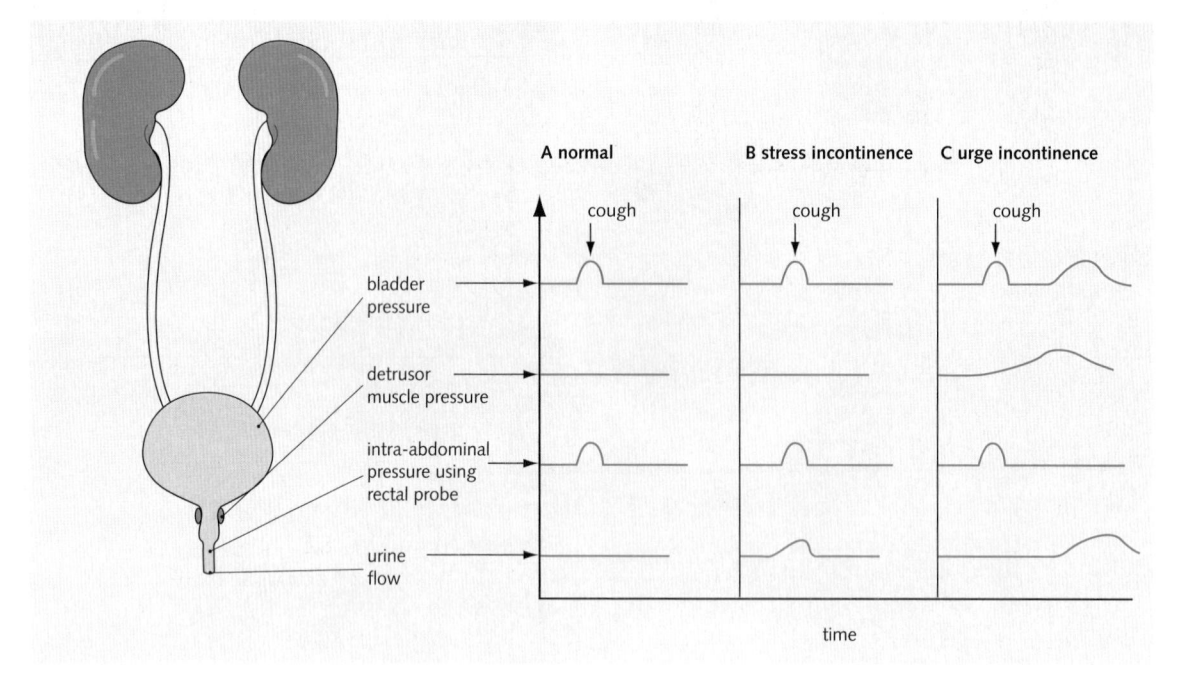

Fig. 8.19 Diagnosing incontinence using urodynamic studies. A, Normal cough; B, identifies stress incontinence, in which urine leakage is seen in response to a raised intra-abdominal pressure; C, shows urge incontinence, in which urine leakage is seen in response to detrusor muscle instability following a rise in intra-abdominal pressure.

- Name five tests that can be performed on a urine sample, and explain the importance of a midstream urine sample.
- Describe the blood tests that can be done to investigate renal function, and give the possible causes of abnormal results.
- Give two reasons why plasma creatinine is a poor indicator of renal function.
- Explain when you would use ultrasonography in preference to plain radiography.
- List four contraindications and four complications of a renal biopsy.
- Explain how you would conduct an IVP.
- Describe the complications of specialist investigations involving the use of contrast medium. How can they be prevented?
- Explain the main differences between a diagnostic and therapeutic cystoscopy.
- Name the main investigation used to stage renal tumors.
- Explain how urodynamic studies can be used to differentiate between genuine stress incontinence and urge incontinence.

Index

A
abdomen, 144–5
abdominal radiograph, 151
abdominal wall
　posterior, 4
abnormal hematuria
　investigation, 133
abnormal junction, 92
acid-base disturbances, 63–8
　classification, 65
　compensation, 65
　identification, 65
acid-base physiology
　basic principles, 60–1
　renal regulation of, 61–2
acidosis
　metabolic, 67
　　acute renal failure, 39
　　chronic kidney disease, 40
　renal tubular
　　classification, 68
　respiratory, 66
active transport
　mechanisms, 23
acute tubular necrosis, 90–1
ADH: see antidiuretic hormone
adrenal adenoma, 136
adrenal hyperplasia, 136
aldosterone, 45–6
　release, 45
alkaline phosphate, 64
alkalosis
　metabolic, 67–8
　respiratory, 66
allopurinol: see xanthine oxidase inhibitors
alternative complement pathway, 83
amino acids, 28
ammonium, 29
　as buffer, 62–3
　in hyperkalemic RTA, 68
amphotericin
　hypomagnesemia, 75
amyloidosis, 88
angiotensin 2, 44–5
　conversion from AT1, 35, 45
angiotensin-converting enzyme, 45, 100

angiotensin-converting enzyme inhibitors, 136
　acute renal failure, 38
　hyperkalemia, 70
anion gap, 67
antegrade pyelography, 155
antibodies
　ANCA, 89, 90
　anti-GBM, 82, 89–90
　cytotoxic, 83
　hepatitis, 141
　HIV, 142
　immune complexes, 82
antidiuretic hormone (ADH), 31, 52–4
　and CHF, 97
　and hyponatremia, 57–9
　and hypernatremia, 59–60
antigen
　prostate specific, 142
　streptococcal, 150
arteriography, renal, 153
aspirin
　metabolic acidosis, 67
　papillary necrosis, 92
auscultation, 145

B
benign prostatic hypertrophy, 125–6
　and ARF, 39
　complications, 126
Berger's disease, 88–9
Bicarbonate
　as buffer, 61
　carbonic anhydrase inhibitors and, 50
　in metabolic acidosis, 67
　in metabolic alkalosis, 67–8
　reabsorption, 28, 62
bladder
　abnormalities, 113
　development, 14
　innervation, 106
　interior, 103–4
　male
　　posterior and interior view, 106
　microstructure, 108
　transitional cell carcinoma, 124
　tumors, 121–4, 153

Index

blood volume, 11
blood pressure, 33
   autoregulation of GFR and RPF, 35
   effective circulating volume, 43
   hypertension, 135–6
body fluid compartments, 3–4
   clinical disorders, 60–76
   composition, 9
   disorders, 46–51
   fluid movement across, 7–8
   measuring, 9–10
   regulation, 43–6
buffers, 60
   bicarbonate system, 61
   physiologic, 61
BUN (blood urea nitrogen). see urea

C

calcium
   homeostasis mechanisms, 74
   kidney stones, 116–17
      urinary investigations, 118
   kidney transport, 73
   regulation and clinical disorders, 70–6
   serum, 142
   thiazides and, 50
cancer
   bladder, 121–4
      cystoscopy, 153
   brain
      and diabetes insipidus, 59
   chemotherapy
      hyperkalemia, 70
   glomerular disease, 86
   hypercalcemia, 74
   hyperuricemia, 76
      urate nephropathy, 92
   lung
      and SIADH, 58
   multiple myeloma
      hypercalcemia, 74
      nephrocalcinosis, 93
      renal failure, 93
      RTA Type II, 68
   nephroblastoma, 96–7
   prostate, 126–7
   renal cell, 95–6
   ureters, 121
   Wilms' tumor, 96–7
carbonic anhydrase inhibitors, 50–1
   proximal RTA and, 68

cardiogenic shock, 99
cardiovascular system
   renal disease, 144–5
CHF. see congestive heart failure (CHF)
Chlamydia trachomatis, 120–3
cholesterol emboli syndrome, 94–5
chronic kidney disease (CKD), 38, 40–3
   acidosis and, 67
   complications, 41
   diagnostic approach, 40
   EPO deficiency and, 76
   hyperkalemia and, 70
   hyperphosphatemia and, 73
   hypocalcemia and, 73
   hyponatremia and, 57–8
   treatment, 40–3
circulating immune complex nephritis, 82
CKD. see chronic kidney disease (CKD)
clearance, 36–7
   creatinine, 37–8
   inulin, 37
collecting ducts, 17
   cortical, 31–2
      ammonium, 62–3
      potassium, 69
   medullary, 32
      natriuretic peptides, 46
computed tomography, 155
   renal cell carcinoma, 96
   renal stones, 117
congenital abnormalities
   urinary tract, 111
congestive heart failure (CHF), 97–8
   ARF, 38
   compensatory mechanisms, 98
   expanded ECF, 47–8
   hyponatremia, 57–8
Conn's Syndrome, 136
continuous ambulatory peritoneal dialysis (CAPD), 42
cortical necrosis, 95
countercurrent multiplier, 55
creatinine, 37–8
   clearance, 37–8
   serum, 38, 39, 150
crescentic glomerulonephritis, 89
cyclosporine
   acute renal failure, 38
   chronic kidney disease, 40
cystic disease, renal, 79–82
   adult autosomal dominant, 79–81

cystic disease, renal (*Continued*)
    acquired, 82
    childhood autosomal recessive, 81
    medullary, 82
cystic renal dysplasia, 82
cystitis, 119
    acute, 119
    chronic, 119
    interstitial, 119
    presentation and treatment, 120
cystoscopy, 153–4
    hematuria, 133
    transitional cell bladder cancer, 124

D

diabetes insipidus, 59–60
diabetes mellitus, 87
    glucosuria, 27
    incontinence, 110–11
    hyponatremia, 56–57
    ketoacidosis, 67
    urinary tract infection, 118, 121
diabetic ketoacidosis, 67
diabetic nephrosclerosis, 87–8
digital rectal examination, 145–6
dilution principle for measuring body volumes
    constant infusion method, 10
    single injection method, 10
distal convoluted tubule, 17, 29–31
    thiazide diuretics, 51
diuretics, 48–51
    causing hyponatremia, 58–9
    causing hypovolemia, 47
    renogram for diagnosing obstruction, 157
    treatment of diabetes insipidus, 60
dopamine, 46
dysfunctional voiding, 137–40
    causes, 140
    diagnostic approach, 140
    obstructive bladder symptoms, 141
dysuria, 137
    causes, 139–42
    female patient investigation, 138
    male patient, 138

E

ectopic kidney, 79
edema, 47–9
    etiology, 49
    treatment, 48–51
embryology, renal, 13–14

endothelial cells, glomerular, 20
epithelial cells, glomerular (podocytes)
    electron micrographs, 21
erythropoiesis
    renal regulation, 76
erythropoietin (EPO), 19–20
    action and synthesis, 76
    clinical use, 19, 41
    deficiency in CKD, 40, 76
ethylene glycol
    metabolic acidosis, 67
exstrophy of bladder, 113
extracellular fluid (volume), 4–6, 11
    clinical disorders, 46
    composition, 9
    depletion, 47
    expansion, 47–8
    hyponatremia, 57–8
    regulation, 43–6
    treatment, 48
extracellular volume (ECV): *see* extracellular fluid

F

Fabry's syndrome, 86
fibromuscular dysplasia, 94
filtration fraction, 38
fluid compartments, 3–11
focal segmental glomerulosclerosis (FSGS), 86
fractional excretion, 38–9

G

Gibbs–Donnan effect, 7
glomerular basement membrane, 20
    GFR, 33–4
    glomerular disease, 82
    nephrotic syndrome, 84
glomerular diseases, 82–91
    clinical manifestations, 83–6
    mechanisms, 82–3
    specific types, 86–91
glomerular filtration, 21
glomerular filtration rate, 33–8
    age-related changes, 36, 37
    determinants, 34
    forces governing, 33–4
    regulation, 35–6
glomerular injury
    mechanisms, 82–3
glomerulonephritis, 82–91
    chronic, 85
    membranoproliferative, 87

glomerulonephritis (Continued)
  post infectious, 88
glomerulopathy
  membranous, 86
glomerulosclerosis
  diabetic, 87
  focal segmental, 86
glomerulus, 16, 20–1
  structure, 20–1
glucose
  osmolality, 5
  hyponatremia, 56
  tubular reabsorption, 25–7
  urine dipstick, 149
GN. see glomerulonephritis
gold, 86, 92
Goodpasture's syndrome, 89–90

H
hematuria, 131, 133
  diagnostic approach, 131
  investigation, 133
  nephritic syndrome, 85
  urine dipstick, 149
hemodialysis, 41–2
hemolytic uremic syndrome (HUS), 94
Henoch–Schönlein purpura (HSP), 89
  rash, 144
hepatorenal syndrome, 99
horseshoe kidney, 79, 80
HSP. see Henoch–Schönlein purpura (HSP)
hydrochlorothiazide. see thiazides diuretics
hydroureter, 112
hyperaldosteronism
  hyperkalemia, 70
  hypertension, 136
hypercalcemia, 74–5
  nephrogenic diabetes insipidus, 59
hyperkalemia, 70
  investigation, 72
  renal tubular acidosis, 68
hypernatremia, 59–60
hyperparathyroidism, 40
  nephrocalcinosis, 93
hyperphosphatemia, 75
hypertension, 135–7
  diabetic glomerulosclerosis, 87–8
  essential, 135
  lupus nephritis, 89
  malignant, 93
  management, 136–7

  measurement, 143–4
  nephritic syndrome, 85
  nephrosclerosis, 93
  polycystic kidney disease, 81
  renal artery stenosis, 135
  RPGN, 89
  secondary, 135–6
hypertensive nephrosclerosis, 93
hypertonic solutions, 6
  treating hyponatremia, 59
hyperuricemia, 76
  investigation, 77
hypoaldosteronism
  hyperkalemia, 70
  hyperkalemic RTA, 68
hypocalcemia, 73
  chronic kidney disease, 39
  hypomagnesemia, 75
hypokalemia, 70
  investigation, 71
  metabolic alkalosis, 68
  nephrogenic diabetes insipidus, 59
  renal tubular acidosis, 68
hypomagnesemia, 75
  and hypocalcemia, 75
hyponatremia, 54, 56–9
  chronic, 59
  symptoms, 56
  thiazides, 50
  treatment, 59
hypophosphatemia, 75
hypoplasia, renal, 79
hypotonic solutions, 6
hypovolemic shock, 99

I
IgA nephropathy, 88–9
immune complexes
  glomerular injury, 82–3
  mechanisms, 83
incontinence, urinary, 110–11
  urodynamic studies, 158
infarction, renal 95
infection
  glomerulonephritis, 88
  pyelonephritis, 91
  septic shock, 99
  urethritis, 120–3
  urinary tract, 117–18
    cystitis, 119–20
    dysuria, 137–9

infection (*Continued*)
    dysfunctional voiding, 140–1
    hematuria, 131–4
    polycystic kidney disease, 81
    obstruction, 116
    prostatitis, 124–5
    pyelonephritis, 91
    pyuria, 134
    stones, 116–17, 151
    urine culture, 149
    urinalysis, 141
intercalated cells
    type A, 31–2
    type B, 32
interstitial fluid, 4, 8–9, 11
interstitium, renal
    diseases, 90–3
intracellular fluid (volume), 3, 8, 11
    composition, 9
intracellular shifting
    potassium, 69
intravenous (IV) fluids
    composition and volume, 48
intravenous (IV) pyelography, 152–3
inulin clearance, 37
ion diffusion
    active transport, 7
    passive transport, 7
ion transport, 9
    loop of Henle, 30
isotonic solutions, 6
IV. *see* intravenous (IV) fluids

J
juxtaglomerular apparatus, 19
    effective circulating volume, 43
    histology, 19

K
kidney
    abdominal radiograph, 151
    agenesis, 79
    anatomy, 14
    anterior relations, 15
    arteriogram, 153
    blood circulation, 18
    blood supply, 17–19
    development, 14
    disease, 79–101. *see also* chronic kidney disease (CKD)
    functions, 3
    glomerular structure and function, 20
    internal structure, 15–20
    intravenous pyelogram, 153
    macroscopic organization, 13–15
    morphology, 15–20
    neoplastic disease, 95–7
    organization, 13–20
    stones. *see* nephrolithiasis
    structural organization, 3
    vascular structure, 17–19
kinins, 46

L
lactic acid
    metabolic acidosis, 67
    shock, 98
lead, 92
loop diuretics, 50
loop of Henle, 17
    ion transport, 30
    role, 29
    structure, 29
lower urinary tract, 103–48
    female anatomy, 104
    male anatomy, 104
lymphatic vessels
    fluid exchange, 8–9

M
macula densa, 35
magnesium, 75
    clinical disorders, 75
magnetic resonance imaging (MRI), 155
malignant hypertension, 93
medullary collecting ducts, 32
medullary interstitium
    concentrating generations, 54
medullary sponge kidney, 82
megaureter, 113
membranoproliferative glomerulonephritis, 87
membranous glomerulopathy, 86
mercury, 92
mesangium, 21
metabolic acidosis. *see* acidosis
metabolic alkalosis. *see* alkalosis
methanol
    metabolic acidosis, 67
microangiopathies
    thrombotic, 94

Index

micturition, 108–10
  abnormal, 108–10
  normal, 108
minimal change disease, 87
MRI. see magnetic resonance imaging (MRI)
multiple myeloma
  hypercalcemia, 74
  nephrocalcinosis, 93
  renal failure, 93
  RTA Type II, 68
multiple sclerosis
  incontinence, 109–10

N

nafcillin, 92
natriuretic peptides, 46
  edema, 48
neoplastic disease. see cancer
nephritic syndrome, 85–6
  diseases, 88–90
  hematuria, 85
nephritis, interstitial, 90–3
nephroblastoma, 96–7
nephrocalcinosis, 93
nephrolithiasis, 116–17
  hematuria, 131–3
  treatment, 117
nephron, 15–16
  transport, 22
  structure, 16
nephropathy, sickle cell, 95
nephrosclerosis, hypertensive, 93
nephrotic diseases
  primary, 86
  secondary, 87–9
nephrotic syndrome, 84–5, 134
  complications, 85
  edema, 47
  treatment, 85
nonsteroidal anti-inflammatory drugs (NSAIDS)
  acute renal failure, 38
  interstitial nephritis, 92
  minimal change disease, 86–7

O

obstruction, urinary tract, 114–16
  acute renal failure, 89
  bladder symptoms, 139
  diagnosis
    antegrade pyelography, 155
    CT scanning, 155
    renogram, 157
    retrograde pyelography, 154
    ultrasonography, 147
  dysfunctional voiding, 137
  nephrolithiasis, 117
  prostate cancer, 126
  prostatic hypertrophy, 125–6
  ureteropelvic junction, 111, 114
osmolality, 4–6
  clinical disorders, 54–60
  plasma, 5
  regulation, 51–4
  serum, 51
  urine, 52, 57
    diagnosing hypernatremia, 60
    diagnosing hyponatremia, 57–8
osmolarity, 4–6. also see osmolality
osmoreceptors, 51, 53
osmotic diuretics, 48
overflow incontinence, 110–11

P

parathyroid hormone, 73
  chronic kidney disease, 40
penicillamine, 86
pericarditis
  in CKD, 40
  pericardial rub, 144
peritoneal dialysis, 41
phenacitin, 92
phosphate
  buffer, 61–2
  disorders, 75
  homeostasis, 73
  reabsorption, 28
  titratable acid, 62
plasma volume, 4, 8, 11
  composition, 9
podocytes. see epithelial cells, glomerular
polyarteritis nodosum, 90
polycystic kidney disease, 79–82
  adult, 79–81
  childhood, 81
  enlarged kidneys, 144
post infectious glomerulonephritis, 88
post streptococcal glomerulonephritis, 88
potassium
  cellular shifting, 69
  clinical disorders, 68–72
  diuretics, 50
  transport, 69

164

potassium (*Continued*)
    ATPase, 24
        reabsorption, 28
        secretion, 31
    regulation, 68–70
    serum, 150
principal cells, 31
prostaglandins, 36, 46
prostate, 104, 106–7
    cancer, 126–7
    disorders, 124–8
    microstructure, 108
    physical exam, 145
prostatic hypertrophy, 125–6
prostatitis, 124–5
    chronic, 125
    treatment, 126
proteinuria, 83–5, 131–4
    causes and investigation, 134
proximal tubule, 16, 24–8
    bicarbonate reabsorption, 28, 62
    cell features, 25
    Fanconi syndrome, 27, 68
    glucose reabsorption, 27
    reabsorption, 24–8
    renal tubular acidosis, 68
    secretion, 28–9
    sodium reabsorption, 24–5
pyelography
    antegrade, 155
    intravenous, 152–3
    retrograde, 154–5
pyelonephritis, 91
pyuria, 134, 138–9, 149
    female, 138
    male, 139

R
radionuclide scanning, 155
rapidly progressive glomerulonephritis (RPGN), 89
reflux, vesicoureteral, 92
renal artery stenosis, 93–4, 154
    hypertension, 135–6
renal biopsy, 149
renal blood flow, 33
    measurement, 36–7
    regulation, 35
renal blood vessels, 17–19
    diseases, 93–5
renal calculi. *see* nephrolithiasis

renal failure. *also see* chronic kidney disease (CKD)
    acute, 38–40
renal medulla, 15–16
    cystic disease, 82
renal pelvis, 15
    urothelial carcinoma, 97
renal plasma flow
    measurement, 36–7
renal stones. *see* nephrolithiasis
renal transplantation, 42
renal tubular acidosis, 67–8
    types, 68
renin, 19, 43–5
renin-angiotensin-aldosterone system, 43–5
    potassium, 69
respiratory acidosis. *see* acidosis
respiratory alkalosis. *see* alkalosis
retrograde pyelography, 154–5
RPGN. *see* rapidly progressive glomerulonephritis (RPGN)

S
Schistosoma hematobium, 120–1
schistosomiasis, 119
shock, 98
sickle cell anemia
    diabetes insipidus, 60
    nephropathy, 95
SLE. *see* systemic lupus erythematosus (SLE)
sodium, 7–8
    ATPase, 23–4
    disorders, 46–51
    extracellular volume, 43
    regulation, 43–4
    reabsorption
        collecting ducts, 31–2
        distal convoluted tubule, 29, 31
        Loop of Henle, 29–30
        proximal tubule, 24–6
spina bifida, 110
squamous cell carcinoma, 124
stones, renal. *see* nephrolithiasis
stress incontinence, 110
systemic disorders
    renal responses to, 97–101
systemic lupus erythematosus (SLE)
    glomerulonephritis, 89

T
thiazide diuretics, 50
    diabetes insipidus treatment, 60

Index

thiazide diuretics (*Continued*)
  hypercalcemia, 74
  hyponatremia, 57–8
  nephrolithiasis treatment, 117–18
thrombotic microangiopathies, 94
titratable acid, 62
tonicity, 5–6
transcellular fluid, 4, 11
transitional cell carcinoma, bladder, 124
transplantation, renal, 42
tubular necrosis, acute, 90–1
tubuloglomerular feedback, 35
tubulointerstitial diseases, 90–3
tubulointerstitial nephritis
  drug and toxin induced, 92
tumors. *also see* cancer
  adrenal, 136
  mechanism, 136
  Wilms', 96–7
type A intercalated cells, 31–2
type B intercalated cells, 32

U

urate nephropathy, 92–3
urea, 28
  BUN/Cr ratio, 39–40
  diabetes insipidus, 60
  measurement (BUN), 150
  medullary osmolality, 54
  prerenal ARF, 39–40
  proximal reabsorption, 28
uremia, 38
ureteric peristalsis, 105
ureteritis, 118–19
ureteropelvic junction obstruction, 111, 114
ureters, 103–8
  abnormalities, 111, 113
  anatomy, 105
  development, 14
  neoplastic disease, 121
  reflux. *see* vesicoureteral reflux
  tumors, 121, 155
urethra
  abnormalities, 113–14
  female, 106
  male, 105–6, 107, 108
urethral discharge, 120–1
  diagnosing, 122
urge incontinence, 110

uric acid
  nephropathy, 76, 92
  regulation and clinical disorders, 76
  secretion, 29
  stones, 76, 116–17
urinary incontinence. *see* incontinence
urinary tract
  congenital abnormalities, 111
  infection, 117–21
  lower, 103–48
    female anatomy, 104
    male anatomy, 104
  obstruction, 114–16. *also see* obstruction
  structure, 3
urinalysis, 134, 147–9
  renal disease, 83, 134, 147–9
  renal failure, 39–40
urodynamic studies, 156
  incontinence diagnosis, 158
urothelial carcinoma, renal pelvis, 97
urothelium, 107–8

V

vasa recta, 17, 18, 54
vasculitis, renal, 89–90
  rash 144
vasopressin. *see* antidiuretic hormone
vesicoureteral reflux, 91–2
  focal segmental glomerulosclerosis, 86
  pyelonephritis, 91
  voiding cystourethrogram, 153–4
vitamin D, 20
  renal conversion to 1,25-dihydroxy-, 20
  therapy with 1,25-dihydroxy- in CKD, 41
voiding cystourethrogram, 153

W

water
  daily intake and output, 9
  disorders, 54–60
  reabsorption, 24–5, 29, 31, 52
  regulation of excretion, 51–4
  total body water, 3, 11
Wegner's granulomatosis, 90
Wilms' tumor, 96–7

X

xanthine oxidase inhibitors, 77